Neurobiology of Mood Disorders

Editors

Bruno P. Guiard

Faculty of Pharmacy
University Paris South XI
Châtenay-Malabry
France

&

Eliyahu Dremencov

Institute of Molecular
Physiology and Genetics,
Slovak Academy of Sciences,
Bratislava, Slovakia, and
Neuroken Consulting
Healthy Ageing Campus Netherlands
Groningen, the Netherlands

Bentham Science Publishers
Executive Suite Y - 2
PO Box 7917, Saif Zone
Sharjah, U.A.E.
subscriptions@benthamscience.org

Bentham Science Publishers
P.O. Box 446
Oak Park, IL 60301-0446
USA
subscriptions@benthamscience.org

Bentham Science Publishers
P.O. Box 294
1400 AG Bussum
THE NETHERLANDS
subscriptions@benthamscience.org

CONTENTS

CHAPTERS

PART I: RESEARCH METHODS IN PSYCHOPHARMACOLOGY

PART II: PATHOPHYSIOLOGY OF MOOD DISORDERS

PART III: NEW STRATEGIES FOR THE TREATMENT OF MOOD DISORDERS

PREFACE: NEUROBIOLOGY OF MOOD DISORDERS

It was our honor and pleasure to prepare this ebook entitled "Neurobiology of Mood Disorders". The World Health Organization considers mood disorders as fourth major reason for disability and they will become the second major reason for disability by 2020. Mood disorders have complex etiology with variable clinical symptoms. This may result from the involvement of abnormalities at the genetic, molecular and cellular levels. As a result, multidisciplinary research approaches have been used to investigate the pathophysiology of mood disorders and the mechanism of action of antidepressant drugs and mood stabilizers.

This ebook is divided to introduction and three parts. The first part addresses different research methods employed by modern neuropsychopharmacology. Several multidisciplinary approaches, from genetically-modified animal models to, neuroimaging in human are considered with a particular attention on optogenetic method. The second part aims to address the molecular and neuronal aspects of mood disorders. The third part focuses on the current genetic, pharmacological and non-pharmacological strategies used to improve the treatment of mood disorders.

This ebook might be out of interest for broad spectrum of researchers and clinicians working in the area of neuroscience and mental health. Undergraduate and graduate students studying life and medical science disciplines, and postdoctoral trainees and young physicians in training, specializing in basic or clinical neuroscience, may found this book beneficial for their education programs.

We would like to thank Bentham Science Publishers for their kind invitation, to the authors for their contributions, and for the reviewers that helped us to prepare this ebook. A very warm acknowledgement should be given Prof. Jakob Korf (University of Groningen Medical Center) for writing introduction to this ebook, to Mr. Sergey Nikolsky (Daatz, Groningen), for his help with preparation of this ebook to print, and to Mrs. Aniza Naveed (Bentham Science e-Books Publication Manager), who coordinated this project.

Bruno P. Guiard
Faculty of Pharmacy
University Paris South XI
Châtenay-Malabry
France

Eliyahu Dremencov
Institute of Molecular Physiology and Genetics
Slovak Academy of Science
Bratislava, Slovakia, and
Neuroken Consulting
Groningen, the Netherlands

LIST OF CONTRIBUTORS

Adell, Albert	Instituto de Investigaciones Biomédicas de Barcelona, CSIC (IDIBAPS), and Centro de Investigación Biomédica en Red de Salud Mental (CIBERSAM), Barcelona, Spain
Blier, Pierre	University of Ottawa Institute of Mental Health Research, Ottawa, Ontario, Canada
Blok, Samanha G.	University of Miami Miller School of Medicine, Miami, Florida, USA
Bosker, Fokko J.	University of Groningen Medical Center, Groningen, The Netherlands
Chernoloz, Olga	Toronto, Ontario, Canada
David, Denis J.	University Paris South, Châtenay-Malabry, France
David, Indira	University Paris South, Châtenay-Malabry, France
den Boer, Johan A.	University of Groningen Medical Center, Groningen, The Netherlands
Dierckx , Rudi A.	University of Groningen Medical Center, Groningen, The Netherlands
Dremencov, Eliyahu	Department of Neuroscience, University of Groningen Medical Center, Neuroken Consulting, Healthy Ageing Campus Netherlands, Groningen, the Netherlands, and Institute of Molecular Physiology and Genetics, Slovak Academy of Sciences, Bratislava, Slovakia.
el Mansari, Mostafa	University of Ottawa Institute of Mental Health Research, Ottawa, Ontario, Canada
Fabbri, Chiara	Institute of Psychiatry, University of Bologna, Bologna, Italy
Gardier, Alain M.	University Paris South, Châtenay-Malabry, France
Guiard, Bruno P.	University Paris South, Châtenay-Malabry, France
Hen, René	University Paris South, Châtenay-Malabry, France
Jiménez-Sánchez, Laura	Instituto de Investigaciones Biomédicas de Barcelona, CSIC (IDIBAPS), and Centro de Investigación Biomédica en Red de Salud Mental (CIBERSAM), Barcelona, Spain
Kheirbek, Mazen A.	Columbia University, New York, NY 10032, USA
Korf, Jakob	University of Groningen Medical Center, Groningen, The Netherlands
La Riche, Christopher L.	University of Miami Miller School of Medicine, Miami, Florida, USA
López-Gil, Xavier	Instituto de Investigaciones Biomédicas de Barcelona, CSIC (IDIBAPS), and Centro de Investigación Biomédica en Red de Salud Mental (CIBERSAM), Barcelona, Spain
Manta, Stella	Laval University, Institut Universitaire en Santé Mentale de Québec (IUSMQ), Québec-City, Québec, Canada
Nemeroff, Charles B.	University of Miami Miller School of Medicine, Miami, Florida, USA
Porcelli, Stefano	Institute of Psychiatry, University of Bologna, Bologna, Italy
Prestia, Davide	University of Miami Miller School of Medicine, Miami, Florida, USA
Quesseveur, Gaël	University Paris South, Châtenay-Malabry, France
Rainer, Quentin	University Paris South, Châtenay-Malabry, France
Samuels, Benjamin A.	University Paris South, Châtenay-Malabry, France
Serretti, Alessandro	Institute of Psychiatry, University of Bologna, Bologna, Italy
van Waarde, Aren	University of Groningen Medical Center, Groningen, The Netherlands
Visser, Anniek K.D .	University of Groningen Medical Center, Groningen, The Netherlands

INTRODUCTION: THE DEPRESSED PATIENT IN A NEUROBIOLOGICAL WORLD: HISTORY, NEUROPHILOSOPHY AND EVIDENCE BASED PSYCHIATRY

JAKOB KORF

Abstract: This essay analyzes possible underlying assumptions and provides bridge laws between various levels of complexity of brain processes. A short historical introduction on the main trends in neuropsychiatry over the last century is given. Then Kendler's philosophical agenda are discussed. The central question is: what kind of relationships between mental and neurobiological levels of complexity is or could become useful in the psychiatric practice? The philosophical analysis based on general systems theory and on Searle's concept, assuming the mind as a biological property of the brain. Consequently the individually unique mind exists in a similarly unique brain, containing all information acquired during life. Clinical investigations show that the occurrence and time course of some psychiatric conditions, such as depression, can best be described in stochastic models. Diagnostic systems and research agenda's should take into account for such uncertainties, that are not due to a lack of scientific knowledge, but might be inherent to the neurobiology of the brain, instead. The probabilistic nature of the brain, together with the possible involvement of multiple genes and other molecules may pose limitations on both the biological understanding of mental disorders and evidence based psychiatric practice.

1. AN HISTORICAL INTRODUCTION

From an historical point of view, mental disorders or any other used denominations to madness and insane persons, have always referred to both mental and materialistic concepts. In Ancient Greece, disease was thought due to an imbalance in the four basic bodily fluids (humors). Melancholia was described as a distinct disease with particular mental and physical symptoms by Hippocrates in his Aphorisms, where he characterized all "fears and despondencies, if they last a long time" as being symptomatic of the ailment. Melancholia was a far broader concept than today's depression; prominence was given to a clustering of the symptoms of sadness, dejection, and despondency, and often fear, anger, delusions and obsessions were included.

In the 19th century there was a movement in Germany, initiated by the internist and later psychiatrist Wilhelm Griesinger, stating that psychiatric illnesses are brain diseases ('Geisteskrankheiten sind Gehirnkrankheiten'). Sigmund Freud's psychoanalytic theory may also been considered as an early attempt to understand mental disorders in terms of bodily functioning. Indeed Freud his ideas were based in part on the notion that psychic processes depend on the functioning of neuronal circuitry: for instance suppression of thoughts or desires was considered the consequence of inhibitory neuronal processes. The 20th century introduced a new psychiatry into the world [1]. Different perspectives of looking at mental disorders began to be introduced. The career of Emil Kraepelin reflects the convergence of different disciplines in psychiatry. Kraepelin initially was very attracted to psychology and ignored the ideas of anatomical psychiatry. Following his appointment to a professorship of psychiatry and his work in a university psychiatric clinic, Kraepelin's interest in pure psychology began to fade and he introduced a plan for a more comprehensive psychiatry. Kraepelin began to study and promote the idea of disease classification for mental disorders. The initial ideas behind biological psychiatry, stating that the different mental disorders were all biological in nature, evolved into a new concept of "nerves" and psychiatry became a rough approximation of neurology and neuropsychiatry. However, Kraepelin was criticized for considering schizophrenia as a biological illness in the absence of any detectable histological or anatomical abnormalities. While Kraepelin tried to find organic causes of mental illness, he adopted many theses of positivist medicine, but he favored the precision of nosological classification over the indefiniteness of etiological causation as his basic mode of psychiatric explanation

Biological psychiatry reemerged in the second at the turn of the 20th century. During the first halve of the 20th century treatments such as insulin coma treatment, drug- or electro-convulsive treatment and lobotomy have been practiced [1]. A breakthrough was the successful treatment of syphilis, often considered a mental disorder, supporting the idea that indeed mental disorders are primarily diseases of the brain (body). The causative organism, Treponema pallidum, was firstly identified in 1905. It was observed that some patients who develop high fevers could be cured of syphilis. Julius Wagner-Jauregg (Austrian physician, Nobel Laureate) tried in 1917 the inoculation of malaria parasites, which proved to be successful in the case of dementia paralytica caused by neurosyphilis, at that time a terminal disease. Later penicillin was explored and its effectiveness confirmed in 1943. Lobotomy (leucotomy) consists of cutting the connections to and from the prefrontal cortex, the anterior part of the frontal lobes of the brain and has been applied for severe psychosis, manic-depressions and compulsive disorders. Half of the Nobel Prize for Physiology or Medicine of 1949 was awarded to António Egas Moniz (Portuguese) for the "discovery of the therapeutic value of leucotomy in certain psychoses". Such interventions were prescribed for psychiatric conditions until the mid-1950s when modern neuroleptic (antipsychotic) and a little later antidepressive medication (monoamine inhibitors and tricyclic antidepressants, *e.g.*, imipramine) were introduced [1, 2]. The discovery of chlorpromazine's effectiveness in treating schizophrenia in 1952 revolutionized treatment of the disease, as did lithium carbonate's ability to stabilize mood highs and lows in bipolar disorder in 1948. Psychopharmacology became an integral part of psychiatry starting with Otto Loewi's discovery of the first-known neurotransmitter, acetylcholine. Later, particularly in the 1950ties, other neurotransmitters, including noradrenalin (nor-epinephrine; initially also epinephrine or adrenaline), dopamine and serotonin began to play their role in psychiatry, both in searching for the cause of mental disorders and in the development of new (psycho) pharmacological treatment options. Nobel prizes to Julius Axelrod (US American, 1970) and Arvid Carlsson (Swedish, 2000), Paul Greengard and Eric Kandel (both US American, 2000) illustrate the scientific recognition of neurobiology and psychopharmacology in the previous 5 decades. In the last 3 decades the position of the psychopharmacology has become very prominent, too prominent according to some. Indeed, criticasters have concluded that drug companies have invented psychiatric diseases that matches the pharmacological profile of their drugs, rather than the reverse: dugs were developed to cure diseases [2]. Genetics were once again (this following previous American investigations and after Nazi-Germany supported eugenetic practice) thought to play a role in mental illness. Other new approaches were developed, essentially to better understand mental disorders at a biological level, which may eventually assist the diagnostic procedures and imply more effective and rationale therapeutic interventions. For instance the analysis of body fluids, such as cerebrospinal fluid (as a direct derivative of the brain), blood and urine became prominent already in the 1950ties. In the sixties and seventies challenge tests were proposed to assess the receptors functioning or the responsively of the organism or some particular subsystem and associated receptors to stress or specific drugs. The dexamethasone suppression test (DST) and its more recent modifications are prominent examples [3, 4]. Molecular biology of the 1980ties opened the door to search for specific genes contributing to mental disorders. Psychotherapy in various formats was and is still utilized, in particular as a treatment for psychosocial issues. Standardization of the diagnosis and assessment of the profile and severity of mental disorders was achieved with the introduction of diagnostic systems (such as the DSM, diagnostic and statistical manual, and the ICD, international classification of diseases) and with rating scales (*e.g.*, Hamilton rating scale for depression and anxiety) [1]. *In vivo* neuroimaging of the intact functioning brain was firstly utilized as a tool for psychiatry in the mid 1980s and abnormal patterns of both anatomical and functional features in various psychiatric disorders have been and are still claimed. Current neurocognitive approaches [5], making use of a variety of neuroimaging techniques, have contributed to the understanding of brain processes underlying normal and psychopathological mental activity.

2. THE PATIENT

The clinical management, and in particular the treatment options of most psychiatric disorders have improved during the last decades. And yet, despite the introduction and application of a wide variety of novel scientific approaches, methods and machineries, current knowledge of the basic underlying neuropathology is still poor. In the following sections I discuss some major obstacles hindering progress in biological psychiatry firstly in more general terms, and subsequently to illustrate my point of view on major depressive disorder (MDD) in more detail. Parts of the present exposé were published as abstracts [6, 7, 8]. Psychiatry is a medical discipline where the conceptualization of the mind and the brain determines to a large extent diagnostic and therapeutic approaches. Accordingly, the psychotherapeutic approaches are often considered to be opposed to or may perhaps even exclude neurobiological therapeutic interventions, for instance drug treatment. In addition, current psychiatric research literature witnesses a vast arsenal of efforts to relate biomarkers, such as hormones, neurotransmitters or genes and their variants, directly or indirectly to psychiatric disorders or some of their prominent characteristics or symptoms. In addition the neuroimaging modalities developed in the past decades have stimulated the search for brain processes essential in the manifestation of psychiatric pathology. Relatively simple and rather deterministic relationships or correlations between the (neuro-)biological parameters and psychological phenomena are presumed.

In his proposal for a philosophy of psychiatry Kendler [9] gives 8 basic presumptions to which modern psychiatry should adhere. These include: 1) psychiatry is grounded in mental, first-person experiences; 2) Cartesian dualism is false; 3) epiphenomenalism is false; 4) both brain—mind and mind–brain causality are real; 5) psychiatric disorders are complex; 6) explanatory pluralism is preferable; 7) embrace empirically rigorous and pluralistic explanatory models; 8) accept piecemeal integration of complex etiological pathways to psychiatric illness a little bit at a time. The issues raised provide a pragmatic albeit attractive summation of what psychiatry is, should be or might become. However useful these presumptions may be, I discuss whether or not Kendler's agenda does indeed offer a coherent philosophical and scientific framework.

I will discuss several assumptions underlying Kendler's philosophy [9], based in part on the previous philosophical discussion, and will emphasize the necessity of bridge laws linking the neurobiological and mental levels. Or formulated in practical terms: what kind of relationships between psychiatrically and neurobiologically relevant items is, could or should become useful in the psychiatric practice where a diagnosis has to be made and a therapeutic intervention has to be chosen. Central is the question whether there might exist an emerging property of the brain that is directly associated (or perhaps identical) with the mind. Important is also the notion that we experience ourselves as a single autonomous person. Our conscious attention is focused on one or a few issues only and, moreover, our brain becomes more personal during life. Hence we experience ourselves as a unity, as a single person. Firstly I discuss these issues from a philosophical perspective. Next I show that fast processes in the brain, necessary to execute higher brain functions, including memory, do not directly depend on brain energy metabolism, and remain therefore invisible with current neuro-imaging technologies. These observations have led to the concept of isoenergicity as an emerging property of the brain [7, 8], that will be summarized here too. The basic concept defended here is that of a physically emergent, subjective, qualitative, unified feature of the brain, or which amounts to the same thing, that the mind is a mental, and therefore biological, and therefore physical, feature of the brain. The implications of this concept for disease, therapeutic interventions and psychiatric research strategies are discussed, with an emphasis on depression.

3. PHILOSOPHICAL PERSPECTIVES

This section considers some philosophical ideas relevant for psychiatry and is particularly focused on the mind-brain relationship. Firstly I approach this question from the point of view of the general systems theory, and subsequently from a monistic, materialistic angle.

3.1. GENERAL SYSTEMS THEORY

Even if one does not adhere to a dualistic brain/mind concept, the psychiatric practice is often dualistic. So the mind (psyche) and the brain (or body) are considered basically as different and non-overlapping entities. In this section systems (*e.g.*, body, brain) are entities that consist of elements (*e.g.*, particles, cells, molecules, neurons) and have a boundary, so it can be recognized from the outside. Systems, as used in the general systems theory [10, 11], might not only be considered as physical entities, but also as ideas or conceptions, so it might help to understand the relation and development of epistemological concepts. Stavenga [10] distinguishes 4 possible relationships between two systems (schematically depicted in figure 1 upper panel). Important is to note that interactions do occur only when the systems belong to the same domain, in the present case the physical or biological domain. Moreover, the current general systems theory does not imply that physical systems belong to only to one kind of system: instead any physical entity or system belongs to many (perhaps an infinitive number) of other systems. In the present analysis I consider the mind and the brain as 2 systems, provided that the mind can be conceptualized as a physical system. The first possible distinction is that the 2 systems are completely separated and have no interaction (the R0 relationship). In the context of system theory this contention is meaningful only if we regard the mind as material otherwise the mind has no causative power. Hence I reject substance dualism, as an impossible option. Having thus concluded, I discuss the other possible relationships. An R1 relationship means that the 2 systems have a common boundary, and this is the only site for possible interactions. For instance Cartesian dualism is an example of an R1 relationship, where the "seat" of the mind is the epiphysis (pineal), the organ that controls the brain. But this idea leaves us with the problem that the mind must anyhow invade the pineal and exert physical energy on the brain. The second possible relationship between mind and brain are the hypotheses that the mind is a product of the brain, like urine of the kidneys, and that all causative power is limited to the brain. These series of ideas (to be discussed in more detail later) might be recognized as R2 relationships. Although the mind may be considered in a R2 relationship as a materialistic system, it has little if any causative power by its own. Neuroscientist have questioned the mind or free will as causing behavior, because decisions (often in laboratory experiments) have already been made before the subjects became aware of their decision or, alternatively, the subjects gave irrelevant arguments for their behavior. This conclusion

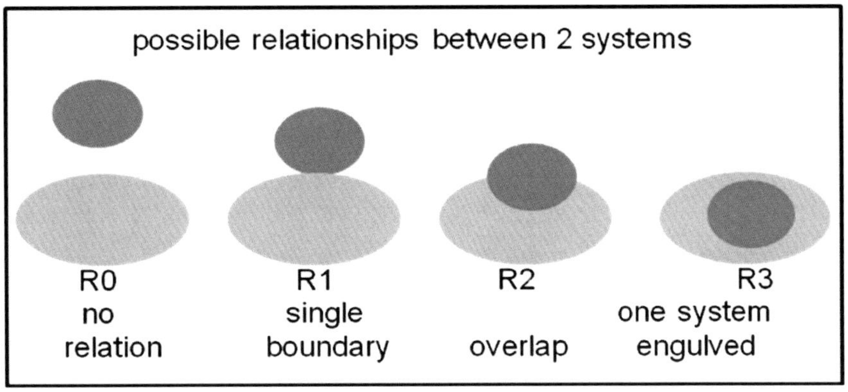

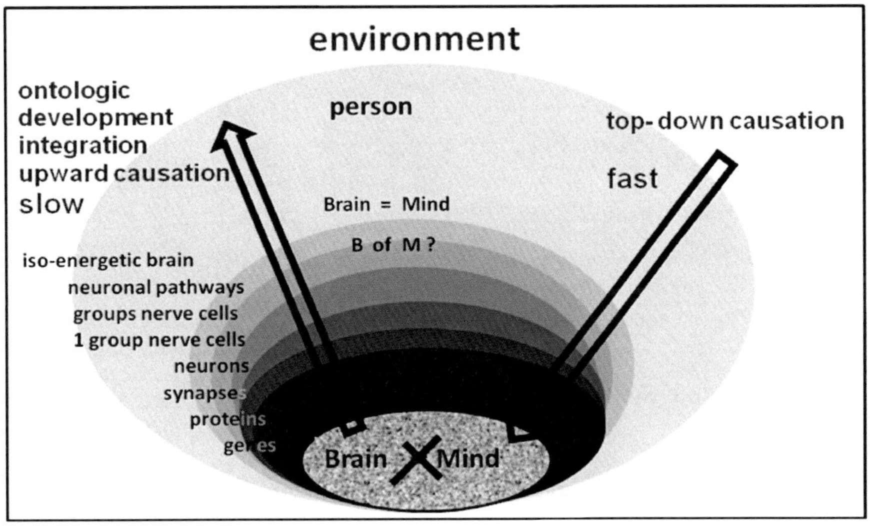

Figure 1: Cartoons of philosophical models on mind-brain relationships. Upper figure shows possible relationships of 2 systems according to systems theories. Accordingly the mind-brain theories may be described as R1-R3 relationship. Lower figure shows the levels of organization (or complexity) of the brain largely based on Searle his concepts. The lowest levels are molecules, whereas the higher levels are formed by aggregates of neurons and neuronal networks. Notice that the next higher level in the lower figure has an R3 relationship with its underlying level, as defined with the systems theory. Whereas the underlying levels has their own dynamics, it is also subject to top-down causation. On the other hand, from an ontological point of view, the higher complexity is an emerging property of the lower level.

may also have implications for psychiatry, as many behavioral therapies and psychotherapies are based on the information of the patient. The 3rd possible relationship between systems is that the 2 systems overlap each other, so that the state of one system is accompanied by a related state of the other. Stavenga [10] illustrated the R3 relationship as the condition of pregnancy: the embryo (system 1) is completely surrounded by the (pregnant) mother (system 2), although both the fetus and the mother have lives of their own. I consider the mind-brain systems as an R3 relationship: the mind is not only part of the brain and depends on that, but also that the mind has its own causative power. In parallel to this reasoning I summarize some philosophical concepts in the following section.

3.2. MIND-BRAIN PHILOSOPHY

The philosophical answer to eliminate dualism is materialism, that assumes that the personal mind (the subjective, qualitative, conscious mind) is reducible to or identical with objective phenomena such as neurobiological, behavioral or functional states, and that, therefore, the conscious mind is, more or less, an illusion (*e.g.*, "The ghost in the machine", the "Cartesian Theatre"). The mind has also been regarded as an epiphenomenon or, alternatively, as an emerging (non-physical) property of the brain ([12] and references therein). Considering the mind as an epiphenomenon tends to deny its importance for functioning and survival of an organism. The question with the emerging mind is: how can a non-materialistic mind (without matter and energy) affect a physical (causally closed) brain [12] [13]? A crucial issue with the "ghost" and the "dualist" concepts is how to imagine that a mind can emerge from a "nutshell filled with proteins, genes and other molecules". Or to put it in more refined terms, how can a splendid mind be the "product" of a neuronal or synaptic network? [14, 15] And how is it possible that even an interactive network of several (perhaps all) brain regions could give a unifying mind with a single focus of attention (the problem of binding? [15, 16]

One solution of such dilemmas is offered by assuming that the mind is an emerging but physical property that is in essence irreducible to all the underlying neurobiological processes. An emergent property is created by the interaction of several elements, but cannot be described as (or reduced to) the additive effects (or properties) of these elements. Formulated as a straightforward question: what is emerging from what? Does it mean that the mind as an apparently non-physical entity could emerge from an apparently physical brain? The issue has been discussed in detail by many philosophers including John Roger Searle [15, 17, 18] and Jeagwon Kim [13]. Kim discussed the concept supervenience "In this is the claim that what happens in our mental life is wholly dependent on, and determined by, what happens with our bodily processes" ([13] p. 14). Searle [15, 17, 18] argued that the supervenience stance leads to over-determination: the mind must be equated with a brain state, but to go to another state of the mind the brain has to change its state. I follow the reasoning of Searle: the only thing that can emerge (or supervene) from a physical (biological) configuration is another physical (biological) configuration. In neurobiological terms, either one has to explain (or reduce) the mind as (to) a property of a collection of any of the constituents of the brain (*e.g.*, proteins, genes, cells, aggregates of cells or neuronal networks), or there is an emerging property that cannot be conceptualized as or reduced to properties of these underlying brain constituents (Fig. 1, lower panel). Then the issue comes down to the question whether there might exist an emerging property of the brain that is directly associated with (or perhaps identical to) the mind. In Searle's terms [18]: there exist emerging properties of the brain that are both physical and mental (opposed to conceptual dualism: it is either physical or mental). The resulting mind-brain concept is indicated as biological naturalism [18] and is characterized "as bottom-up micro macro no time gap, where cause and effect are simultaneously realized and effect (macro) is realized as a macro-feature of the system made out of that microstructure (micro) that in turn explains the existence and causal powers of higher-level or system features" ([18] p. 54). This formulation is nearly identical with the R3 relationship of the general systems theory. Following Searle's analysis a major challenge the neurobiologist is confronted with, is to define a brain configuration that equals the mind. Particularly relevant here is the position of psychiatry in such conceptualization.

4. FAST BRAIN PROCESSING

This section pursues on the idea as formulated as an R3 relationship, as an element of the general systems theory, and as supported by the conceptualization of the mind/brain relationship by Searle, where "cause and effect are simultaneously realized". I summarize some current ideas to illustrate the speed of processing of -what are conventionally denoted as- higher (psychological) functions. Neuronal transmission of information throughout the brain is based on the generation and propagation of action potentials and on fast neurotransmission between neurons, each lasting 2-5 msec. These neuronal processes are initiated by transitions of protein configurations within nanoseconds (more information in [19, 20]). As compared to the neural processes, how fast proceed higher brain functions, such as memory? This has for instance been assessed with psycho-physiological experiments. In linguistic experiments, done together with EEG recordings, it appeared that visually offered words can be recognized and subsequently vocalized within 50 msec [21]. Non-conscious cerebral processing of auditory and visual stimuli of less than 50 msec duration, are the basis of subliminal perception and masking experiments (and of related advertisements). Such experiments show that unconscious processing of information is very fast and requires only about 10 sequential neural processes (action potentials + neurotransmissions). But the millisecond range does not appear the fastest processing of information. For instance, binaural discrimination of sounds in the human brain is achieved already within 100 microseconds, *i.e.*, more than 10 times faster than glutamate neurotransmission [19, 20]. It should be realized that it takes far more time for (unconscious) information to become conscious; according to Libet's experiments at least 0.4 s [22], *i.e.*, about 10x slower than memory recognition and more than 4000x slower than binaural discrimination.

Interpersonal communication is essential for the expression and assessment of a psychiatric disorder. One criterion is whether or not the disorder can empathically be understood, as defined by Dilthey and Jaspers ("Erklären oder Verstehen"; understanding versus explanation) [23]. Such distinction is strongly supported by the discovery of mirror neurons, which are groups of neurons that become active during watching related motor activity of littermates. In particular mirror neurons in the frontal cortex appear to be involved in empathetic processes; they may be less or inactive in autism. The prefrontal mirror neurons have no direct connection with sensory information, so the question is how they get the input (information) necessary for firing. This can best be understood in terms of unconscious brain activity preceding the activation of the mirror neurons. Considering the speed of (higher) neural processes the brain may "recognizes" empathically relevant environmental clues and subsequently "shapes" the activity into a format to activating prefrontal mirror neurons in a few milliseconds. It takes several hundreds of milliseconds before mirror neurons become active after watching behavior of a littermate. This delay is remarkably similar to that for a sensory stimulus to become conscious [20, 22].

Fast brain processes are essential to achieve a unitary action (also termed binding) of the brain and may eventually evoke conscious perception and activity. fMRI and any other neuro-imaging technique, all based on the detection of differences of local brain energy consumption, do not visualize these initial very fast and most often diffuse information processing of the brain. Being apparently independent on brain energy metabolism led us to the idea [19, 20] that the energy required for fast neural activity depends only on the potential energy (*i.e.*, rest membrane potentials) and such potential energy is distributed more or less evenly over the brain, *i.e.*, the brain can be considered as an isoenergetic configuration. Isoenergicity means that there are no or little energy barriers to distribute information over the brain and that is possible because brain energy metabolism is aimed to maintain or restore isoenergicity after neuronal activity. In the ideal isoenergetic brain there are no energy barriers to propagate and distribute information. Isoenergicity therefore facilitates unitary (binding) activity of the various neuronal subsystems. This is not to say that in addition to isoenergicity many more conditions (and structures) are necessary to form the mind. We mentioned already the easy access to memory, but also the embodiments of somatic functions should be emphasized as well. Of interest may also the notion that the time period necessary to develop a fMRI signal following a sensory stimulus is close to that required for an unconscious stimulus to becoming conscious, suggesting that consciousness is closely related to focused brain activity (see also our previous comments on mirror neurons).

We explored the philosophical ideas based on systems theory and the philosophical concepts of Searle that cause and effect are simultaneously realized. I describe some experiments that brain processes are indeed faster than neurotransmission processes, often considered as the fastest possible way to distribute information over the brain. Hence modern brain physiology approaches the philosophical propositions, in terms of simultaneousness. These processes are too fast to depend on brain energy metabolism. Hence brain energy metabolism and associated blood flow is a restorative process, and the brain might be considered as isoenergetic, allowing information processing down to the sub-millisecond range.

5. THE PERSONAL BRAIN

In this section I propose the existence of a personal time-space configuration of the brain that is continuously formed during life. This idea conforms to the concept of the mind (and -perhaps counter intuitively- also the person) as a process, rather than as a static entity. Personal memories do not disappear after a night of sleep, or during ECT (electroconvulsive therapy; except recent memories), when the brain is damaged (by stroke or cardiac arrest) or after awakening from a deep coma (although brain damage may impair memory processing). The inefficacy of insulin coma once used to treat schizophrenia and some other psychiatric conditions ([1], p. 208-213) may be seen in this context. So even when the brain is damaged, hence becoming in part dysfunctional and the formation of memory is affected, far most memories do not disappear. We do never regress to a naïve child. Memory problems associated with electroconvulsive interventions or Alzheimer's dementia illustrate that personal memories disappear in a time-dependent manner: the more recent traces disappear before old memories. To summarize, one's perception of the world, one's social network and cultural environment, in other words what makes us a person, is primarily confined to the brain and is virtually independent of the actual electrophysiological state of the brain. Apparently, it is the morphology of the brain -but considered at a micro level- that guarantees continuity of -or perhaps better formulated that creates- the person. Recent memories should be seen as new additions to brain micro-morphology. On the other hand one should not see the cerebral micro-morphology as hardware as opposed to electrophysiological processes being the software [20]. The micro-morphology and electrophysiology together create continuously (or -if preferred in the present context - cause the continuous emergence) a new personal time-space configuration.

The proposed time-space configuration can be generated from an iso-electric brain (when *e.g.,* all electrophysiological activity has disappeared because of ischemia) provided that some (possibly brainstem pacemaker) neurons are still active and that the brain regains its iso-energetic state. Such proposed time-space configuration of the brain changes continuously because of storing new information, so its configuration does never become the same again during life. The alluded time-space configuration is a requisite for consciousness of the person. Such personal brain configuration is unique and can therefore not be reduced to any other entity (or brain) in the universe nor to a scientific (deterministic) model.

In this section I argue that the information that the individual collects during life is -in a way-morphologically - in spatial dimensions- stored. This together with the dimension time, *i.e.,* electrophysiological activity, create a functioning brain. Such proposed time-space configuration is personal and does never become the same again during life. This conclusion supports Kendler's presumption that psychiatry should be grounded in mental, first-person experiences, and is in line with the current neurobiological analysis.

6. DEPRESSION AND THE BRAIN

Stated briefly, a psychiatric disorder is the collective consequence of external challenges, cultural and social environment, personal experiences and biological disposition. To take depression as an example: external challenges (*e.g.,* severe life events, bereavement) together with personal experiences (*e.g.,* misuse in the youth, previous depressive episodes) and biological dispositions (*e.g.,* gene variants, hypothyroid, hypercortisolaemia, interferon treatments, viral infections) are considered risk factors to develop a depression. Just like in somatic illness an essential characteristic of a psychiatric disorder is the duration of the condition. Short periods of depression are considered as normal and may not deserve psychiatric attention. Many symptoms essential for a psychiatric diagnosis are unspecific, as they are present in the general population as well. In psychiatric patients, however, more symptoms aggregate, they are more severe and last longer. The DSM classification [1, 24] of major depressive disorder is illustrative; 2 essential (sad mood, loss of interest in social interactions) and 4 out of 7 optional symptoms should be present for at least 2 weeks. The structure of a psychiatric condition does not differ from somatic disorders, although the relative contribution of the various symptoms may differ. Unique in psychiatry is that the cultural and social environment and the personal experiences are more prominent, which are -as argued- predominantly if not exclusively linked to the personal time-space configuration of the brain. Life-events considered so important in depression have often been considered to equal stress. This idea has led to vast amount of reports on the physiology of stress in depressive patients (*e.g.,* the DST). But stress and live events should conceptually be distinguished: the impact of a life event depends on its perception and hence on its interpretation of the subject. Such interpretation depends on memory, thus on the constellation of the time-space configuration of that person's brain. Unlike a life event, a stressor affects any subject in a non-specific manner; essentially independent of the person's history. Psychiatric interventions are also focused on the symptoms contributing to the diagnosis: so psychotherapies are aimed to help coping with external challenges and social (sometimes cultural) environment.

Often brain stem neurons containing monoamine neurotransmitters, such as dopamine, serotonin and noradrenalin (norepinephrine) are considered hyper- or hypoactive in various psychiatric conditions. Noradrenergic neurons of the locus coeruleus, projecting to many forebrain regions are presumed to be overactive following stress and in anxiety disorders, and possibly subfunctoning in depression. Similarly brain serotonin neurons have been postulated to be hypoactive in depression [25-28]. Monoamine systems are no autonomous islands in the brain (stem) but are part of a network, instead. So the hypo- or hyperactivity of such systems are not necessarily causally predisposed by a gene variant or defect in the various monoamine neurons, but may be the consequence of the (unconscious) activity of the presumed time-space brain configuration, instead. If indeed the latter is the case, then it is meaningless to search for aberrant genes, but it might be more relevant to investigate the personal history of the patient.

We [29, 30] investigated the time course of recovery from depression. The length of the depressive episodes was determined in each subject of a cohort of 250 depressed subjects of the general population. In this cohort about 20% did not recover during the observation period. In the remainder the distribution of the length of the depressive episodes could be modeled very precisely as an exponential distribution (and not as a mean with Gaussian distribution). The exponential function

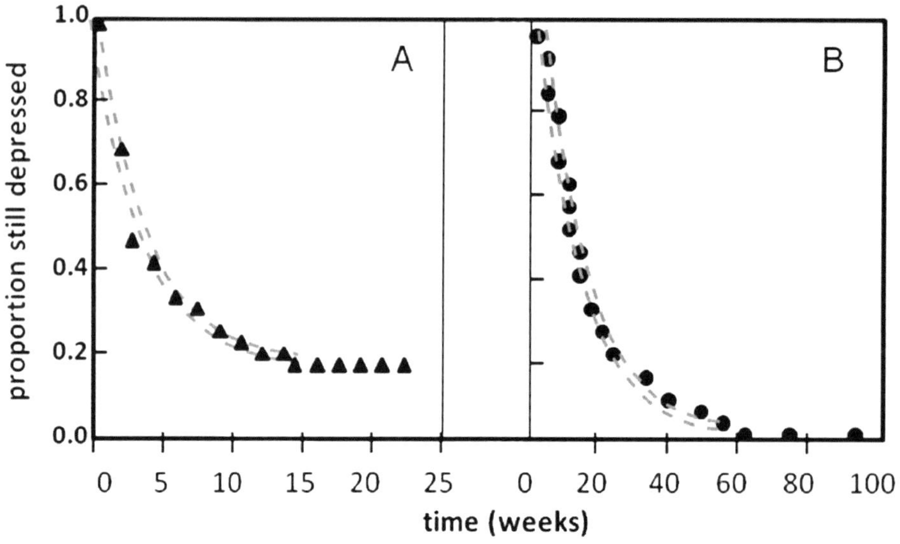

Figure 2: Time course of recovery from depression in MDD diagnosed patients. (A) shows data from a cohort identified in the general population. (B) shows the data from recurrent depression. The grey broken lines are the best fitting exponential decline function. The exponential character of the fits suggest that the mood transitions occur randomly (similar to radioactive decay in labile atomic nuclei). (A) from data of [29]; (B) was composed from data of [30]. Data of cohorts of 250-400 subjects.

signifies that that the recovery is the result of a random (or more precisely stochastic) transition from the depressed to the non-depressed state Fig. **2A**. This stochastic mood model applied to all sub-cohorts: male/female subjects, with or without co-morbid psychiatric or somatic pathologies, severe and non-severe depressed patients. Close inspection of the data indicated that the DSM inclusion criterion for major depressive disorder of 2 weeks was also found, indicating that this criterion is pragmatic and probable not a "property" of depression. In another study with recurrent depressions [30] we showed, that there was no correlation between the lengths of the depressive episodes, or between the length of the non-depressed periods and the depressive episodes in a single subject (illustrated in Fig. **2B**. These findings together suggest that MDD might primarily be viewed as due to failing mood-transitions. In daily life we may experience fast mood transitions as well, for instance after receiving good or bad news.

Fast depressiogenic and anti-depressive state transitions have also been noticed in patients recovering from depression following one night of sleep deprivation: within a nap of about 5 minutes they may become depressed again [31, 32]. In some (non-depressed) patients electrical stimulation of the subthalamic nucleus, aimed to alleviate tremor in Parkinson's disease, evokes within 5 seconds depressed mood that has disappeared within 30 seconds after cessation of the stimulation [33, 34]. Electrical stimulation does not imply that the stimulated neuronal pathway become more active: rather it impairs the integration of the stimulated pathway in a functional neuronal network. Hence, electrical stimulation might be seen as a reversible method to block neuronal pathways.

Mood transitions can be fast and might occur stochastically. Depressive mood might be considered as more or less normal state of the brain; the pathology is the inability to evoke anti-depressive transitions. Isoenergicity of the brain facilitates stochastic mood transitions.

7. THERAPEUTIC INTERVENTIONS

In this section I discuss the stochastic transitions in an attempt to understand therapeutic interventions. In somatic medicine at least 4 types of interventions might be distinguished. The type 1 intervention aims to remove the disease-causing agent either by direct challenging its existence in the patient's body or to assist the disease-eliminating activity. Antibiotic therapy is the classical example. Compensation is the type 2 intervention: a component with a similar or identical activity is prescribed or measures are taken to enhance the production of the missing compound. Many anti-diabetic treatments or the L-DOPA therapy and dopamine agonists in Parkinson's disease are examples. The 3rd type intervention aims to remove a pathological agent with non-specific toxins, mechanical devices or irradiation. Cancer may serve as an example. And finally, type 4 treatment is primarily aimed to reduce suffering by, for instance, palliative treatment. Each of these treatments is rational and possibly evidence-based.

To what category do antidepressant interventions belong? In depression the most prevailing treatments are cognitive behavioral therapies and medication. Other regimens include physical exercise, sleep deprivation, light exposure therapy and -in severe cases- electroconvulsive treatment, alone or combined with the routine treatments. Medication has often been thought as type 1 or type 3 interventions, but there is as yet little evidence that deficiencies of brain monoamines cause depression. It appeared that low brain serotonin (due to low plasma tryptophan) is associated with failing impulse-control and aggression rather than with depression [26, 27]. Cognitive therapies have been developed to correct misconceptions associated with the depression (*i.e.*, to reduce the impact of life events). Whether their effects are due to a type 4 rather than a type 1 (or perhaps type 3) effect remains to be proven. Interventions, such as physical exercise, sleep deprivation, light exposure therapy and electroconvulsive treatment are certainly not type 1, 2 or 3 treatments. The latter are perhaps type 4 treatment (alleviating suffering), but that indexation may feel as artificial. In the previous section we described the time-morphology of depression with a stochastic mood model suggesting that major depressive disorders might primarily be viewed as a condition of failing mood-transitions. In view of the transition hypothesis the anti-depressive interventions may seen as to facilitate switching from the depressive to the non-depressed state. Sleep deprivation and electroconvulsive treatments are treatments that could show early antidepressant effects. But their effects are unstable; illustrative are the rapid mood transitions in sleep deprived and responsive patients following short naps [32]. Exercise and light therapy may also improve mood or serve as prophylactic. Their effects could be seen as type 1 therapies, as hypo-activity is often a prominent symptom of depression, whereas exposure to light activates or compensates failing mechanisms in seasonal affective disorders, respectively. Alternatively, these treatments may facilitate mood (and so brain) transitions. Therefore, I suggest to adding another type of treatment. So the type 5 treatment is to facilitate brain transitions. This idea might be seen as an extension of type 1 as that they assist the organism to battle the ailment, but that is a rather artificial formulation for randomly occurring brain states.

There is an ongoing debate on the therapeutic efficacy of antidepressants [35, 36]. In several meta-analyses their effects appear to be modest as compared to placebo. Two comments: 1st the response of depressed subjects to medication varies widely: both fast en clear-cut responses, and no response at all have been reported, and 2nd the placebo response is relatively high and variable. Apparently no meaningful distinction can be made between subjects who need medication and those who recover without medication (or placebo). Is this a matter of lack of knowledge or is this inherent of the current conception of depression? The placebo-drug controversy may serve as another argument supporting the random-mood concept and if so drug treatment is a type 5 intervention.

In short: we argued that -except perhaps cognitive psychotherapy- none of the current anti-depressive interventions treats underlying patho-psychological mechanisms directly. So an anti-depressive treatment is often not aimed to influence the depressive feelings, but to influence the course and severity of depression. Considering the stochastic-mood concept, thus assuming random brain transitions, a strict causality and possibly a strong prediction between diagnosis and therapeutic response in depression may not always be evident. Therapeutic consequences of mood transitions must also be seen in the context of the micro-morphology of the brain. It can be argued that not only biological therapies but also psychotherapies should change brain micro-morphology to become effective. Or as a research paradigm: how to optimize the effect of a therapy on the change of the brain's micro-morphology.

8. DIAGNOSTIC SYSTEMS

Emil Kraepelin was the founder of the present diagnostic approaches and his ideas were the basis of current classification proposals [1]. It was well realized from the onset onwards that any classification needs a firm scientific basis. The current version of the DSM distinguishes nearly 300 diagnostic entities enabling about 170 different combinations to fulfill the criterion MDD. Such number may be considered as exuberant, but there is as yet no scientific argumentation whether such number is too much, too little or just perfect. The question arises whether or not it is possible to make a rational decision about the treatment of the individual patient and this is in fact challenging the concept of evidence based treatment regimens and -in a broader perspective- strict causality as the usefulness of the medical model for MDD.

The current classification systems (such as the DSM) are formulated to a large extent ex cathedra (by consensus) and are therefore not well amenable to scientific falsification [37]. In other words: a biological or any other parameter or marker will never be sufficiently strong to falsify and reject the DSM. Consider for instance the DST: this test may be found to be abnormal in approximately 70% (at best) of the depressive subjects and in 30% of –perfectly- matched controls [3, 4]. But has the dexamethason test challenged the DSM-classification of MDD? It might -of course- be argued that the dexamethason test is not included in the DSM definition of depression, so it cannot be used as an argument against the DSM. But if that is so, than the question arises what then could be the scientific justification of the DSM? Another example referring to the response to therapies. An intervention may prove to be therapeutically effective in only in 60% of a cohort, as is the case with antidepressants, including SSRI's [35, 36]. Would this partial efficacy (together with a substantial placebo response) ever challenge a clinical classification? The limited therapeutic efficacy is, instead, attributed to such factors as heterogeneity of depression, to patient specific characteristics or to ineffective drugs. But we think there are no criteria to verify or reject classification systems, and as argued in this essay there are no biologically founded parameters to do that, and more generally: such parameters (genes, biomarkers, time-courses of symptoms) will never persuade for changing a classification. Finally another obstacle to challenge the DSM has to be mentioned here: publication bias. It is generally discouraged to publish psychiatric investigations without adherence to some classification system (*i.e.,* the DSM).

A diagnosis identifying MDD should lead to an effective therapy, which is a prerequisite of evidence-based psychiatric practice. We have examined the strengths and weaknesses of causal relationship between diagnosis and therapy of MDD. Three major obstacles for a rational evidence-based praxis were discerned 1st current classification systems are scientifically non-falsifiable, 2nd mood transitions (and so cerebral processes) are -at least to some extent-non-deterministic, *i.e.,* they are random, stochastic and /or chaotic, and 3rd the relatively weak efficacy and specificity of current anti-depressive interventions. These considerations together indicate that a scientific foundation of the DSM or any other ex cathedra classification is practically unreachable. Our arguments encourage the search for alternative approaches.

9. FINAL REMARKS

The main theme of this chapter is how we conceive the psychiatric patient in a neurobiological context. To appreciate the origins of the current research and conceptualizations, I gave a short overview of the developments of the last 100 years or so. Moreover some philosophical thoughts about neurobiology and psychiatry were discussed. I have argued that the assumption of a unitary mind requires a concomitant configuration of the brain. Such time-space conformation contains all information of the subject has collected during live. We may simplify the concept of a personal brain by saying that: it is not that you have your memories, but you are your memories, instead. The concept of the individual space-time configuration of the brain acknowledges the individual expression of a psychiatric disorder and offers a neurobiological platform of first-person psychiatry.

Psychiatric therapies should be seen as an attempt to reshape the personal time-space configuration. An obstacle might be that new memories and experiences are built in the existing configuration, and not necessarily erasing them. This conclusion might also be seen as a challenge for future research to optimize the efficacy of (psycho)therapeutic interventions. In fact, reshaping the proposed time-space configuration might be the basis of both legal and illegal brainwashing. Possibly the combination of biological and psychotherapeutic treatments might offer new therapeutic avenues. Desensitization exposure therapies as used in phobic disorders might lead to rewiring of the brain, thereby suppressing phobia provoking thoughts.

Another aspect of the here proposed space-time configuration of the brain is its stochastic character, as illustrated with studies on fast mood transitions. Stochastic processes are nearly unpredictable in the individual, and can only be described and understood in a population or cohort. Stochastic processes are a threat for conventional medicine, where the ideal diagnosis guarantees therapeutic success. In depression we questioned whether such an ideal can ever be reached.

In the last decade genetic approaches have changed from relating single genes to psychiatric disorders, usually defined by classification systems, such as the DSM, to the possible involvement of multiple genes. Current investigations suggest that many genes are involved in depression. And even if the underlying multi factorial cause of the disorder is precisely known, for an external observer (clinician, scientist) depression might appear as a stochastic process. A (psychiatric) disorder such as major depression is characterized by features such as duration, recurrence and severity and it might well be that these are better associated with the genetic makeup or with some other biomarkers, than the mood itself. If so, than for instance a gene variant or biomarker may erroneously become linked to MDD, whereas, the gene variant prolongs the diseased state only. Another approach is to recognize endo-phenotypes as subject vulnerable to develop a psychiatric disorder. For instance subjects prone to depression are exposed to stress, concomitant with measuring local brain activity with functional neuroimaging (fMRI). As emphasized, fMRI is unable to show neural processing preceding the development of the imaging signal: so the bias of fMRI is possibly on the execution of tasks or functions, rather than on the initial unconscious psychopathological processes.

The present analysis conforms many items of the agenda of Kendler [9]: that psychiatry is grounded in mental, first-person experiences; Cartesian dualism and epiphenomenalism are false and both brain—mind and mind–brain causality are real, psychiatric disorders are complex and explanatory pluralism is preferable. The present exposé emphasizes that the various psychiatric approaches force to abandon some brain concepts. By doing so, the present conceptualization reconciles both psychotherapeutic and biological approaches in psychiatry. But it illuminates also the limitations of these approaches: one question is how to influence the brain micro-morphology with current psychiatric interventions. The 7th item of Kendler's agenda is to embrace empirically rigorous and pluralistic explanatory models. I may emphasize here again, that in psychiatry rigorous explanatory models may perhaps be impossible anyway. The last item of Kendler's agenda, accept piecemeal integration of complex etiological pathways to psychiatric illness a little bit at a time, is fully acknowledged.

REFERENCES

[1] Shorter E. A history of psychiatry. Wiley & Son, New York, 1997, pp 1-436.

[2] Healy D. The creation of psychopharmacology. Harvard university Press Cambridge Massachusetts. 2002, pp 1-469.

[3] Carroll BJ, Feinberg M, Greden JF, Tarika J, Albala AA, Haskett RF, James, NM, Kronfol Z, Lohr N, Steiner M, de Vigne JP, Young E. A specific laboratory test for the diagnosis of melancholia. Standardization, validation, and clinical utility. Archives of General Psychiatry 1981, 38:15-22.

[4] Nierenberg, AA, Feinstein, AR. How to evaluate a diagnostic marker test. Lessons from the rise and fall of dexamethasone suppression test. Journal of the American Medical Association 1988, 259:1699-1702.

[5] Broom MR Bortlotti L (Eds). Psychiatry as cognitive neuroscience: philosophical perspectives. Oxford University Press. Oxford OX2 6DP, 2009, pp 1-382.

[6] Korf J. On causality in psychiatry. Psychiatry and Freedom: conference for philosophy and mental health. Dallas. Texas USA. www.utsouthwestern.edu/psychiatryandfreedom, 2008.

[7] Korf J. You are your memory: Neurobiological reflections on a personal brain and on the nature of psychiatric disorders, including depression. Abstract. 13th International Conference of the International Network for Philosophy and Psychiatry (INPP). Manchester, 2010.

[8] Korf J. A stochastic and personal brain versus evidence based psychiatry Abstract 14th International Conference of the International Network for Philosophy and Psychiatry (INPP) Gothenburg, 2011.

[9] Kendler K. S. Toward a philosophical structure for psychiatry. Am J Psychiatry 2005 , 162:433-440.

[10] Stavenga GJ. Verheldering van de werkelijkheid (Elucidation of the Reality by a systems theoretical approach). Het Zuiden Vught the Nederlands, 2011, pp 14-364.

[11] Plessner H. Die Stufen des Organischen und der Mensch. Einleitung in die philosophische Anthropologie, Walter de Gruyter. Berlin Berlin / Leipzig. (ed .1975), 1928.

[12] Den Boer JA. den. Neurofilosofie: hersenen, bewustzijn, vrije wil (Neurophilosophy:, brain, consciousness, free will) Boom Publ Amsteram, 2003, pp 19-302.

[13] Kim J. Physicalism, or something near enough. Princeton University Press. Princeton and Oxford, 2005, pp 1-174.

[14] LeDoux. J. Synaptic Self How Our Brains Became Who We Are. Paperback Penguin Books, 2003, pp 1- 250.

[15] Searle JR. Dualism Revisited. J Physiology (Paris), 2007, 101:168-178.

[16] Stam CJ. Characterization of anatomical and functional connectivity in the brain: a complex networks perspective. Int J Psychophysiol 2010, 77:186-194.

[17] Searle JR, Consciousness. Annual Review Neurosciences 2000, 23:557-578.

[18] Vicari G. Beyond Conceptula Dualism: Ontology of consciousness, mental causation, and holism in John R Searle's Philosophy of mind. Value Inquiry Book Series Vol 196. Rudolphi Amsterdam, New York NY, 2008, pp 1-192.

[19] Korf J, Gramsbergen JB. Timing of potential and metabolic brain energy. J Neurochem. Dec; 2007, 103:1697-708.

[20] Korf J. (2010) The isoenergetic brain: the idea and some implications. Neuroscientist. 16:118-124.

[21] Turennout M, Hagoort P, Brown CM. Brain activity during speaking: from syntax to phonology in 40 milliseconds. Science 1998; 280:572-574.

[22] Libet B. Reflections on the interaction of the mind and brain. Progress Neurobiology. Feb-Apr; 2006, 78:322-326.

[23] Phillips J. Understanding/explanation. In: The philosophy of psychiatry: a companion. Ed Jennefer Radden. Oxford University Press Oxford 2004, Chapter 12 pp 180-190.

[24] American Psychiatric Association. Diagnostic and statistical manual of mental Disorders (4th and following editions) (DSM IV). Washington DC: APA, 1994.

[25] aan het Rot M, Mathew SJ & Charney DS. Neurobiological mechanisms in major depressive disorder. Canadian Medical Association Journal 2009, 180:305-313.

[26] Russo S, Kema IP, Bosker F, Haavik J & Korf J. Tryptophan as an evolutionarily conserved signal to brain serotonin: Molecular evidence and psychiatric implications. World Journal of Biological Psychiatry 2009, 10:258-268.

[27] Russo S, Kema IP, Fokkema MR, Boon JC, Willemse PH, de Vries EG, den Boer JA & Korf J. Tryptophan as a link between psychopathology and somatic states. Psychosomatic Medicine 2003, 65:665-671.

[28] Bosker FJ, Hartman CA, Nolte IM, Prins BP, Terpstra P, Posthuma D, van Veen T, Willemsen G, DeRijk RH, de Geus EJ, Hoogendijk WJ, Sullivan PF, Penninx BW, Boomsma DI, Snieder H & Nolen WA. Poor replication of candidate genes for major depressive disorder using genome-wide association data. Molecular Psychiatry 2010b, 15:1-17.

[29] van der Werf SY, Kaptein KI, de Jonge P, Spijker J, de Graaf R, Korf J. Major depressive episodes and random mood. Archives of General Psychiatry. 63 2006, (5):509-518.

[30] de Jonge P, Conradi HJ, Kaptein KI, Bockting CL, Korf J, Ormel J. Duration of subsequent episodes and periods of recovery in recurrent major depression. J Affective Disorders 2010, 125:141-145.

[31] Wirz-Justice A & Van den Hoofdakker RH. Sleep deprivation in depression: what do we know, where do we go? Biological Psychiatry 1999, 46:445-453.

[32] Riemann D, Wiegand M, Lauer CJ, Berger M. Naps after total sleep deprivation in depressed patients: are they depressiogenic? Psychiatry Res. 1993 Nov; 1993, 49:109-120.

[33] Bejjani BP, Damier P, Arnulf I, Thivard L, Bonnet AM, Dormont D, Cornu P, Pidoux B, Samson Y & Agid Y. Transient acute depression induced by high-frequency deep-brain stimulation. New England Journal of Medicine 1999, 1340:1476-1480.

[34] Tommasi G, Lanotte M, Albert U, Zibetti M, Castelli L, Maina G & Lopiano L. Transient acute depressive state induced by subthalamic region stimulation. Journal of Neurological Sciences 2008, 273:135-138.

[35] Moncrieff J, Kirsch I. Efficacy of antidepressants in adults. British Medical Journal 16; 2005, 155-157.

[36] Turner EH, Matthews AM, Linardatos E, Tell RA, Rosenthal R. Selective publication of antidepressant trials and its influence on apparent efficacy. New England Journal of Medicine 17; 2008, 358:252-260.

[37] Stoyanov D, Korf J, de Jonge P & Popov G. The possibility of evidence-based psychiatry: depression as a case. Clinical Epigenetics 2011, 2:7-15.

1

Send Orders for Reprints to reprints@benthamscience.net
Neurobiology of Mood Disorders, 2014, 3-22

CHAPTER 1

BRAIN MICRODIALYSIS IN KNOCKOUT MICE: DRAWBACKS AND ADVANTAGES TO STUDY THE ROLE OF 5-HT$_{1A}$ AND 5-HT$_{1B}$ AUTORECEPTORS IN THE MECHANISM OF ACTION OF ANTIDEPRESSANTS

ALAIN M. GARDIER*

Faculty of Pharmacy, University Paris South IV, Paris, France

Abstract: From anesthetized rats in the 90s to conscious wild-type or knockout mice today, intracerebral *in vivo* microdialysis provided important information about the brain mechanism of action of psychotropic drugs such as antidepressants. The principle of microdialysis technique is based on the balance between the release of neurotransmitters (*e.g.*, serotonin 5-HT, norepinephrine, dopamine) and re-uptake by selective transporters (*e.g.*, SERT for 5-HT). Complementary to electrophysiology, this technique reflects presynaptic monoamines release and intrasynaptic events corresponding to ≈ 80% of whole brain tissue content. It has been proposed that the inhibitory role of 5-HT$_{1A}$ and 5-HT$_{1B}$ serotonergic receptor sub-types that limit somatodendritic and nerve terminal 5-HT release, respectively, plays a key role in the mechanism of action of Selective Serotonin Reuptake Inhibitors (SSRI). This hypothesis is based partially on results of microdialysis experiments performed in naïve, non stressed Rodents. Examples from our own experience and from relevant publications from key investigators in this field will illustrate this statement. The present chapter will first remind the principle and methodology of the microdialysis technique when performed in mice. We will also underline the crucial need of developing animal models displaying behavioral, neurochemical and brain morphological phenotypes reminiscent of depression and anxiety in Human. Recently developed genetic mouse models have been generated to independently manipulate 5-HT$_{1A}$ autoreceptor and heteroreceptor populations and microdialysis helped to clarify the role of the presynaptic component, i.e., by measuring extracellular levels of neurotransmitters in serotonergic nerve terminal regions and raphe nuclei. The last two paragraphs will summarize main advantages and drawbacks of using microdialysis in mice through recent examples obtained in knockouts or alternatives such as infusion of a small-interfering RNA (siRNA) suppressing receptor functions in the mouse brain. Finally, by using drug infusion through the probe, correlation of microdialysis changes with behavioural data can be obtained, *e.g.*, with the antidepressant-like activity.

Keywords: Serotonin (5-HT), serotonin-1A/1B (5-HT1A/5-HT1B) receptors, serotonin transporter (SERT), depression, antidepressant drugs, selective serotonin reuptake inhibitors (SSRIs), animal models, knockout mice, microdialysis, small-interfering RNA (siRNA).

1. INTRODUCTION

Most of the antidepressants such as Selective Serotonin Reuptake Inhibitors (SSRI) act as indirect agonists of monoamine receptors. While SSRI drugs produce relatively rapid blockade of serotonin (5-hydroxytryptamine, 5-HT) transporters (SERT) *in vitro*, the onset of clinical benefits usually takes several (4-6) weeks to occur [1]. This gap in timing between SSRI near-immediate effect on neurotransmitter systems and the slow symptomatic recovery is a paradox that has not been completely

***Address correspondence to Alain M. Gardier:** Faculty of Pharmacy, University Paris South IV, Paris, France; E-mail: alain.gardier@u-psud.fr

Bruno P Guiard and Eliyahu Dremencov (Eds)

solved yet. At presynaptic level, SSRI-induced blockade of SERT results in a rapid suppression of the firing activity of 5-HT neurons in the brainstem [2]: these results have been obtained by using an electrophysiological technique in anesthetized animals.

1.1. FIRST IN RATS:

Another technique has provided complementary information about the mechanism of action of SSRIs : intracerebral *in vivo* microdialysis performed in awake, freely moving animals (first in rats, now in mice). Information included in this chapter was drawn from our own experience in this field and relevant publications from other investigators.

When it was first used in rat brain in the mid-80s, this technique measured, for example, extracellular concentrations of monoamines such as serotonin (5-hydroxytryptamine, 5-HText), which reflect presynaptic release of 5-HT and intrasynaptic events. With its coupling to very sensitive analytical techniques, it has provided much information regarding changes in the local presynaptic release of monoamines following acute drug administration. Thus, it has been possible to obtain two major arguments supporting the hypothesis that somatodendritic 5-HT_{1A} autoreceptors located in the raphe nuclei play an important role in the mechanism of action of SSRIs in rats [3]. At first, we have learned that a single administration of SSRIs at low doses comparable to those used therapeutically, increased 5-HText in the vicinity of the cell body and the dendrites of serotoninergic neurones of the dorsal raphe nucleus (DRN) [4]. This effect was more pronounced than that observed in regions rich in nerve endings (frontal cortex, ventral hippocampus: [5]), probably due to a higher SERT density [6]. Hence, the magnitude of the activation of the serotonergic neurotransmission depends on the brain area studied and the dose of the SSRIs administered to rats. This difference has been attributed to the activation activation of somatodendritic 5-HT_{1A} autoreceptors by endogenous 5-HT in the raphe nuclei, thereby limiting the corticofrontal effects of the antidepressant. Microdialysis technique demonstrated that, despite SSRI-induced 5-HT reuptake inhibition also taking place at nerve terminals, there is a decrease in 5-HT release *via* activation of 5-HT_{1A} (somatodendritic) or 5-HT_{1B} (nerve terminal) autoreceptors [7]. Thus, depending on the terminal 5-HT brain area, only a small increase or no change at all in the synaptic availability of 5-HT occurs [5, 8]. These microdialysis results obtained in rats, have then been extended to measure SSRI-induced changes in DRN 5-HText in awake, freely moving knockout mice [9, 10].

Next, we have learned from microdialysis performed in rats that SSRIs cause a larger increase in 5-HText at nerve endings following an acute treatment *versus* a chronic one. As the treatment is prolonged, a robust and time-dependent downregulation of the 5-HT transporter SERT was observed [11, 12], while 5-HT_{1A} autoreceptors gradually desensitize leading to a progressive recovery to normal of the firing rate of 5-HT neurons [13, 14, 15]. However, these molecular events seem to depend on 5-HT_{1A} autoreceptor internalization [16]. Indeed, we studied the function of the 5-HT system in the raphe nuclei and hippocampus by using repeated *in vivo* microdialysis sessions in awake freely moving mice. We assessed the degree of 5-HT_{1A} autoreceptor desensitization by using a local infusion of the 5-HT_{1A} receptor antagonist, WAY 100635 in the raphe *via* reverse microdialysis. We found that the anxiolytic-like effects of fluoxetine correlate in time and amplitude with 5-HT_{1A} autoreceptor desensitization, but neither with the basal extracellular levels of 5-HT in the raphe nuclei, nor in the hippocampus. These results suggests that the beneficial anxiolytic/antidepressant-like effects of chronic SSRI treatment depend on 5-HT_{1A} autoreceptor internalization, but do not require a sustained increase in extracellular 5-HT levels in a territory of 5-HT projection such as hippocampus. Several studies of patients with depression appear to confirm these experimental results, suggesting that co-administration of a 5-HT_{1A} autoreceptor antagonist (pindolol) and a SSRI accelerated the onset of the antidepressant effect [17]. However, given the complex pharmacology of pindolol, new drug developments may help to discover either selective and silent 5-HT_{1A} receptor antagonists to be prescribed in combination with SSRIs, or dual action agents (SSRI+5-HT_{1A} receptor blockers [18].

1.2. NEXT IN WILD-TYPE AND KNOCKOUT MICE:

The mouse genome can be specifically manipulated to produce the targeted deletion, replacement of genes or down-/over-expression of related proteins in the brain [19]. This was first obtained in embryonic stem cells, but more recently, temporal and spatial controls of gene expression were possible in adult mice. In the field of anxiety and depression, preclinical studies such as those described above, have been mostly performed in healthy, "not depressed" animals. In the mid-90s, genetically manipulated mice became available. It complicated the experimental protocol because it was necessary to include littermates as wild-type (WT) control mice. Great hopes were placed in mutant lines, some of them being considered as putative animal models of anxiety or depression. Several lines of transgenic (Tg) mice (carrying a human gene) or knockout (KO) mice (i.e., homozygous mice lacking the two copies of a gene coding for a receptor or transporter of neurotransmitter or neuropeptide) were generated between 1994 and 1998. The first KO mice were generated by homologous recombination in the laboratory of S. Tonegawa at MIT [20].

The mouse is a model organism of choice in the field of Neurosciences because: (i) numerous genes have a human equivalent, (ii) many biological and biochemical functions of the mouse are similar to those of humans, and (iii) the genome mouse is easily manipulated by homologous recombination. This technique allowed the creation of animal-related patterns of human brain pathologies. The genetic background is a fundamental parameter for analyzing the phenotype of KO mice. Historically, the mutant mice were established using embryonic stem (ES) line 129/Sv. However, creating new lines of mutant mice on a genetic background C57BL/6 is now preferred, although there are limits on the use of this strain in some behavioral tests (see [21] for a review).

At that time, the procedure of intracerebral *in vivo* microdialysis needed to be quickly adapted to perform experiments in an animal model having a smaller brain size than rats. Microdialysis experiments were first performed in Tyrosine hydroxylase Tg mice by Nakahara *et al.*, (1993) [22]. Then, it was applied to 5-HT_{1B} receptor KO mice [23, 24], to dopamine transporter DAT KO mice [25], and so on. Of course, at the end of the experiments, the precise location of the microdialysis probe must be macroscopically verify according to the stereotaxic coordinates given by the mouse brain atlas [26].

Regarding the pharmacological knowledges of antidepressants, the choice of KO mice as experimental models of anxiety – depression was remarkably appropriate because it is now well recognized that major depressive disorders result from a combination of genetic and environmental factors. In addition, knowing that anxiety and depression have a high co-morbidity [27, 28], it is critical for basic research to develop animal models that present behavioral, neurochemical and brain morphological phenotypes reminiscent of depression and anxiety. Some "serotonergic" KO mice display important changes in their basal phenotype. For example, constitutive 5-HT_{1A} receptor KO mice were simultaneously described by three different laboratories as an animal model of anxiety-related disorder [29, 30, 31]. They display decreased exploratory activity and increased fear of aversive environments and exhibited a decreased immobility in the forced swim test, an effect commonly associated with antidepressant treatment. Brain microdialysis performed in 5-HT_{1A} receptor KO mice have proven to be a valuable technique to address key questions regarding the mechanism of action of antidepressants. One of the most interesting applications of microdialysis is to allow the study of basal extracellular levels of neurotransmitters for example in 5-HT_{1A} receptor KO mice. While conventional microdialysis does not allow reliable measurements of these basal levels (see § 2.1), the no-net-flux (or zero-net-flux) method of quantitative microdialysis in mutants allows the direct and accurate determination of basal extracellular levels of neurotransmitters (see § 2.3). The dorsal raphe nucleus (DRN) is a brain region where 5-HText is known to regulate serotonergic transmission through activation of 5-HT_{1A} autoreceptors. When microdialysis was performed in the DRN, it was found that baseline DRN 5-HText did not differ between wild-type control and KO mice. This result suggests a lack of tonic control of 5-HT_{1A} autoreceptors on DR 5-HT release [9, 32].

Furthermore, microdialysis helped to decipher the brain region-dependent effects of antidepressants. Both a saline injection and handling for 3 min increased DRN 5-HText in 5-HT_{1A} receptor KO mice, but not in control mice. Fluoxetine, a serotonergic antidepressant, induced a dose-dependent increase in DRN 5-HText in both genotypes, but this effect was markedly more pronounced in 5-HT_{1A} KO mice. These results suggest that the increased responsiveness of dialysate 5-HText in the DRN of 5-HT_{1A} receptor KO mice at least in part explain the anxious phenotype of these mutants. Such information can help to define a better treatment of anxiety-related disorders.

The inhibitory 5-HT_{1A} receptor exists in two separate populations with distinct effects on serotonergic signaling, i.e., an autoreceptor that limits 5-HT release throughout the brain and a heteroreceptor that mediates inhibitory responses to release 5-HT. Traditional pharmacologic and transgenic strategies have tried to separate the distinct roles of these two receptor populations. Recently, Richardson-Jones *et al*., (2010) [33] developed a new strategy to manipulate presynaptic 5-HT_{1A} autoreceptors in serotonergic raphe neurons without affecting 5-HT_{1A} heteroreceptors, generating mice with higher (1A-High) or lower (1A-Low) autoreceptor levels. In this latter line, it was thus possible to examine the brain 5-HT system by partially turning off 5-HT_{1A} autoreceptors at a specific time point and to study correlations between changes in 5-HT transmission and antidepressant-like activity of SSRIs in various behavioral tests. This strategy robustly affects raphe firing rates, but has no effect on either basal extracellular 5-HT levels as measured by *in vivo* microdialysis in the frontal cortex and ventral hippocampus. Interestingly, following 8 days of fluoxetine treatment, a difference in 5-HT levels was found in the hippocampus, with higher levels in the 1A-low mice. In addition, 1A-Low mice displayed a larger increase in 5-HT in response to an acute challenge of fluoxetine in both brain regions. Together with electrophysiology data showing an increased spontaneous neuronal activity in the dorsal raphe of 1A-Low mice under stressful conditions, the microdialysis results were consistent with an increased serotonergic tone in these animals in response to an SSRI. Compared to 1A-Low mice, 1A-High mice show a blunted physiological response to acute stress, increased behavioral despair, and no behavioral response to antidepressant, thus modeling what we can find in patients with the 5-HT_{1A} risk allele. Indeed, human studies implicate a polymorphism in the promoter of the 5-HT_{1A} receptor gene in increased susceptibility to depression and decreased treatment response [34]. These mice may thus be conceived as a human equivalent to SSRI response (1A-Low) and resistance (1A-High) [35]. These results establish a causal relationship between 5-HT_{1A} autoreceptor levels and response to antidepressants.

The same group of researchers used a recently developed genetic mouse system to independently manipulate 5-HT_{1A} autoreceptor and heteroreceptor populations. They found that 5-HT_{1A} autoreceptors affect anxiety-like behavior, while 5-HT_{1A} heteroreceptors affect responses to forced swim stress, without effects on anxiety-like behavior [36]. These results establish distinct roles for the two receptors' populations, providing evidence that signaling through endogenous 5-HT_{1A} autoreceptors is necessary and sufficient for the establishment of normal anxiety-like behavior.

Taken together, these data obtained in KO mice brought a lot of information about the pathophysiology of psychiatric disorders and their treatments.

Thus, in 2012 we have at our disposal a large number of genetically engineered mice, some of them being interesting animal models of anxiety and depression. These mice are very helpful to discover the underlying pathological mechanisms that limit the effects of current treatments of major depressive episodes and to identify the nature of the molecular cascades leading to the installation of disorders such as anxiety and depression. In addition, KO mice help to study the effects of acute and chronic treatment with antidepressants.

Changes in the amount of neurotransmitters (mainly monoamines such as serotonin, 5-hydroxytryptamine, 5-HT, norepinephrine, NE, and dopamine, DA) in synapses can be viewed as near-immediate effects of SSRI on brain neurotransmitter systems. *In vivo* brain microdialysis allows to measure basal extracellular levels of these neurotransmitters giving an idea of neurochemical events occurring at nerve terminals in brain regions of awake, freely moving rodents. In our laboratory, we extensively applied this technique in genetic and pharmacological studies aimed at investigating the relationship between neurotransmitters and brain regions, or between neurochemical changes and animal behaviors (see examples below). Among the main interests of microdialysis application is the infusion of drugs through the microdialysis probe (reverse dialysis) in conscious KO mice as well as in WT mice used as controls in these pharmacological experiments [*e.g.*, intra-raphé perfusion of substance P in Guiard *et al.*, 2007 [37]; BDNF in Deltheil *et al.*, 2009 [38].

Recent advances in experimental approaches using genetically manipulated mice have already been summarize in the literature [19]. Knowing the large number of KO mice generated to date, it is not possible to detail the findings of each putative model interesting in the anxiety and depression field of research (SERT KO mice: [39]; NK1 receptor KO mice: [10, 40]; ß-arrestin 2 KO mice: [41]). Therefore, the remainder of the present chapter will only describe some examples, which explain these statements.

As already mentioned, most prescribed serotonergic antidepressants show limited efficacy and delayed onset of action, partly due to the activation of somatodendritic 5-HT_{1A} autoreceptors by the excess extracellular 5-HT produced by SSRI in the raphe nuclei. A group of scientists in Spain recently addressed this problem using an original strategy. Bortolozzi *et al.*, (2012) [42] administered a small-interfering RNA (siRNA) to suppress acutely 5-HT_{1A} autoreceptor-mediated negative feedback mechanisms in the mouse brain. They developed a conjugated siRNA (C-1A-siRNA) by covalently binding siRNA targeting 5-HT_{1A} receptor mRNA with the SSRI sertraline in order to concentrate it in serotonin axons, rich in serotonin transporter (SERT) sites. The intracerebroventricular (i.c.v.) infusion of C-1A-siRNA to mice resulted in its selective accumulation in serotonin neurons. This was associated with anti-depressant-like effects in the forced swim and tail suspension tests, but did not affect anxiety-like behaviors in the elevated plus-maze. In addition, C-1A-siRNA administration markedly decreased 5-HT_{1A}-autoreceptor expression and suppressed 8-OH-DPAT-induced hypothermia (a pre-synaptic 5-HT_{1A} receptor effect in mice) without affecting postsynaptic 5-HT_{1A} receptor expression in the hippocampus and prefrontal cortex. Moreover, i.c.v. C-1A-siRNA infusion augmented the increase in cortical dialysate 5-HT levels induced by fluoxetine to the level measured in 5-HT_{1A} receptor KO mice. Hence, C-1A-siRNA represents a new approach to treat mood disorders as monotherapy or in combination with SSRI.

To learn whether or not the *in vitro* affinity of SSRIs towards monoamine transporters can predict *in vivo* microdialysis data, we studied whether a single administration of a range of doses (1, 4 and 8 mg/kg, given i.p.) of paroxetine, citalopram or venlafaxine may simultaneously increase dialysate 5-HText and norepinephrine (NEext) by using *in vivo* microdialysis in the frontal cortex of awake, freely moving mice [43]. We found that citalopram and paroxetine have the highest potency to increase cortical 5-HText and NEext, respectively. In addition, the rank of order of efficacy of these antidepressant drugs to increase cortical 5-HText *in vivo* in mice was as follows: venlafaxine>citalo pram>paroxetine, while the efficacy to increase cortical NEext in mice of paroxetine and citalopram is similar, and greater than that of venlafaxine. Thus, the highest doses of the very selective SSRI citalopram, and the very potent SSRI paroxetine were able to increase cortical NEext. Surprisingly, the SNRI venlafaxine increased cortical 5-HText to a greater extent rather than NEext in the range of doses studied in mice.

We recently confirmed these data with escitalopram, the S(+)-enantiomer of citalopram. To analyze the mechanisms by which SSRIs activate noradrenergic transmission in the brain, we compared the effects of escitalopram, on both 5-HText and NEext in the frontal cortex of wild-type (WT) *versus* mutant mice lacking the 5-HT transporter (SERT(-/-) (44). In particular, the possibilities that escitalopram enhances NEext either by a direct mechanism involving the inhibition of the low- or high-affinity NE transporters, or by an indirect mechanism promoted by 5-HText elevation were explored. The forced swim test (FST) was used to investigate whether enhancing cortical 5-HText and/or NEext affected the antidepressant-like activity of escitalopram. As expected, a single systemic administration of escitalopram increased cortical 5-HText and NEext in WT mice. However, escitalopram failed to increase cortical 5-HText in SERT(-/-) mice, whereas its neurochemical effects on NEext persisted in these mutants. In WT mice, these neurochemical changes induced by escitalopram were associated with increased swimming parameter in the FST. Finally, escitalopram, at relevant concentrations, failed to inhibit cortical NE and 5-HT uptake mediated by low-affinity monoamine transporters (i.e., organic cation transporters such as OCT1, 2 or 3. These experiments suggest that escitalopram enhances, although moderately, cortical NEext *in vivo* by a direct mechanism involving the inhibition of the high-affinity NE transporter (NET). Such *in vivo* effects of SSRIs couldn't be predict by measuring the *in vitro* affinity of SSRIs towards SERT and NET in brain synaptosomes.

These results are not surprising. Indeed, experimental conditions (rat *versus* mice; whole brain *versus* cortical membranes; cell bodies *versus* nerve terminal regions; etc.....) highly influence the values of binding parameters of ligands to neurotransmitter receptors or transporters obtained *in vitro* (Bmax, K_D) GTP-gammaS binding, *etc...* The potency and selectivity of SSRIs as determined *in vitro* do not take into account noradrenergic projections and others which obviously interfer *in vivo*, but not *in vitro*. Thus, function of monoamines transporters are much more complex than previously thought. *In vivo* experiments help to depict this complexity when it is possible to measure correlation between neurochemical parameters and behavior.

2. MICRODIALYSIS: PRINCIPLE AND METHODOLOGY IN MICE

The principle of microdialysis technique is based on the balance between the release of neurotransmitters (*e.g.*, 5-HT) and its re-uptake (*e.g.*, by SERT). Usually, male 3 to 4-months old wild-type or mutant mice (25-30 g in body weight) are used for microdialysis experiments.

2.1.CONVENTIONAL INTRACEREBRAL *IN VIVO* MICRODIALYSIS

Whole brain tissue measurements represent a mixture of the intracellular (≈20%) and extracellular (≈80%) content. To obtain a measurement more directly related to synaptic transmission, it is interesting to sample specifically the content of the extracellular space, which is the site of exchanges between neurons, glial cells and blood vessels [45]. It contains various monoamines, excitatory and inhibitory amino acids, neuropeptides and their metabolites as well as precursors of these neurotransmitters. In the mid-80s, the development of very sensitive analytical techniques such as liquid chromatography and electrochemical detection (LC-ED) had made possible to perform *in vivo* microdialysis first in anesthetized rodents, then in awake, freely moving animals.

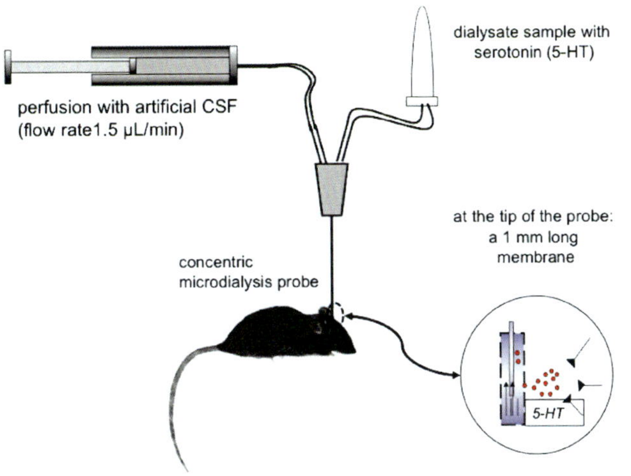

Figure 1: Principle of intracerebral microdialysis in awake, freely moving mice.

In vivo microdialysis technique, in anesthetized or awake animals, was developed by the group of Delgado in 1972 in monkeys [46], then improved in rats by the group of Ungerstedt in the early 80s. It is based on the law of passive diffusion of low molecular weight compounds through a porous membrane from the compartment with the highest concentration of neurotransmitters (the synaptic extracellular space) to the less concentrated compartment (i.e., the dialysis probe perfused with a buffer solution at physiological pH that does not contain neurotransmitters) (Figure **1**). This technique, now currently applied in our laboratory in awake, freely moving WT control or knockout (KO) adult mice, allows the collection of samples (named 'dialysates') every 10 or 20 minutes with a flow rate from 0.5 to 1.5 µl / min depending on the experimental protocol and the brain region studied. These samples contain, among other molecules, serotonin (5-HT), its major metabolite (5-HIAA) and noradrenaline (NA), dopamine (DA) and their metabolites. These molecules are then quantified by using high-performance liquid chromatography coupled to an amperometric detector (*e.g.*, 1049A, Hewlett-Packard, Les Ulis, France). The limit of sensitivity for 5-HT is ~ 0.5 fmol/sample (signal-to-noise ratio = 2).

The concentrations of neurotransmitters reflect the physiological balance between the calcium-dependent neurotransmitter release and its reuptake by the selective carrier (*e.g.*, SERT or 5-HTT for 5-HT) located on the membrane of presynaptic neurons. A comprehensive study of intracerebral microdialysis has four phases: (1) surgical stereotaxic implantation of the probe under anesthesia, (2) the collection of dialysates (first to measure baseline value of extracellular neurotransmitter levels before and 2-3 hours after drug treatment), (3) the collection of brains for the accurate verification of the implantation site of the microdialysis membrane and (4) of chromatographic analysis of dialysate samples. See [10] and [47] for details.

2.2.DRUG ADMINISTRATION BY REVERSE MICRODIALYSIS

A major advantage of the microdialysis technique is to infuse a drug locally into the brain to confirm central effects on dialysates first measure following a peripheral injection of the drug. Thus, drugs with a high molecular weight can be dissolved in artificial cerebrospinal fluid (aCSF) and administered locally, for example into the ventral hippocampus *via* a silica catheter glued to the microdialysis probe (flow rate : 0.2 µL/min for 2 min), at the dose of 10 to 100 ng [37, 48]. For each experiment, a control group must receive the appropriate vehicle.

2.3.ZERO NET FLUX METHOD OF QUANTITATIVE* INTRACEREBRAL MICRODIALYSIS

The zero net flux method of quantitative microdialysis is used to quantify basal extracellular neurotransmitter concentrations and the extraction fraction of this neurotransmitter (Ed), which provides an index of the functional status of the neurotransmitter uptake *in vivo*. Usually, four samples are collected to determine basal hippocampal 5-HT levels (as in [49] in NK1 receptor KO mice), before local perfusion of increasing concentrations of 5-HT (0, 5, 10 and 20 nM). The dialysate 5-HT concentrations (Cout) obtained during perfusion of the various concentrations of 5-HT (Cin) are used to construct a linear regression curve for each animal [50]. The net change in 5-HT (Cin-Cout) is plotted on the y-axis against Cin on the x-axis. Extracellular 5-HT levels ([5-HT]ext) and the extraction fraction of the probe (Ed) are determined as described by Parsons *et al.* (1991) [51]. The concentration of 5-HT in the extracellular space is estimated from the concentration at which Cin-Cout=0 and corresponds to point at which there is no net diffusion of 5-HT across the dialysis membrane. The extraction fraction (Ed) is the slope of the linear regression curve and has been shown to provide an estimate of changes in transporter-mediated 5-HT uptake [51, 52].

As an example of the relevance of the zero-net-flux method of quantitative microdialysis, we have recently shown the critical impact of a neuropeptide, Brain-Derived Neurotrophic factor (BDNF) on serotonergic neurotransmission under basal conditions and following SSRI treatment. In a series of experiments, we examined the consequences of either a constitutive decrease [50] or increase in brain BDNF protein levels [38, 48, 53] on hippocampal extracellular levels of 5-HT in conscious mice. The no-net-flux method allow unveiling differences in basal extracellular 5-HT levels in heterozygous BDNF +/- mice [50]. Indeed, this neurotrophic factor is known to play a role in mood disorders and the mechanism of action of antidepressant drugs. However, the relationship between BDNF and serotonergic signalling is poorly understood. BDNF +/- mice were used to investigate the influence of BDNF on the 5-HT system and the activity of the serotonin transporter (SERT) in the hippocampus. The zero net flux method revealed that these mutants have increased basal extracellular 5-HT levels in the hippocampus and decreased 5-HT reuptake capacity. These results are coherent with the lack of effect of paroxetine to increase hippocampal 5-HText levels in BDNF +/- mice, while it produced robust effects in wild-type littermates. As expected, *in-vitro* autoradiography and synaptosome techniques in BDNF +/- mice revealed a significant decrease in [3H]citalopram-binding-site density in the CA3 subregion of the ventral hippocampus and a significant reduction in [3H]5-HT uptake in hippocampal synaptosomes. Taken together, these results provide evidence that constitutive reductions in BDNF modulate SERT function reuptake in the hippocampus.

2.4.STATISTICAL ANALYSIS AND EXPRESSION OF RESULTS OF MICRODIALYSIS EXPERIMENTS IN KO MICE

Usually, microdialysis data are reported as means ± SEMs. For conventional microdialysis experiments, we used to perform statistical analyses on areas under the curve (AUC) values for the amount of 5-HT outflow collected during the 0-120 min post-treatment period. To compare different

AUC values in each group of mice, a two-way ANOVA with genotype factor and treatment factor is performed.. We used to present microdialysis data as histograms because statistical analysis on AUC values better reflects the pharmacological properties of a compound than the kinetics. We strongly believe that the interpretation of these data is more appropriate when performed on AUC values in dialysate 5-HT levels [44, 54] as well as for dopamine levels [55, 56] when changes induced by drugs are compared between WT versus KO mice.

Using intracerebral microdialysis in the hippocampus and cortex in mice, measuring statistically significant changes in dialysate 5-HT levels induced, for example, by a given drug between t30 min and t45 min offers little interest. We feel that these information make the message more difficult to interpret and do not fundamentally improve the study. These time courses are strongly dependent on the experimental conditions and consequently not reproducible between laboratories. By contrast, our experience reveals that comparable results from distinct laboratories can be obtained from the analysis of AUC values. The inclusion of the data showing the time course for the microdialysis is oftten superfluous. Microdialysis is a neurochemical technique not sensitive enough to explore precisely (i.e., sample by sample) the time course of drug effects.

However, in some cases, it is interesting to show the time course analysis of the microdialysis data:
1)- when we need to express time course data in microdialysis experiments as concentrations (in fmol/sample, not as % changes) because the baseline dialysate levels of the neurotransmitter are statistically different between two groups of mice, *i.e.,* in Table **1** and Figures **2** and **3** in Guiard *et al.*, (2008) [50] : heterozygous BDNF +/- mice had a higher basal 5-HText levels in the hippocampus compared to WT mice. See also in Table **1** and Figure **6** in Guilloux *et al.*, (2011) [54], in which double 5-$HT_{1A/1B}$ -/- mice display a higher basal 5-HText levels in the frontal cortex and DRN compared to WT mice.
2)- when it is sometimes important to collect some pharmacokinetic information about the short term or long lasting effect of a new drug in rodents. AUC analysis of microdialysis data disregards information about differences in Cmax and duration of the drug effects.
3)- when a grey line (Figure **3** in Guilloux *et al.*, 2006 [32]: Figures **1** and **2** in Nguyen *et al.*, 2012 [44]) indicates the duration time of the forced swim test (i.e., 6 minutes), which was performed, in a separate group of animal, at the maximum effect of the antidepressant on cortical extracellular 5-HT levels in mice. It emphasizes that microdialysis and behavioral experiments were carried out by using the same experimental protocol.

3. SEROTONIN, KO MICE AND MICRODIALYSIS

Depressive disorders result from a combination of genetic and environmental factors. To date, several genes appear to have in humans and animals, a greater influence than the other and emerge from the literature. Among them, the presence of a polymorphism of either the carrier of 5-HT, SERT [39, 57], 5-HT_{1A} receptor (34), the tryptophan hydroxylase type 2 (TPH-2; [58]), BDNF [59], is associated with the occurrence of depression related to stress, or to a response to behavioral tests predictive of the antidepressant-like activity of a molecule [60, 61].

3.1. ADVANTAGES OF USING MICRODIALYSIS IN KO MICE

In these KO mice, we can measure for example the paradigms of stress to predict the antidepressant potential of a molecule and the selectivity of behavioral responses in comparison with non mutated control animals: if these responses are diminished or absent in KO mice deprived of a gene encoding a neurotransmitter receptor, we may conclude that this receptor plays a major part either in the antidepressant-like effect and/or of the molecule. Regarding microdialysis, changes in dialysate levels of neurotransmitters following acute [47] or chronic [52] SSRI treatment can highlight the mechanism of action of these drugs.

Thus, we combined KO mice and receptor antagonist strategies to investigate the contribution of the 5-HT_{1B} receptor sub-type in mediating the effects of a SSRI, paroxetine in mice [47]. Using microdialysis, we found that a single systemic administration of paroxetine (1 or 5 mg/kg by the i.p. route) increased 5-HText in the ventral hippocampus and frontal cortex of WT control and mutant mice. However, in the ventral hippocampus, the SSRI induced a larger increase in dialysate 5-HT levels in KO 5-HT_{1B} mice than in control mice. In addition, either the absence of the 5-HT_{1B} receptor (in KO 5-HT_{1B} mice) or its pharmacological blockade with the mixed 5-$HT_{1B/1D}$ receptor antagonist, GR 127935 (in WT mice) potentiated the effect of a single administration of paroxetine on extracellular 5-HT levels in the ventral hippocampus. Thus, these data underline several points:
- complementary results were obtained by combining KO mice and receptor antagonist strategies.
- there were already *in vitro* studies showing the role of terminal 5-HT_{1B} autoreceptors *in vivo* to control 5-HT release and reuptake (in slices: [62]). Our microdialysis data in KO 5-HT_{1B} mice brought additional information by suggesting that 5-HT_{1B} autoreceptors limit the effects of SSRIs on dialysate 5-HT levels at serotonergic nerve terminals and revealed the importance of a particular brain region, the ventral hippocampus. It is interesting to notice that recently, many experimental arguments have accumulated to suggest that antidepressants exert their behavioral activity in adult rodents, at least in part, by inducing of cellular and molecular changes in the adult hippocampus (see the Chapter on "*Hippocampal neurogenesis in adult rodents*" by David *et al.*, in the present text book).

By using microdialysis, we can also study changes in dialysate 5-HT levels in the dorsal raphe nucleus (see Introduction). Data described above in 5-HT_{1A} receptor KO mice illustrated this important contribution. This experiment can give further information when combined with measurements of the electrical activity of 5-HT neurons. Again, the comparison of results between a KO mice model and WT mice is very informative.

Neurochemical changes as measured by using microdialysis can have functional consequences since they correlated with behavioural data obtained, for example, in the forced swim test (FST). Three examples can illustrate these benefits.

The first example in wild-type mice: the antidepressant-like activity of paroxetine as measured on swimming behavior was potentiated by BDNF. These data suggest an interesting synergy between BDNF and SSRI on 5-HT neurotransmission, thus such a co-administration improved the antidepressant-like activity of the SSRI [38].

The second example, in 5-HT_{1A} receptor KO mice: As described in Guilloux *et al.*, 2006 [32], paroxetine (1 and 4 mg/kg) dose-dependently increased cortical 5-HText in both WT and KO genotypes, but the effects were greater in mutants. Paroxetine administration also dose-dependently decreased the immobility time in both strains of mice, but the response was much greater in $5HT_{1A}$ -/- mice. Overall these results suggest that the genetic inactivation of 5-HT_{1A} receptors, abolished the inhibitory feedback control exerted by somatodendritic 5-HT_{1A} autoreceptors, thus enhancing the response of mutant mice to stressful conditions such as the FST. Thus, following SSRI administration, an indirect activation of presynaptic 5-HT_{1A} receptors by endogenous 5-HT may limit its antidepressant-like effects in the FST in wild type mice.

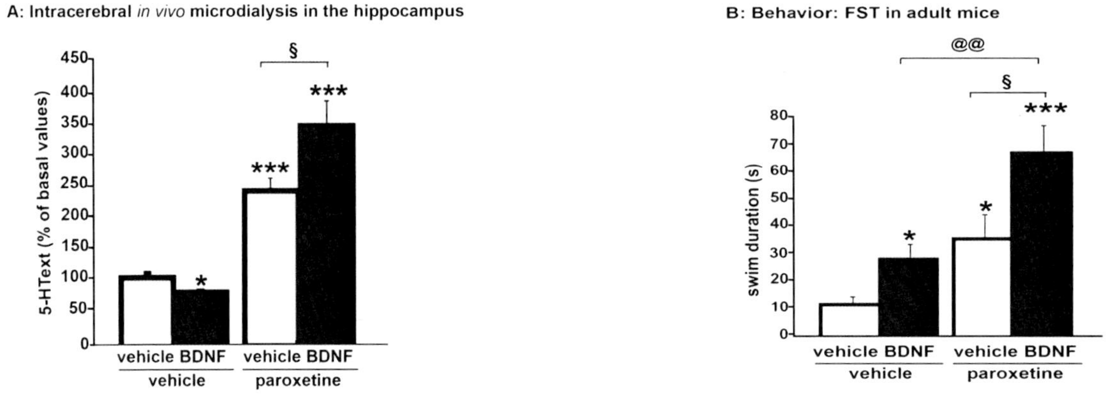

Figure 2: (A) Microdialysis data showing that an acute intra-hippocampal injection of BDNF (100 ng) potentiated the effects of the systemic administration of an SSRI, paroxetine (4 mg/kg; i.p.) on dialysate 5-HText in the hippocampus of freely moving wild-type mice. Results are expressed as AUC values (means ± S.E.M.) calculated for the amount of 5-HText collected during the 0–120 min post-treatment period. (B) Antidepressant-like activity of paroxetine as measured on swimming behavior in the Forced Swim Test (FST) was potentiated by BDNF. Thus, neurochemical changes correlated with behavioral data in this protocol, suggesting that a BDNF + SSRI combination may offer new alternatives to treat mood disorders (From [38]).

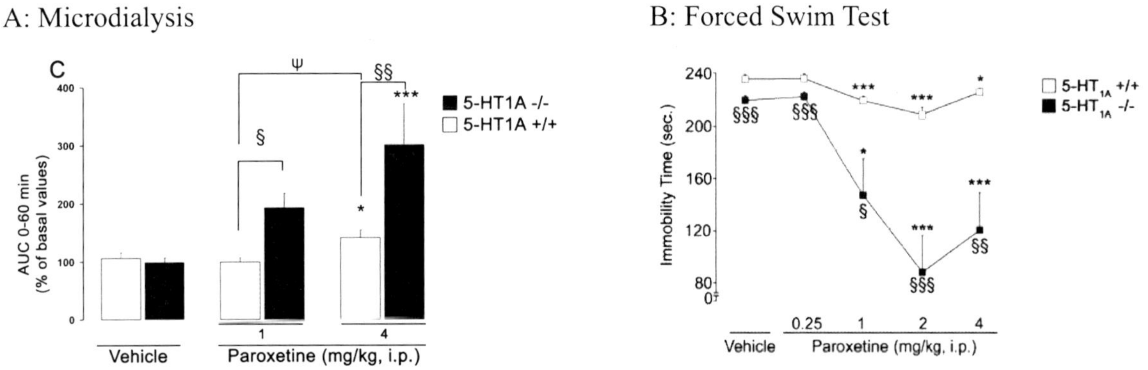

Figure 3: (A) Microdialysis data showing the effects of paroxetine on cortical 5-HText in 5-HT_{1A} +/+ wild-type and 5-HT_{1A} -/- mice. Results are expressed as AUC values (means ± S.E.M.) calculated for the amount of 5-HText collected during the 0–60 min post-treatment period. (B) Antidepressant-like effects of paroxetine on the immobility time in the mouse forced swimming test (FST) in 5-HT_{1A} +/+ and 5-HT_{1A} -/- mice. FST and microdialysis experiments have been performed separately. Microdialysis and behavioral experiments were carried out by using the same experimental protocol. The duration time of the FST was 6 min, performed at the maximum effect of paroxetine on dialysate 5-HText, i.e., 30 min after its administration (From [32]).

The third example, in SERT KO mice: Another interest of brain microdialysis is to allow the measurements of several neurotransmitters in the same sample. Thus, we recently examined the effects of escitalopram, the S(+)-enantiomer of citalopram, on both [5-HT]ext and extracellular levels of norepinephrine [NE]ext in the frontal cortex (FCx) of freely moving WT and mutant mice lacking the 5-HT transporter ($SERT^{-/-}$) by using intracerebral microdialysis [44]. In WT mice, a single systemic administration of escitalopram produced a significant increase in cortical [5-HT]ext and [NE]ext. As expected, escitalopram failed to increase cortical [5-HT]ext in SERT-/- mice, whereas its neurochemical effects on [NE]ext persisted in these mutants. In addition, in WT mice submitted to the FST, escitalopram increased swimming parameter without affecting climbing behavior.

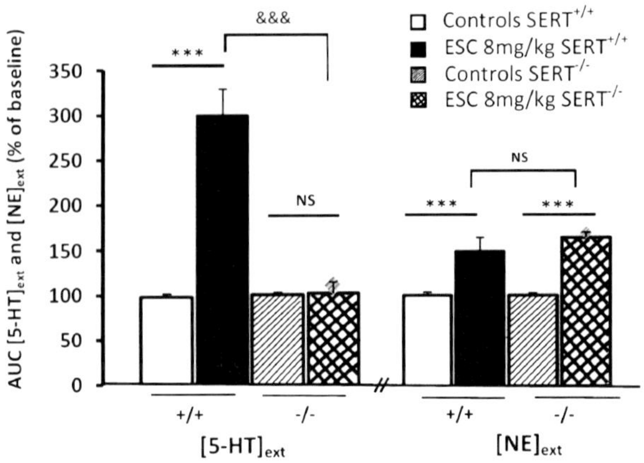

Figure 4: Effect of systemic administration of escitalopram (ESC) on extracellular levels of 5-HT and noradrenaline (NE) in the frontal cortex in WT (SERT$^{+/+}$) and KO (SERT$^{-/-}$) mice. AUC values (means ± S.E.M.) were calculated for the amount of 5-HT and NE outflows collected during the 0–120 min post-treatment period (From [44]).

Thus, the following text summarizes the main advantages of the microdialysis technique:

- *In vivo* presynaptic test to study consequences of autoreceptor of transporter blockade on release and reuptake of neurotransmitters.
- Home made microdialysis probe with different membranes (and different cut off).
- Provide exogenous molecules directly into the brain tissue, with minimal damage.
- It is possible to implant two probes in the same mouse: a probe at the vicinity of cell bodies (*e.g.*, into the raphe nuclei for the neuronal 5-HT system), and a probe into a serotonergic nerve terminal region (hippocampus, frontal cortex), thus evaluating a neural circuit.
- It is an ideal approach to confirm central effects observed following the systemic administration of the drug. Even more interesting when the drug do not cross easily the blood brain barrier (such as molecules with a high molecular weight:

neurotrophic factors, *e.g.*, BDNF [38, 53]

substance P [37]

- Measurements of several neurotransmitters in the same sample [44].
- Study the same animal for two consecutive days, each one being used as its own control, *e.g.*, on Day 1 following administration of the vehicle, and on Day 2 following the pharmacological treatment.
- When using a guide cannula, it's possible to collect samples in the same animal once a week for several weeks [16].
- When applied in awake, freely moving animals, functional consequences of SSRI-induced increases in extracellular neurotransmitter levels can be studied, *e.g.*, correlation between changes in brain 5-HText and behavioral data (the swimming time in the FST [38, 44].

3.2. DRAWBACKS OF USING MICRODIALYSIS IN KO MICE

There are also limits regarding the use of constitutive KO mice. Compensatory events may occur when mice are generated by homologous recombination [21]. For example, 5-HT$_{1B}$ receptor KO mice exhibit a higher efficacy of 8-OH-DPAT-induced hypothermia suggesting that an adaptive thermoregulatory process involving the functional activity of somatodendritic 5-HT$_{1A}$ receptors is altered in 5-HT$_{1B}$ receptor KO mice [63]. By contrast, Bouwknecht *et al.*, 2002 [64] found no indications for adaptive changes in presynaptic 5-HT$_{1A}$ receptor function in 5-HT$_{1B}$ receptor KO mice as measured telemetrically on body temperature and heart rate responses.

Indeed, to study the direct consequences of alterations in the targeted gene, constitutive KO mice are very valuable tools because of compensatory processes that have taken place in reaction to life-long changes in gene expression [65]. The constitutive deletion of the noradrenaline transporter (NET), for example, induced an up-regulation of two other monoamine transporters, dopamine and serotonin (DAT and SERT, respectively) [66]. An increase in the binding of [(3)H]paroxetine to the SERT and [(3)H]GBR12935 to the DAT was observed in various brain regions of NET-KO mice, without alterations of mRNA encoding these transporters, as measured by *in situ* hybridization. This important finding obviously impacts the interpretation of previous data. Similarly, in SERT KO mice, Zhou *et al.*, (2002) [67] reported that 5-HT was found in DA neurons of homozygous (-/-), but not of heterozygous (+/-) mutant mice. DA neurons containing 5-HT have been observed in the substantia nigra and ventral tegmental area (VTA), but not in other brain areas of SERT KO mice. To verify the role of the DA transporter in such ectopic uptake, SERT KO mice were treated with DA uptake blocker GBR-12935 : ectopic 5-HT in DA neurons was disappeared. These data indicate that 5-HT can be taken into DA neurons in rodents when SERT is not functionally adequate to remove extracellular 5-HT levels, and (c) the DA transporter is responsible for the 5-HT uptake into DA neurons. Thus, cross neuronal type uptake exists and serves as a compensatory backup when a specific transporter is dysfunctional. Thus, when using mice lacking an important protein from the earliest period of their existence, one has to be aware that compensatory alterations may occur in the brain as well as at the periphery. This point must be considered when it comes to interpretation of the experimental results.

Other critical points of the microdialysis technique are summarized below:
- During microdialysis experiments, we used to collect the samples every 15 to 20 minutes (in the hippocampus and frontal cortex), every 10 minutes in raphe nuclei. This is due to the slow flow rate of the perfusion medium (≈1 μl/min), which leads to a poor temporal resolution compared to the technique of reference, electrophysiology (400 milliseconds).
- Classically, 1 experimenter, 2 mice, 1 day; 10 to 12 animals per group; delayed results (HPLC). Possible improvement with more sensitive analytical methods such as capillary electrophoresis with a laser-induced fluorescence detection [68, 69], but it remains a very complex technique.
- 3 to 6 months to complete an experiment, i.e., to evaluate the effects of several doses of an agonist - antagonist compared to mice treated with the vehicle or wild-type (WT) mice (a control groups). Even longer when using transgenic mice (breeding, genotyping, selection of age, sexe, and so on ...).
- Effect of stress, delicate animal handling, so it requires an experienced experimenter
- Cost of commercially available microdialysis probes. Large outer diameter of the probe (0.2 mm).
- Fairly approximative location of the membrane: at the end of the experiment, especially in mice, it is necessary to verify the exact location of the probe implantation, macroscopically on brain coronal sections [70].
- Poor prognostic value of <u>basal</u> extracellular concentrations of 5-HT, DA and NA.
- Extracellular concentrations of metabolites in dialysates (*e.g.*, 5-HIAA):

Under basal conditions: it reflects intracellular metabolism of 5-HT, and not release or utilization [71, 72].

Following pharmacological treatment: it has little interest because we know that dialysate 5-HIAA levels decrease, independently of the dose of the indirect 5-HT receptor agonist administered. These changes are not related to the neuronal activity [4, 73].

CONCLUSION

These past 25 years, different strains of KO mice became extremely valuable tools in Neuropharmacology. They help to identify in animals susceptibility genes and proteins involved in the pathological processes leading to anxiety and depression. These biological markers could then be helpful to pose the diagnosis of the disease in human. They also give information on their functional role, thus offering opportunities to develop new drug treatments. When performed in KO mice, and together with other techniques, brain microdialysis was very useful to define central monoaminergic dysfunctions having behavioral consequences similar to those associated with endogenous depression in humans. Some KO mice with mutations of serotonin targets (*e.g.*, the 5-HT transporter SERT, 5-HT_{1B}, 5-HT_{1A} and 5-HT_4 receptors) display changes in phenotypes similar to those induced by chronic treatment with antidepressants in WT control mice.

Chronic antidepressant treatment may regulate the expression of neurotrophic factors such as BDNF and stimulate the process of adult neurogenesis in the dentate gyrus of the hippocampus in rats [74] and adult mice [75, 76]. Changes in adult neurogenesis are only seen after chronic, but not acute, antidepressant treatment. Microdialysis studies in heterozygous mice for BDNF [38, 48, 50, 77] contributed to this knowledge by exploring the relationship between the hippocampal 5-HT system (i.e., the function of its transporter, one of the main targets of antidepressants), and brain BDNF levels.

In the future, our efforts to understand the pathophysiology of mood disorders, especially anxiety/depression, will focus on the antidepressant responses, especially in non-stressed and stressed rodents. Microdialysis technique in young or adult KO mice will continue to decipher region-dependent relationships between brain neurotransmitters and circuits involved in the mechanism of action of an antidepressant drugs' polytherapy, soon available on the market. Furthermore, original strategies are now available to rescue the expression of a particular receptor sub-type in a tissue specific and temporally controlled manner in mice. For example, it well known that agonists of the 5-HT_{1A} receptor such as buspirone have anxiolytic properties, and KO mice lacking this receptor show increased anxiety-like behavior (as indicated above). However, the relevant brain regions involved in anxious phenotype have not been delineated. Using such a tissue-specific, conditional rescue strategy for the 5-HT_{1A} receptor, Gross *et al.* [78] engineered mice in which the expression of the 5-HT_{1A} receptor gene was under the control of the antibiotic doxycycline. The gene of interest was switched off when the mice were fed with the antibiotic. They used autoradiography to demonstrate that high levels of postsynaptic 5-HT_{1A} receptor expression in the hippocampus and cortex of the rescue mice, but the presynaptic 5-HT_{1A} autoreceptor, was undetectable in the raphe nuclei. By using mice in which the 5-HT_{1A} receptor can be knocked out at will, they show that the absence of the receptor in newborns lead to anxiety-like behavior, whereas its knockout during adult life has no effect. In addition, they found that postnatal developmental processes help to establish adult anxiety-like behavior. Generating such a rescue mice is a long lasting process, but each animal can be used as its own control.

Another strategy can be used to rescue a gene of interest, in which the KO mice line previously generated was used as the control group. To our knowledge, this strategy has not already been applied to the serotonin field of research: it was recently described to study the role of beta2-subunit of the nicotinic acetylcholine receptor (nAChR) (55) in the ventral tegmental area (VTA) in mediating the reinforcement properties of drugs: a gene of interest was re-expressed into the midbrain of ß2-KO mice by stereotaxically injecting a lentiviral vector carrying this gene coding for a receptor to test for the selectivity of the effects. In this example, microdialysis experiments were performed to confirm the rescue of nicotine effects in the vectorized line of mice compared to WT and KO lines.

These techniques allow greater precision and flexibility to generate KO rodents for understanding neurotransmitter function, No doubt that such novel and powerful tools, together with techniques of knock-in or SiRNA recently applied to the field of 5-HT receptors, will continue to give unexpected information on molecular and cellular mechanisms involved in mood disorders and their treatments.

REFERENCES

[1] Blier P, de Montigny C, Chaput Y. Modifications of the serotonin system by antidepressant treatments: implications for the therapeutic response in major depression. J Clin Psychopharmacol 1987, 7:24S-35S.

[2] Blier P. Pharmacology of rapid-onset antidepressant treatment strategies. J Clin Psychiatry 2001, 15:12-17.

[3] Gardier A, Malagié I, Trillat A-C, Jacquot C, Artigas F. Role of $5HT_{1A}$ autoreceptors in the mechanism of action of serotoninergic antidepressant drugs: recent findings from *in vivo* microdialysis studies. Fundamental and Clinical Pharmacology 1996, 10:16-27.

[4] Malagié I, Trillat AC, Jacquot C, Gardier AM. Effects of acute fluoxetine on extracellular serotonin levels in the raphe: an *in vivo* microdialysis study. Eur J Pharmacol 1995, 286:213-217.

[5] Malagié I, Trillat AC, Douvier E, Anmella MC, Dessalles MC, Jacquot C, Gardier AM. Regional differences in the effect of the combined treatment of WAY 100635 and fluoxetine: an *in vivo* microdialysis study. Naunyn Schmiedebergs Arch Pharmacol 1996, 354: 785-790.

[6] Hrdina PD, Foy B, Hepner A, Summers RJ. Antidepressant binding sites in brain: autoradiographic comparison of [3H]paroxetine and [3H]imipramine localization and relationship to serotonin transporter. J Pharmacol Exp Ther 1990, 252:410-8.

[7] Rutter JJ, Gundlah C, Auerbach SB. Systemic uptake inhibition decreases serotonin release *via* somatodendritic autoreceptor activation. Synapse 1995, 20:225-233.

[8] Romero L, Hervas I, Artigas F. The $5\text{-}HT_{1A}$ antagonist WAY-100635 selectively potentiates the presynaptic effects of serotonergic antidepressants in rat brain. Neurosci Lett 1996, 219:123-126.

[9] Bortolozzi A, Amargós-Bosch M, Toth M, Artigas F, Adell A. *In vivo* efflux of serotonin in the dorsal raphe nucleus of $5\text{-}HT_{1A}$ receptor knockout mice. J Neurochem 2004, 88:1373-9.

[10] Guiard BP, Przybylski C, Guilloux JP, Seif I, Froger N, De Felipe C, Hunt SP, Lanfumey L, Gardier AM. Blockade of substance P (neurokinin 1) receptors enhances extracellular serotonin when combined with a selective serotonin reuptake inhibitor: an *in vivo* microdialysis study in mice. J Neurochem 2004, 89:54-63.

[11] Pineyro G, Blier P, Dennis T, de Montigny C. Desensitization of the neuronal 5-HT carrier following its long-term blockade. J Neurosci 1994, 14:3036-47.

[12] Benmansour S, Owens WA, Cecchi M, Morilak DA, Frazer A. Serotonin clearance *in vivo* is altered to a greater extent by antidepressant-induced downregulation of the serotonin transporter than by acute blockade of this transporter. J Neurosci 2002, 22:6766-72.

[13] Blier P, de Montigny C, Azzaro AJ. Modification of serotonergic and noradrenergic neurotransmissions by repeated administration of monoamine oxidase inhibitors: electrophysiological studies in the rat central nervous system. J Pharmacol Exp Ther 1986, 237:987–994.

[14] Chaput Y, Blier P, de Montigny C. *In vivo* electrophysiological evidence for the regulatory role of autoreceptors on serotoninergic terminals. J Neurosci 1986, 6:2796–2801.

[15] El Mansari M, Sánchez C, Chouvet G, Renaud B, Haddjeri N. Effects of acute and long-term administration of escitalopram and citalopram on serotonin neurotransmission: an *in vivo* electrophysiological study in rat brain. Neuropsychopharmacology 2005, 30:1269-1277.

[16] Popa D, Cerdan J, Repérant C, Guiard BP, Guilloux JP, David DJ, Gardier AM. A longitudinal study of 5-HT outflow during chronic fluoxetine treatment using a new technique of chronic microdialysis in a highly emotional mouse strain. Eur J Pharmacol 2010, 628:83-90.

[17] Portella MJ, de Diego-Adeliño J, Ballesteros J, Puigdemont D, Oller S, Santos B, Álvarez E, Artigas F, Pérez V. Can we really accelerate and enhance the selective serotonin reuptake inhibitor antidepressant effect? A randomized clinical trial and a meta-analysis of pindolol in nonresistant depression. J Clin Psychiatry 2011, 72:962-9.

[18] Artigas F, Adell A, Celada P. Pindolol augmentation of antidepressant response. Curr Drug Targets 2006, 7:139-47.

[19] Sotnikova TD and Gainetdinov RR. Microdialyis in genetically altered animals. Chapter 5.1, pages 399-417. In Volume 16: Handbook of Microdialyis: Methods, applications and clinical aspects, by Ben H.C. Westerink and Thomas F.H. Cremers (Ed.). Academic Press 2007.

[20] Silva AJ, Paylor R, Wehner JM, Tonegawa S. Impaired spatial learning in alpha-calcium-calmodulin kinase II mutant mice. Science 1992, 257:206-11.

[21] Gardier AM. Mutant mouse models and antidepressant drug research: focus on serotonin and brain-derived neurotrophic factor. Behav Pharmacol 2009, 20:18-32.

[22] Nakahara D, Hashiguti H, Kaneda N, Sasaoka T, Nagatsu T. Normalization of tyrosine hydroxylase activity *in vivo* in the striatum of transgenic mice carrying human tyrosine hydroxylase gene: a microdialysis study. Neurosci Lett 1993, 158:44-6.

[23] Saudou F, Amara DA, Dierich A, LeMeur M, Ramboz S, Segu L, Buhot MC, Hen R. Enhanced aggressive behavior in mice lacking 5-HT_{1B} receptor. Science 1994, 265:1875-8.

[24] Trillat AC, Malagié I, Scearce K, Pons D, Jacquot C, Hen R, Gardier AM. Regulation of serotonin release in the frontal cortex and ventral hippocampus of homozygous mice lacking 5-HT_{1B} receptors: *in vivo* microdialysis studies. J Neurochem 1997, 69:2019-25.

[25] Gainetdinov RR, Fumagalli F, Jones SR, Caron MG. Dopamine transporter is required for *in vivo* MPTP neurotoxicity: evidence from mice lacking the transporter. J Neurochem 1997, 69:1322-5.

[26] Paxinos G, Franklin KBJ. The mouse brain in stereotaxic coordinates. 2001, 2nd Edition. Academic Press.

[27] Gorman JM, Coplan JD. Comorbid depression and anxiety spectrum disorders. J Clin Psychiatry 1996, 57:34-41;

[28] Leonardo ED, Hen R. Genetics of affective and anxiety disorders. Annu Rev Psychol 2006, 57:117-37.

[29] Ramboz S, Oosting R, Amara DA, Kung HF, Blier P, Mendelsohn M, Mann JJ, Brunner D, Hen R. Serotonin receptor 1A knockout: an animal model of anxiety-related disorder. Proc Natl Acad Sci U S A. 1998, 95:14476-81.

[30] Heisler LK, Chu HM, Brennan TJ, Danao JA, Bajwa P, Parsons LH, Tecott LH, Elevated anxiety and antidepressant-like responses in serotonin 5-HT_{1A} receptor mutant mice. Proc Natl Acad Sci U S A 1998, 95:15049-54.

[31] Parks CL, Robinson PS, Sibille E, Shenk T, Toth M. Increased anxiety of mice lacking the serotonin1A receptor. Proc Natl Acad Sci U S A. 1998, 95:10734-9.

[32] Guilloux JP, David DJ, Guiard BP, Chenu F, Repérant C, Toth M, Bourin M, Gardier AM. Blockade of 5-HT_{1A} receptors by (+/-)-pindolol potentiates cortical 5-HT outflow, but not antidepressant-like activity of paroxetine: microdialysis and behavioral approaches in 5-HT_{1A} receptor knockout mice. Neuropsychopharmacology 2006, 31:2162-72.

[33] Richardson-Jones JW, Craige CP, Guiard BP, Stephen A, Metzger KL, Kung HF, Gardier AM, Dranovsky A, David DJ, Beck SG, Hen R, Leonardo ED. 5-HT_{1A} autoreceptor levels determine vulnerability to stress and response to antidepressants. Neuron 2010, 65:40-52.

[34] Lemonde S, Turecki G, Bakish D, Du L, Hrdina PD, Bown CD, Sequeira A, Kushwaha N, Morris SJ, Basak A, Ou XM, Albert PR. Impaired repression at a 5-hydroxytryptamine 1A receptor gene polymorphism associated with major depression and suicide. J Neurosci 2003, 23:8788-99.

[35] Blier P. Altered function of the serotonin 1A autoreceptor and the antidepressant response. Neuron 2010, 65:1-2.

[36] Richardson-Jones JW, Craige CP, Nguyen TH, Kung HF, Gardier AM, Dranovsky A, David DJ, Guiard BP, Beck SG, Hen R, Leonardo ED. Serotonin-1A autoreceptors are necessary and sufficient for the normal formation of circuits underlying innate anxiety. J Neurosci 2011, 31:6008-18.

[37] Guiard BP, Guilloux JP, Reperant C, Hunt SP, Toth M, Gardier AM. Substance P neurokinin 1 receptor activation within the dorsal raphe nucleus controls serotonin release in the mouse frontal cortex. Mol Pharmacol 2007, 72:1411-8.

[38] Deltheil T, Tanaka K, Reperant C, Hen R, David DJ, Gardier AM. Synergistic neurochemical and behavioural effects of acute intrahippocampal injection of brain-derived neurotrophic factor and antidepressants in adult mice. Int J Neuropsychopharmaco 2009, 12:905-915.

[39] Bengel D, Murphy DL, Andrews AM, Wichems CH, Feltner D, Heils A, Mössner R, Westphal H, Lesch KP. Altered brain serotonin homeostasis and locomotor insensitivity to 3, 4-methylenedioxymethamphetamine ("Ecstasy") in serotonin transporter-deficient mice. Mol Pharmacology 1998, 53:649-655.

[40] Froger N, Gardier AM, Moratalla R, Alberti I, Lena I, Boni C, De Felipe C, Rupniak NM, Hunt

SP, Jacquot C, Hamon M, Lanfumey L. 5-hydroxytryptamine 5-HT_{1A} autoreceptor adaptive changes in substance P (neurokinin 1) receptor knock-out mice mimic antidepressant-induced desensitization. J Neurosci 2001, 21:8188-97.

[41] Beaulieu JM, Marion S, Rodriguiz RM, Medvedev IO, Sotnikova TD, Ghisi V, Wetsel WC, Lefkowitz RJ, Gainetdinov RR, Caron MG. A beta-arrestin 2 signaling complex mediates lithium action on behavior. Cell 2008, 132:125-136.

[42] Bortolozzi A, Castañé A, Semakova J, Santana N, Alvarado G, Cortés R, Ferrés-Coy A, Fernández G, Carmona MC, Toth M, Perales JC, Montefeltro A, Artigas F. New antidepressant strategy based on acute siRNA silencing of 5-HT_{1A} autoreceptors. Mol Psychiatry 2012, 17:567.

[43] David DJ, Bourin M, Jego G, Przybylski C, Jolliet P, Gardier AM. Effects of acute treatment with paroxetine, citalopram and venlafaxine *in vivo* on noradrenaline and serotonin outflow: a microdialysis study in Swiss mice. Br J Pharmacol 2003, 140:1128-36.

[44] Nguyen Hai T, Guiard BP., Bacq A, David DJ, David I, Quesseveur G, Gautron S, Sanchez C, Gardier AM. Blockade of the high-affinity norepinephrine transporter (NET) by the selective serotonin reuptake inhibitor escitalopram: an *in vivo* microdialysis study in mice. British J Pharmacol 2012, (in press).

[45] Zetterström T, Sharp T, Marsden CA, Ungerstedt U. *In vivo* measurement of dopamine and its metabolites by intracerebral dialysis: changes after d-amphetamine. J Neurochem 1983, 41:1769-73.

[46] Delgado JM, DeFeudis FV, Roth RH, Ryugo DK, Mitruka BM. Dialytrode for long term intracerebral perfusion in awake monkeys. Arch Int Pharmacodyn Ther 1972, 198:9-21

[47] Malagié I, Trillat AC, Bourin M, Jacquot C, Hen R, Gardier AM. 5-HT_{1B} Autoreceptors limit the effects of selective serotonin re-uptake inhibitors in mouse hippocampus and frontal cortex. J Neurochem 2001, 76:865-71.

[48] Deltheil T, Guiard BP, Cerdan J, David DJ, Tanaka KF, Repérant C, Guilloux JP, Coudoré F, Hen R, Gardier AM. Behavioral and serotonergic consequences of decreasing or increasing hippocampus brain-derived neurotrophic factor protein levels in mice. Neuropharmacology 2008, 55:1006-1014.

[49] David DJ, Froger N, Guiard B, Przybylski C, Jego G, Boni C, Hunt SP, De Felipe C, Hamon M, Jacquot C, Gardier AM, Lanfumey L. Serotonin transporter in substance P (neurokinin 1) receptor knock-out mice. Eur J Pharmacol 2004, 492:41-8.

[50] Guiard BP, David DJ, Deltheil T, Chenu F, Le Maître E, Renoir T, Leroux-Nicollet I, Sokoloff P, Lanfumey L, Hamon M, Andrews AM, Hen R, Gardier AM. Brain-derived neurotrophic factor-deficient mice exhibit a hippocampal hyperserotonergic phenotype. Int J Neuropsychopharmacol 2008, 11:79-92.

[51] Parsons LH, Smith AD, Justice JB Jr. Basal extracellular dopamine is decreased in the rat nucleus accumbens during abstinence from chronic cocaine. Synapse 1991, 9(1):60-5.

[52] Gardier AM, David DJ, Jego G, Przybylski C, Jacquot C, Durier S, Gruwez B, Douvier E, Beauverie P, Poisson N, Hen R, Bourin M. Effects of chronic paroxetine treatment on dialysate serotonin in 5-HT_{1B} receptor knockout mice. J Neurochem 2003, 86:13-24.

[53] Benmansour S, Deltheil T, Piotrowski J, Nicolas L, Reperant C, Gardier AM, Frazer A, David

DJ. Influence of brain-derived neurotrophic factor (BDNF) on serotonin neurotransmission in the hippocampus of adult rodents. Eur J Pharmacol 2008, 587:90-8.

[54] Guilloux JP, David DJ, Xia L, Nguyen HT, Rainer Q, Guiard BP, Repérant C, Deltheil T, Toth M, Hen R, Gardier AM. Characterization of 5-$HT_{1A/1B}$-/- mice: an animal model sensitive to anxiolytic treatments. Neuropharmacology 2011, 61:478-88.

[55] Maskos U, Molles BE, Pons S, Besson M, Guiard BP, Guilloux JP, Evrard A, Cazala P, Cormier A, Mameli-Engvall M, Dufour N, Cloëz-Tayarani I, Bemelmans AP, Mallet J, Gardier AM, David V, Faure P, Granon S, Changeux JP. Nicotine reinforcement and cognition restored by targeted expression of nicotinic receptors. Nature 2005, 436:103-107.

[56] Reperant C, Pons S, Dufour E, Rollema H, Gardier AM, Maskos U. Effect of the alpha4beta2* nicotinic acetylcholine receptor partial agonist varenicline on dopamine release in beta2 knock-out mice with selective re-expression of the beta2 subunit in the ventral tegmental area. Neuropharmacology 2010, 58:346-50.

[57] Kuzelova H, Ptacek R, Macek M. The serotonin transporter gene (5-HTT) variant and psychiatric disorders: review of current literature. Neuro Endocrinol Lett 2010, 31:4-10.

[58] Invernizzi RW. Role of TPH-2 in brain function: news from behavioral and pharmacologic studies. J Neurosci Res 2007, 85:3030-5.

[59] Chen ZY, Jing D, Bath KG, Ieraci A, Khan T, Siao CJ, Herrera DG, Toth M, Yang C, McEwen BS, Hempstead BL, Lee FS. Genetic variant BDNF (Val66Met) polymorphism alters anxiety-related behavior. Science 2006, 314:140-3.

[60] Porsolt RD, Le Pichon M, Jalfre M. Depression: a new animal model sensitive to antidepressant treatments. Nature 1977, 266:730-732.

[61] Steru L, Chermat R, Thierry B, Simon P. The tail suspension test: a new method for screening antidepressants in mice. Psychopharmacology (Berl) 1985, 85:367–370.

[62] Pineyro G, Castanon N, Hen R, Blier P. Regulation of [3H]5-HT release in raphe, frontal cortex and hippocampus of 5-HT_{1B} knock-out mice. Neuroreport 1995, 7:353-9.

[63] Gardier AM, Trillat AC, Malagié I, David D, Hascoët M, Colombel MC, Jolliet P, Jacquot C, Hen R, Bourin M. 5-HT_{1B} serotonin receptors and antidepressant effects of selective serotonin reuptake inhibitors. C R Acad Sci III 2001, 324:433-41.

[64] Bouwknecht JA, Hijzen TH, van der Gugten J, Maes RA, Hen R, Olivier B. 5-HT_{1B} receptor knockout mice show no adaptive changes in 5-HT_{1A} receptor function as measured telemetrically on body temperature and heart rate responses. Brain Res Bull 2002, 57:93-102.

[65] Groenink L, Pattij T, De Jongh R, Van der Gugten J, Oosting RS, Dirks A, Olivier B. 5-HT_{1A} receptor knockout mice and mice overexpressing corticotropin-releasing hormone in models of anxiety. Eur J Pharmacol 2003, 463:185-97.

[66] Solich J, Faron-Gorecka A, Kusmider M, Palach P, Gaska M, Dziedzicka-Wasylewska M. Norepinephrine transporter (NET) knock-out upregulates dopamine and serotonin transporters in the mouse brain. Neurochem Int 2011, 59:185-91.

[67] Zhou FC, Lesch KP, Murphy DL, Serotonin uptake into dopamine neurons *via* dopamine transporters: a compensatory alternative. Brain Res 2002, 942:109-19.

[68] Parrot S, Lambás-Señas L, Sentenac S, Denoroy L, Renaud B. Highly sensitive assay for the measurement of serotonin in microdialysates using capillary high-performance liquid chromatography with electrochemical detection. J Chromatogr B Analyt Technol Biomed Life Sci 2007, 850:303-309.

[69] Denoroy L, Parrot S, Renaud L, Renaud B, Zimmer L. In-capillary derivatization and capillary electrophoresis separation of amino acid neurotransmitters from brain microdialysis samples. J Chromatogr A 2008, 1205:144-149.

[70] Bert L, Favale D, Jego G, Greve P, Guilloux J-P, Guiard BP, Gardier AM, Suaud-Chagny MF, Lestage P. Rapid and precise method to locate microdialysis probe implantation in the rodent brain. J Neurosci Methods 2004, 140:53-57.

[71] Wolf WA, Youdim MB, Kuhn DM (1985) Does brain 5-HIAA indicate serotonin release or monoamine oxidase activity? Eur J Pharmaco 109:381-387.

[72] Bel N, Artigas F. Reduction of serotonergic function in rat brain by tryptophan depletion: effects in control and fluvoxamine-treated rats. J Neurochem 1996, 67: 669-676.

[73] Rocher C, Bert L, Robert F, Renaud B, Jacquot C, Gardier AM. Microdialysis monitoring of variations in extracellular levels of serotonin, GABA and excitatory amino acids in the frontal cortex of awake rats in response to a single peripheral or central administration of dexfenfluramine. Brain Research 1996, 737:221-230.

[74] Malberg JE, Eisch AJ, Nestler EJ, Duman RS. Chronic antidepressant treatment increases neurogenesis in adult rat hippocampus. J Neurosci 2000, 20:9104-10.

[75] Santarelli L, Saxe M, Gross C, Surget A, Battaglia F, Dulawa S, Weisstaub N, Lee J, Duman R, Arancio O, Belzung C, Hen R. Requirement of hippocampal neurogenesis for the behavioral effects of antidepressants. Science 2003, 301:805-9.

[76] David DJ, Samuels BA, Rainer Q, Wang JW, Marsteller D, Mendez I, Drew M, Craig DA, Guiard BP, Guilloux JP, Artymyshyn RP, Gardier AM, Gerald C, Antonijevic IA, Leonardo ED, Hen R. Neurogenesis-dependent and -independent effects of fluoxetine in an animal model of anxiety/depression. Neuron 2009, 62:479-93.

[77] Szapacs ME, Mathews TA, Tessarollo L, Ernest Lyons W, Mamounas LA, Andrews AM. Exploring the relationship between serotonin and brain-derived neurotrophic factor: analysis of BDNF protein and extraneuronal 5-HT in mice with reduced serotonin transporter or BDNF expression. J Neurosci Methods 2004, 140:81-92.

[78] Gross C, Zhuang X, Stark K, Ramboz S, Oosting R, Kirby L, Santarelli L, Beck S, Hen R. Serotonin1A receptor acts during development to establish normal anxiety-like behaviour in the adult. Nature 2002, 416:396-400.

Send Orders for Reprints to reprints@benthamscience.net
Neurobiology of Mood Disorders, 2014, 23-33

CHAPTER 2

OPTOGENETIC INVESTIGATION OF CIRCUITS UNDERLYING AFFECTIVE BEHAVIOR

MAZEN A. KHEIRBEK*

Department of Neurobiology & Behavior, Columbia University, New York, NY, USA

Abstract: There is considerable evidence for circuit dysfunction anxiety disorders, but our basic knowledge of the complex neural pathways that underlie emotional behavior remains incomplete. A more complete understanding of these systems promises both to facilitate a fuller understanding of anxiety disorder pathogenesis as well as suggest novel therapeutic strategies for unmet psychiatric needs. Classically, researchers have used correlational imaging techniques, gross lesion or electrical stimulation to delineated the brain structures involved in generating affective responses. While these studies have provided a wealth of information describing the structures involved in the generation of emotional behavior, in many instances they lack sufficient regional or temporal specificity. This chapter will review recent studies using optogenetic methodologies for delineating the circuits that underlie emotional behavior. First, I will review the suite of available tools for optical inhibition and excitation, and their utility for modulating activity in a cell-type and projection-specific manner. Then, I will highlight recent experiments using these tools to dissect the circuitry that underlies emotional behavior. As anxiety disorders are increasingly being viewed as a circuit-based dysfunction, optogenetics proves to be a powerful method for identifying the circuits that generate emotional responses, and will provide essential insight for development of novel therapies.

Keywords: designer receptors exclusively activated by designer drugs (DREADD), channelrhodopsin-2 (ChR2), eNHpR, Arch, basolateral amygdala (BLA), prefrontal cortex (PFC), step-function opsin (SFO),G-protein-coupled receptor (GPCR), Elevated Plus Maze (EPM), Open Field Test (OFT)

1. INTRODUCTION

Historically, neuroanatomical underpinnings of mental illness have been studied by documenting the behavioral consequences of neuronal damage. Patients with dysfunction in hippocampus, amygdala and prefrontal cortex have provided insight into how these areas contribute to cognitive and emotional behavior [1, 2] With the introduction of advanced brain imaging technologies, clinicians and researchers can now correlate specific changes in neuronal activity with disease state, as well as on-line activity changes during behavior [2]. The ability to lesion specific brain regions in pre-clinical models has refined the subregions involved in motivation, cognition, and mood, while pharmacological interventions and electrical stimulation have added another level of sophistication to understand the circuits and cell types that underlie specific behaviors. Yet, these techniques remain crude and have a number of limitations, most notably, their lack of specificity as within each brain region there are a number of excitatory, inhibitory, modulatory neuronal cell types, as well as glial cells and fibers of passage. Electrical stimulation or lesion studies cannot distinguish between these different cell types, thus complicating any interpretation of results obtained by these methods. Recent advances in optogenetics have allowed researchers for the first time to selectively manipulate specific cells within a neuronal circuit to ask how they contribute to behavior and disease state.

***Address correspondence to Mazen A. Kheirbek:** Department of Neurobiology & Behavior, Columbia University, New York, NY, USA; E-mail: mk3156@columbia.edu

Bruno P Guiard and Eliyahu Dremencov (Eds)

"Optogenetics" refers to the combination of optics and genetics to target light sensitive proteins (opsins) to genetically defined neuronal subtypes in a region-specific manner [3-7]. Expression of these opsins within specific circuit elements allows them to be controlled by light in both *in vivo* and *in vitro* preparations. This chapter will describe the currently available tools and their application, then discuss recent findings using these tools to dissect the circuitry underlying emotional behavior.

2. TOOLS FOR OPTICAL EXCITATION OF NEURONAL ACTIVITY

Recently, a number of approaches have been taken to engineer or isolate proteins that can be used to control neuronal activity. Researchers have successfully used chemical-genetic approaches to control neuronal activity with designer drugs, employing the use of modified receptors that can be activated by a synthetic ligand that does not activate endogenous receptors (DREADDs, designer receptors exclusively activated by designer drugs) [8-11]. These techniques, while lacking the temporal precision of light, have a number of advantages, most notably the ability to control activity through use of drugs, thus making them less invasive than local stimulation or inhibition techniques. Yet, one of the most promising ligands for experimental research in recent years has been light. Due to the wealth of light-sensitive proteins available in nature, as well as the ability to control light pulses within millisecond timescales, this approach has received much attention in the field of behavioral neuroscience. This chapter will focus on two classes of light sensitive proteins, those that when stimulated excite neurons, and those that inhibit them.

Initial studies in invertebrates showed that introduction of a light-sensitive phototransduction cascade in Drosophila neurons could make these neurons sensitive to light [12]. The field of optogenetics was significantly advanced with the discovery that Channelrhodopsin-2 (ChR2), an opsin expressed by the green algae Chlamydomonas reinhardtii to drive phototaxis, could be effectively expressed in mammalian neurons [13-15]. ChR2 is a light-gated cation channel that passes positive ions (such as Na+, H+ and Ca2+]) in response to blue light (peak activation at ~470nm wavelength light)[13,

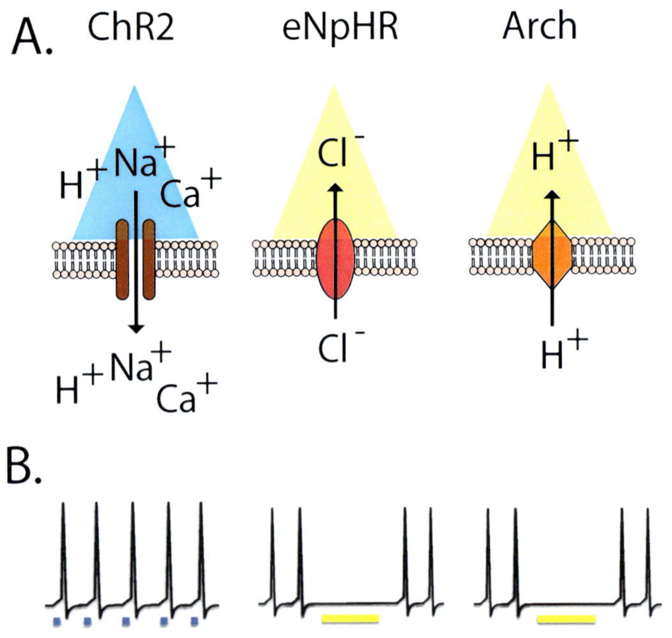

Figure 1: Tools for optogenetic excitation and inhibition. Light activated opsins provide high speed, locally specific control of neuronal function. A. Upon light activation, ChR2 opens and allows for passage of positively charged ions to depolarize the cell to threshold. As shown in B, action potentials are elicited by brief blue light stimulation and spikes are time locked to light presentation. Alternatively eNHpR and Arch may be used for optical silencing of neurons. Upon yellow light activation, eNHpR, a chloride pump, pumps Cl- ions into the cell effectively hyperpolarizing the membrane and reducing spiking ability, as shown in B. Like eNHpR, the yellow light gated Arch can silence activity in cells by pumping positively charged protons out of the cell, effectively hyperpolarizing the cell membrane.

14, 16-18] (Figure **1**). Expression of ChR2 in neurons is well tolerated, efficiently targeted to the membrane, and passes sufficient current to induce spiking of the cell with millisecond time precision [15]. *In vivo*, ChR2 can be targeted to specific neuron populations using viral expression of the opsin under control of specific promoter elements, or with more recently developed transgenic mice [18-21]. Expression of ChR2 in a specific subset of cells allows the experimenter to gain control of just those cells while leaving the cells surrounding it unaffected (Figure **2**). Recently, a number of variants of ChR2 have been developed with altered kinetics of activation and deactivation, as well as those responding to red light [22, 23]. The most recent iteration of ChR2 contains two point mutations, T159C and E123T that substantially increased photocurrents as well as increased channel kinetics allowing for high frequency stimulation at over 100Hz [24]. The red shifted VChR1, and the more recently developed C1V1, are excited by 590 nm light allowing for expression of blue and red light responsive opsins in differing cell types allowing for combinatorial activation of differing circuit elements [25]. For longer periods of activation, recently engineered step-function opsins (SFOs) exhibit long time constants of deactivation, allowing for neuronal excitation of long timescales [25, 26]. Use of the SFO's can be advantageous when longer time periods of stimulation are required. A recently engineered SFO, can be activated with a brief pulse of blue light that depolarizes the cell with a very slow time constant of deactivation of ~30 min, and can quickly deactivated with yellow light. This opsin has been used in rodents to model social dysfunction by manipulating excitation in the prefrontal cortex (PFC) [25].

Engineering chimeras of light sensitive opsins have achieved further control of neuronal activity by modifying G-protein coupled receptors to allow for control of intracellular signaling cascades in response to light. Recently developed "optoXRs" are chimeras of opsin proteins and either the alpha-1 or beta-2 adrenergic receptors, that are stimulated by blue light to regulate the Gq and Gs signaling pathways, respectively [27]. *In vivo* application of these receptors was achieved by expression in the nucleus accumbens and controlling conditioned place preference by activating selectively the Gq mediated signaling pathway [27]. More recently, rhodopsin was tagged with the C-terminal domain of the 5-HT_{1A} receptor, allowing for light-induced control of 5-HT_{1A}-dependent signaling pathways [28]. Loss of 5-HT_{1A} signaling in cultured neurons and slices from the dorsal raphe of 5-HT_{1A}-KO mice could be rescued by introduction of rhodopsin-5-HT_{1A} receptors and activating with light [28]. Future studies *in vivo* will be of great interest to test how stimulation of 5-HT_{1A}-specific signaling pathways in defined cell types can control emotional behavior. As many neuropsychiatric disorders share an underlying dysfunction in monoaminergic systems, future work manipulating the signaling pathways downstream of serotonergic, dopaminergic or noradrenergic receptors in a cell type specific manner will allow for greater resolution and understanding of the substrates underlying these disorder.

3. TOOLS FOR OPTICAL INHIBITION OF NEURONAL ACTIVITY

In addition to the sufficiency provided by optical stimulation experiments linking specific circuits with behavior, one would ideally like to prove that certain circuit elements are necessary for the studied behavior. For this, a number of methods have been classically used, lesion or inactivation of a brain region, genetic ablation or knockout, or pharmacological intervention. As discussed above, while these interventions have been informative, they lack the temporal and spatial precision offered by optogenetics. To tackle this, researchers have isolated opsins that can hyperpolarize the cell membrane and inhibit neuronal firing. One such opsin, isolated from Natronomonas pharaonis, NpHR is a chloride pump activated by yellow (~590 nm) light [29, 30], (Figure **2**). Modification of NpHR by addition of a targeting sequence from Kir2.0, increased surface expression and increased photocurrents suitable for *in vivo* manipulation of neuronal activity [30]. While eNpHR3.0 has provided the majority of behavioral data on optical inhibition, recently developed opsins have expanded the repertoire of available tools for *in vivo* inhibition. One such tool, the yellow- light-driven proton pump archaerhodopsin-3 (Arch, Figure **1**), provides potent neuronal inhibition when alternative methods to modulating chloride levels is required [31].

4. IN VIVO OPTICAL MODULATION OF NEURONAL ACTIVITY

In order to study the neuronal circuits that underlie mood and anxiety, tools for optical manipulation must be applied *in vivo*. For this, one must overcome two hurdles, local delivery of light in a freely moving animal, efficient and selective targeting of opsins to cell-type of interest. Local delivery of light can be achieved by stereotaxic implantation of a fiber optic cable coupled to a laser diode of appropriate wavelength [3, 32]. Detailed protocols for this have been published [32] and allow for *in vivo* manipulation of neuronal activity in a number of assays for testing mood and anxiety. The most popular method for expression of opsins has been using viral based approaches [30]. With viral approaches, one can rapidly express the opsin of interest at very high levels due to high copy number. Spatial selectivity can be limited by location of viral injection, as well as use of cell-type specific promoter elements to drive gene expression [3]. For example, ChR2 can be readily targeted to excitatory neurons of the forebrain by driving expression with calmodulin-dependent protein kinase II promoter elements, thus excluding activation of neighboring inhibitory interneurons [33]. Other promoter elements from genes such as elongation factor type 1-alpha, synapsin, and GFAP have also been used to target opsins to specific neuronal subtypes [34]. In addition, use of conditional, Cre-recombinase mediated opsin expression design provided an added level of refinement to the targeting of opsins [21, 35]. In this design, the double floxed inverted opsin gene has negligible expression due to the inverted open reading frame of the opsin [21, 35]. In cells expressing Cre-recombinase, the ORF is inverted in the proper orientation and the opsin is expressed. This approach allows use of the wide array of cell type specific Cre lines available to selectively target opsin expression [21, 35]. This method can be used to target ChR2 and eNpHR to dopaminergic, serotonergic, cholinergic and noradrenergic neurons, as well as subclasses of inhibitory interneurons. More recently, non-viral based approaches have been used for expression of ChR2 *in vivo*, using transgenic based strategies. Mice have been generated using the tetracycline inducible system (tetO-tTA) to regulate ChR2 gene transcription reversibly with dietary doxycycline to drive expression in medium spiny neurons of the striatum [19]. In principle, these mice can be used to drive expression in any number of tTA-based driver lines. In addition, a number of BAC-transgenic lines have been generated, including TPH-ChR2, CHAT-ChR2 and PV-ChR2, targeting ChR2 to serotonergic, cholinergic and parvalbumin neurons respectively [20]. Use of these lines provides the cell-type specificity, without the variability of viral based approaches.

Using a combination of genetic tools for cell type specificity and local fiber optic implantation can provide unprecedented selectivity of activation or inhibition of neuronal circuit elements. Figure **2** describes three (of many) possible arrangements for this selectivity. For example, expression of ChR2 in only one genetically defined subset of cells [blue cells] allows for selective stimulation of these cells while leaving neighboring cells unperturbed. Alternatively, expression of ChR2 in a subset of cells that project to a region of interest allows for stimulation of the terminals of these cells, while leaving the terminals of neurons from non-ChR2 expressing terminals from other projection zones in the region unperturbed. Using techniques like these, researchers have begun to pinpoint the regions, projections and cell types that underlie anxiety-like behavior.

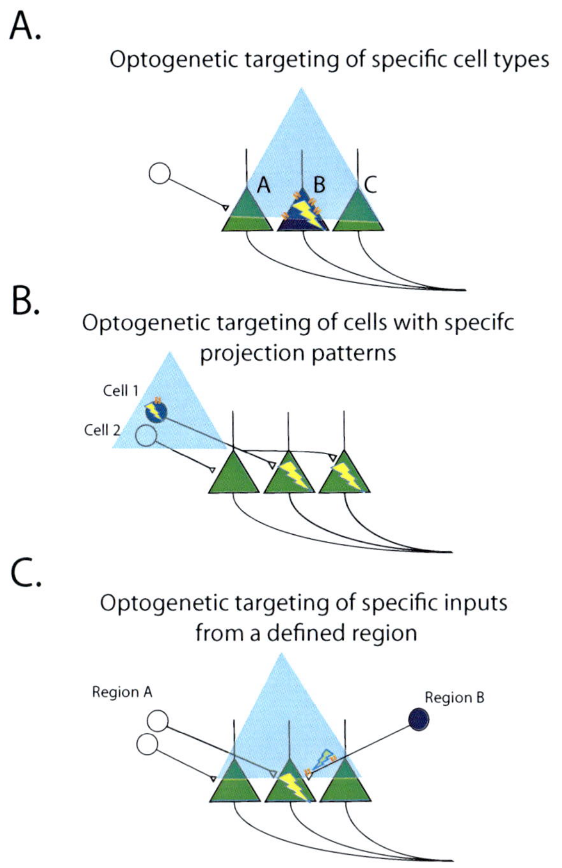

Figure 2: Methods for *in vivo* optical control of specific circuit elements. Using a combination of genetic targeting methods and local optical stimulation, neuronal activity can be controlled in very specific manner to determine the circuits that underlie a specific behavior. In A, using cell-type specific promoters, one can express ChR2 only in a subset of cells (cell B, shown in blue) to allow for control of only these cells, leaving others unperturbed. B. When the projection patterns of a neuron are known, ChR2 can be expressed only in a subset of cells (cell 1, in blue) that project to regions of interest. Then, with local optical stimulation, only the cells projecting to the regions of interest will become excited, leaving neighboring cells unaffected. C. When a specific region receives a number of different inputs, ChR2 can be expressed in only one of the projection fields (region B), then the afferent inputs can be stimulated locally. This allows for dissection of the role of specific inputs to a region on behavior.

5. OPTOGENETIC MODULATION OF AFFECTIVE BEHAVIOR

5.1. OPTOGENETIC CONTROL OF ANXIETY-LIKE BEHAVIOR

While still a relatively new technology for use *in vivo*, a few groups have now begun to use optogenetic techniques to explore the circuits that underlie anxiety and depression-like behaviors in rodents. In these studies, classically used tests of rodent anxiety/depression-like behavior such as the Elevated Plus Maze (EPM), Open Field Test (OFT) and susceptibility to social defeat have been combined with local optical stimulation to determine the circuits that underlie anxiety in these tests. Here, we will highlight a few of these studies.

Deep brain stimulation and imaging in humans has implicated a role for the PFC in depression, and a recent study has used optogenetic stimulation in rodents to model the antidepressant effect of electrical stimulation of the PFC in humans [36]. In these studies, it was revealed that depressed humans or mice that had been socially defeated exhibited decreased activity in the ventral medial PFC [as measured by immediate early gene expression] [36]. The authors expressed ChR2 in only excitatory neurons of the mPFC of socially defeated mice and implanted fiber optics targeted to the mPFC. It was shown that optical stimulation of this region could reverse depression-like behavior exhibited by socially defeated mice, while leaving other behaviors intact. This suggests that optical stimulation of specific subregions of the PFC can have a fast-acting antidepressant-like effect. These studies have provided a new animal model for the rapid onset of deep brain stimulation of the subgenual cingluate area Cg25 seen in some treatment-resistant depressed patients [1]. Future studies with optogenetics, using more refined cell-type and projection specific expression will allow for a delineation of the circuit that underlies this rapid antidepressant effect, providing novel avenues for treatment.

In a more recent study, the role of the amygdala in unconditioned anxiety was tested using the EPM and the OFT. In this study, selective activation or inhibition of the terminals of basolateral amygdala (BLA) neurons in the central nucleus of the amygdala [CeA] could bidirectionally modulate anxiety in mice [37]. The authors expressed ChR2 in the BLA, and then selectively stimulated the BLA terminals in the CeA. This stimulation had a reversible anxiolytic effect in the EPM and the OFT. In a complementary set of studies, the authors used eNpHR3.0 to inhibit these projections. This manipulation induced an anxiety-like state in the EPM and OFT. Electrophysiological experiments revealed that illumination of BLA-CeL synapses could reliably activate CeL neurons, as well as inhibit downstream centromedial [CeM] neurons, suggesting that feed-forward inhibition of the output of the amygdala may underlie the anxiolytic effect seen *in vivo*. This study thus not only revealed a microcircuit in the amygdala that underlies innate anxiety, but reveals the power of optogenetics to activate or silence anatomically distinct terminal fields of a genetically defined population of neurons provides an added level of refinement to study the complex circuits that underlie behavior.

Recently, a number of studies have used optogenetic techniques for mapping the circuitry that underlie fear conditioning, a task classically used to model anxiety disorders such as post-traumatic stress disorder and phobia. A long line of research has implicated the amygdala in the learning and expression of fear, but recent optogenetic techniques have elucidated the neural circuitry within the lateral amygdala (LA) that underlie the fear response. Optogenetic targeting of pyramidal neurons of the LA, leaving GABAergic interneurons intact, revealed that selectively driving these cells is sufficient to condition animals to a neutral stimulus, indicating that activation of glutamatergic neurons in the LA is sufficient to elicit a fear response [38]. In addition, optogenetic targeting of protein kinase Cδ- positive neurons in the central nucleus of the amygdala [CeA] revealed an inhibitory microcircuit that regulates the expression of conditioned fear [39]. In a related study, it was recently shown that acquisition of conditioned fear requires the lateral portion of the CeA, while the medial portion of the CeA drives expression of fear [40]. Finally, using contextual fear conditioning, a role for the hippocampus in remote memory has been revealed with temporally specific eNpHR-mediated silencing of pyramidal neurons in CA1 [41]. Future studies teasing out the neural circuits that underlie fear, and how they go awry in anxiety disorders, will provide novel avenues for the development therapies to alleviate conditions associated with pathological fear.

5.2. OPTOGENETIC CONTROL OF REWARD

Reward-guided behavior has received special attention from researchers using optogenetic tools due to the ability to test inhibition and excitation of specific circuit elements within a framework of well-defined behaviors. As mentioned above, optoXRs have been used to test the role of specific signaling events in the nucleus accumbens underlying context-reward associations using a conditioned place preference task [27]. These studies revealed that stimulation of phospholipase-C dependent pathways could elicit preference for one compartment, while stimulation of Gs dependent pathways could not. Using a similar behavioral assay, in conjunction cell-type specific promoters to drive ChR2 expression in dopaminergic neurons of the ventral tegmental area, it has been shown that phasic stimulation of dopamine neurons can elicit behavioral conditioning to drive preference for the compartment in which stimulation was provided [35]. This could not be attained with tonic stimulation of these cells, supporting a previously described role for phasic dopaminergic neurotransmission in reward-guided behavior. In other studies in mice using an operant task, it has been shown that selective stimulation of the fibers from the basolateral amygdala to the nucleus accumbens is rewarding, as animals will repetitively nosepoke in order to receive future stimulations [33]. Light induced stimulation of PFC-nucleus accumbens fibers could not reinforce the behavior, suggesting that stimulation of inputs from the amygdala to the nucleus accumbens are sufficient to motivate reward-seeking behavior, while those inputs from PFC are not.

Optogenetic tools have also been used to parse out the circuits that underlie drug reward. Optical stimulation of D_1-receptor containing medium spiny neurons has been shown to augment the rewarding effects of cocaine, while stimulation of the D_2-expressing population can inhibit these rewarding effects [42]. Finally, in one of the first studies to demonstrate of the effectiveness of eNHpR3.0 *in vivo*, researchers have shown that silencing the cholinergic interneurons of the nucleus accumbens can block conditioned place preference for cocaine, illuminating the importance of this small population of cells within the nucleus accumbens in regulating the rewarding properties of cocaine [43].

6. CONCLUSIONS AND FUTURE DIRECTIONS

In this chapter, we have covered the basic principles and rationale for use of optogenetic tools to study behavior. The power and promise of these tools is only beginning to be fully understood, and future work will provide essential insight into the circuits that underlie depression. For example, deep brain stimulation in humans can have rapid antidepressant effects, and optogenetic tools are well-suited for understanding the circuitry that underlie this fast acting antidepressant effect. Also, in recent years, the promise of ketamine as a fast-acting antidepressant has led to significant questions speculation on the mechanism of action and the circuits involved [44-47]. With optogenetic tools one can begin to parse this out, by modulating inhibitory and excitatory circuits in a region-specific manner to understand the mechanism for quick antidepressant responses. In addition, with the recently developed optical tools for regulating biochemical signaling pathways, the mechanism of action within the cell can begin to be elucidated. While the viability of optogenetics for the treatment of human disorders requires significant improvements in safety and opsin/light targeting, it has clear applicability to the dissection of the neuronal circuits that underlie these disorders [48]. When used in concert with available imaging technologies and circuit mapping techniques, its translational potential is quite promising. At its core, depression and anxiety are circuit disorders, and use of proper tools to dissect these circuits will provide essential insight into new ways to treat the disease.

REFERENCES

[1] Mayberg HS, Lozano AM, Voon V, McNeely HE, Seminowicz D, Hamani C, *et al.* Deep brain stimulation for treatment-resistant depression. Neuron 2005, 45[5]:651-60.

[2] Small SA, Schobel SA, Buxton RB, Witter MP, Barnes CA. A pathophysiological framework of hippocampal dysfunction in ageing and disease. Nat Rev Neurosci 2011;12:585-601.

[3] Yizhar O, Fenno LE, Davidson TJ, Mogri M, Deisseroth K. Optogenetics in neural systems. Neuron 2011, 71:9-34.

[4] Deisseroth K, Feng G, Majewska AK, Miesenbock G, Ting A, Schnitzer MJ. Next-generation optical technologies for illuminating genetically targeted brain circuits. J Neurosci 2006;26:10380-6.

[5] Gradinaru V, Thompson KR, Zhang F, Mogri M, Kay K, Schneider MB, *et al.* Targeting and readout strategies for fast optical neural control *in vitro* and *in vivo*. J Neurosci 2007, 27:14231-8.

[6] Deisseroth K. Controlling the brain with light. Sci Am 2010, 303:48-55.

[7] Deisseroth K. Optogenetics. Nat Methods 2011, 8:26-9.

[8] Lechner HA, Lein ES, Callaway EM. A genetic method for selective and quickly reversible silencing of Mammalian neurons. J Neurosci 2002, 22:5287-90.

[9] Alexander GM, Rogan SC, Abbas AI, Armbruster BN, Pei Y, Allen JA, *et al.* Remote Control of Neuronal Activity in Transgenic Mice Expressing Evolved G Protein-Coupled Receptors. Neuron 2009, 63:27-39.

[10] Lerchner W, Xiao C, Nashmi R, Slimko EM, van Trigt L, Lester HA, *et al.* Reversible silencing of neuronal excitability in behaving mice by a genetically targeted, ivermectin-gated Cl- channel. Neuron 2007, 54:35-49.

[11] Magnus CJ, Lee PH, Atasoy D, Su HH, Looger LL, Sternson SM. Chemical and genetic engineering of selective ion channel-ligand interactions. Science 2011, 333:1292-6.

[12] Lima SQ, Miesenbock G. Remote control of behavior through genetically targeted photostimulation of neurons. Cell 2005, 121[1]:141-52.

[13] Nagel G, Ollig D, Fuhrmann M, Kateriya S, Musti AM, Bamberg E, *et al.* Channelrhodopsin-1: a light-gated proton channel in green algae. Science 2002, 296:2395-8.

[14] Nagel G, Szellas T, Kateriya S, Adeishvili N, Hegemann P, Bamberg E. Channelrhodopsins: directly light-gated cation channels. Biochem Soc Trans 2005, 33:863-6.

[15] Boyden ES, Zhang F, Bamberg E, Nagel G, Deisseroth K. Millisecond-timescale, genetically targeted optical control of neural activity. Nat Neurosci 2005, 8:1263-8.

[16] Adamantidis AR, Tsai HC, Boutrel B, Zhang F, Stuber GD, Budygin EA, *et al.* Optogenetic interrogation of dopaminergic modulation of the multiple phases of reward-seeking behavior. J Neurosci 2011, 31:10829-35.

[17] Aravanis AM, Wang LP, Zhang F, Meltzer LA, Mogri MZ, Schneider MB, *et al.* An optical neural interface: *in vivo* control of rodent motor cortex with integrated fiberoptic and optogenetic technology. J Neural Eng 2007, 4:S143-56.

[18] Zhang F, Wang LP, Boyden ES, Deisseroth K. Channelrhodopsin-2 and optical control of excitable cells. Nat Methods 2006, 3:785-92.

[19] Chuhma N, Tanaka KF, Hen R, Rayport S. Functional connectome of the striatal medium spiny neuron. J Neurosci 2011, 31:1183-92.

[20] Zhao S, Ting JT, Atallah HE, Qiu L, Tan J, Gloss B, *et al.* Cell type-specific channelrhodopsin-2 transgenic mice for optogenetic dissection of neural circuitry function. Nat Methods 2011, 8:745-52.

[21] Atasoy D, Aponte Y, Su HH, Sternson SM. A FLEX switch targets Channelrhodopsin-2 to multiple cell types for imaging and long-range circuit mapping. J Neurosci 2008, 28:7025-30.

[22] Zhang F, Prigge M, Beyriere F, Tsunoda SP, Mattis J, Yizhar O, *et al.* Red-shifted optogenetic excitation: a tool for fast neural control derived from Volvox carteri. Nat Neurosci 2008, 11:631-3.

[23] Gunaydin LA, Yizhar O, Berndt A, Sohal VS, Deisseroth K, Hegemann P. Ultrafast optogenetic control. Nat Neurosci 2010, 13:387-92.

[24] Berndt A, Schoenenberger P, Mattis J, Tye KM, Deisseroth K, Hegemann P, *et al.* High-efficiency channelrhodopsins for fast neuronal stimulation at low light levels. Proc Natl Acad Sci U S A 2011, 108:7595-600.

[25] Yizhar O, Fenno LE, Prigge M, Schneider F, Davidson TJ, O'Shea DJ, *et al.* Neocortical excitation/inhibition balance in information processing and social dysfunction. Nature 2011, 477:171-8.

[26] Berndt A, Yizhar O, Gunaydin LA, Hegemann P, Deisseroth K. Bi-stable neural state switches. Nat Neurosci 2009, 12:229-34.

[27] Airan RD, Thompson KR, Fenno LE, Bernstein H, Deisseroth K. Temporally precise *in vivo* control of intracellular signalling. Nature 2009, 458:1025-9.

[28] Oh E, Maejima T, Liu C, Deneris E, Herlitze S. Substitution of 5-HT_{1A} receptor signaling by a light-activated G protein-coupled receptor. J Biol Chem 2010, 285:30825-36.

[29] Zhang F, Wang LP, Brauner M, Liewald JF, Kay K, Watzke N, *et al.* Multimodal fast optical interrogation of neural circuitry. Nature. 2007, 446:633-9.

[30] Gradinaru V, Zhang F, Ramakrishnan C, Mattis J, Prakash R, Diester I, *et al.* Molecular and cellular approaches for diversifying and extending optogenetics. Cell 2010, 141:154-65.

[31] Chow BY, Han X, Dobry AS, Qian X, Chuong AS, Li M, *et al.* High-performance genetically targetable optical neural silencing by light-driven proton pumps. Nature 2010, 463:98-102.

[32] Zhang F, Gradinaru V, Adamantidis AR, Durand R, Airan RD, de Lecea L, *et al.* Optogenetic interrogation of neural circuits: technology for probing mammalian brain structures. Nat Protoc 2010, 5:439-56.

[33] Stuber GD, Sparta DR, Stamatakis AM, van Leeuwen WA, Hardjoprajitno JE, Cho S, *et al.* Excitatory transmission from the amygdala to nucleus accumbens facilitates reward seeking. Nature 2011, 475:377-80.

[34] Gradinaru V, Mogri M, Thompson KR, Henderson JM, Deisseroth K. Optical deconstruction of parkinsonian neural circuitry. Science 2009, 324:354-9.

[35] Tsai HC, Zhang F, Adamantidis A, Stuber GD, Bonci A, de Lecea L, *et al.* Phasic firing in dopaminergic neurons is sufficient for behavioral conditioning. Science 2009, 324:1080-4.

[36] Covington HE, 3rd, Lobo MK, Maze I, Vialou V, Hyman JM, Zaman S, *et al.* Antidepressant effect of optogenetic stimulation of the medial prefrontal cortex. J Neurosci 2010, 30:16082-90.

[37] Tye KM, Prakash R, Kim SY, Fenno LE, Grosenick L, Zarabi H, *et al.* Amygdala circuitry mediating reversible and bidirectional control of anxiety. Nature 2011, 471:358-62.

[38] Johansen JP, Hamanaka H, Monfils MH, Behnia R, Deisseroth K, Blair HT, *et al.* Optical activation of lateral amygdala pyramidal cells instructs associative fear learning. P Natl Acad Sci USA 2010, 107:12692-7.

[39] Haubensak W, Kunwar PS, Cai H, Ciocchi S, Wall NR, Ponnusamy R, *et al.* Genetic dissection of an amygdala microcircuit that gates conditioned fear. Nature 2010, 468:270-6.

[40] Ciocchi S, Herry C, Grenier F, Wolff SB, Letzkus JJ, Vlachos I, *et al.* Encoding of conditioned fear in central amygdala inhibitory circuits. Nature 2010, 468:277-82.

[41] Goshen I, Brodsky M, Prakash R, Wallace J, Gradinaru V, Ramakrishnan C, *et al.* Dynamics of Retrieval Strategies for Remote Memories. Cell 2011, 147:678-89.

[42] Lobo MK, Covington HE, 3rd, Chaudhury D, Friedman AK, Sun H, Damez-Werno D, *et al.* Cell type-specific loss of BDNF signaling mimics optogenetic control of cocaine reward. Science 2010, 330:385-90.

[43] Witten IB, Lin SC, Brodsky M, Prakash R, Diester I, Anikeeva P, *et al.* Cholinergic interneurons control local circuit activity and cocaine conditioning. Science 2010, 330:1677-81.

[44] Autry AE, Adachi M, Nosyreva E, Na ES, Los MF, Cheng PF, *et al.* NMDA receptor blockade at rest triggers rapid behavioural antidepressant responses. Nature 2011, 475:91-5.

[45] Li N, Lee B, Liu RJ, Banasr M, Dwyer JM, Iwata M, *et al.* mTOR-dependent synapse formation underlies the rapid antidepressant effects of NMDA antagonists. Science 2010, 329:959-64.

[46] Li N, Liu RJ, Dwyer JM, Banasr M, Lee B, Son H, *et al.* Glutamate N-methyl-D-aspartate receptor antagonists rapidly reverse behavioral and synaptic deficits caused by chronic stress exposure. Biol Psychiatry 2011, 69:754-61.

[47] Duman RS, Li N, Liu RJ, Duric V, Aghajanian G. Signaling pathways underlying the rapid antidepressant actions of ketamine. Neuropharmacology 2011.

[48] Lin SC, Deisseroth K, Henderson JM. Optogenetics: Background and Concepts for Neurosurgery. Neurosurgery 2011, 69:1-3.

Send Orders for Reprints to reprints@benthamscience.net

Neurobiology of Mood Disorders, 2014, 34-57

CHAPTER 3

THE SEROTONERGIC SYSTEM AS A TARGET FOR POSITRON EMISSION TOMOGRAPHY LIGANDS APPLICATIONS IN AFFECTIVE DISORDERS

ANNIEK K.D. VISSER*, AREN VAN WAARDE, FOKKO J. BOSKER, JOHAN A. DEN BOER, RUDI A. DIERCKX

Department of Nuclear Medicine and Molecular Imaging, University of Groningen Medical Center, Groningen, the Netherlands

Abstract: The serotonergic (5-HT) system consists of a complex network of neurons, originating in the midbrain raphe nuclei and projecting to almost every brain region. Serotonin is involved in various processes and behavioural functions through the involvement of at least 15 pre- and postsynaptic receptors belonging to 7 receptor families. Synthesis, vesicular storage and reuptake are crucially involved in the release and extracellular levels of the monoamine 5-HT from nerve terminals.Serotonin has been implicated in many different behaviours and pathologies, which is reflected by the intensive research into this monoamine. Serotonin function is believed to play a pivotal role in the pathology and treatment of affective disorders, but its role is still far from clear. Efficacy of antidepressant and antipsychotic medications is likely related to different aspects of 5-HT function, including synthesis and 5-HT_{1A} and 5-HT_{2A} receptor function. So far Positron Emission Tomography (PET) has the best prospects to investigate these aspects of 5-HT function in humans in a relatively non invasive manner. Through kinetic modelling of the imaging data valuable information like receptor binding potential, enzymatic activity or receptor occupancy can be acquired. PET tracers are available for some of the components of the serotonergic system, but some of them are not optimal and a large part of the system can not yet be visualised with imaging techniques. However, as more tracers become available and imaging techniques improve, PET can play a major role in research and the development of new pharmacological agents.

Keywords: Serotonin (5-HT), serotonin-1A/2A (5-HT1A/5-HT2A) receptors, serotonin transporter (SERT), dorsal (DRN) and median (MRN) raphe nuclei, depression, antidepressant drugs, selective serotonin reuptake inhibitors (SSRIs), brain imaging, positron emission tomography (PET), depression, affective disorders

1. INTRODUCTION

The serotonergic system is a neuromodulatory system, influencing many other neurotransmitter systems through neuronal cells originating in the dorsal (DRN) and median raphe (MRN) nuclei, projecting to almost every division in the brain. Synthesis of serotonin (5-HT) takes place within neurons and especially in serotonergic terminals, and this process includes two enzymatic steps. The first step is the conversion of the precursor molecule, the amino acid tryptophan (Trp), to 5-hyroxytryptophan (5-HTP) by tryptophan hydroxylase (TPH) 1 or 2. The second step in the production of 5-HT involves the enzymatic action of aromatic amino acid decarboxylase (AADC) that has L-DOPA and 5-HTP as a substrate. 5-HT is eventually degraded to 5-hydroxyindole acetic acid (5-HIAA) by monoamine oxidase (MAO).

After synthesis, 5-HT is transported by the vesicular monoamine transporter (VMAT) and stored in vesicles at the neuronal presynaptic endings. When neurons fire, these vesicles fuse with the synaptic

*Address correspondence to Anniek K.D. Visser: Department of Nuclear Medicine and Molecular Imaging, University of Groningen Medical Center, Groningen, the Netherlands; E-mail: visserakd@ngmb.umcg.nl

Bruno P Guiard and Eliyahu Dremencov (Eds)

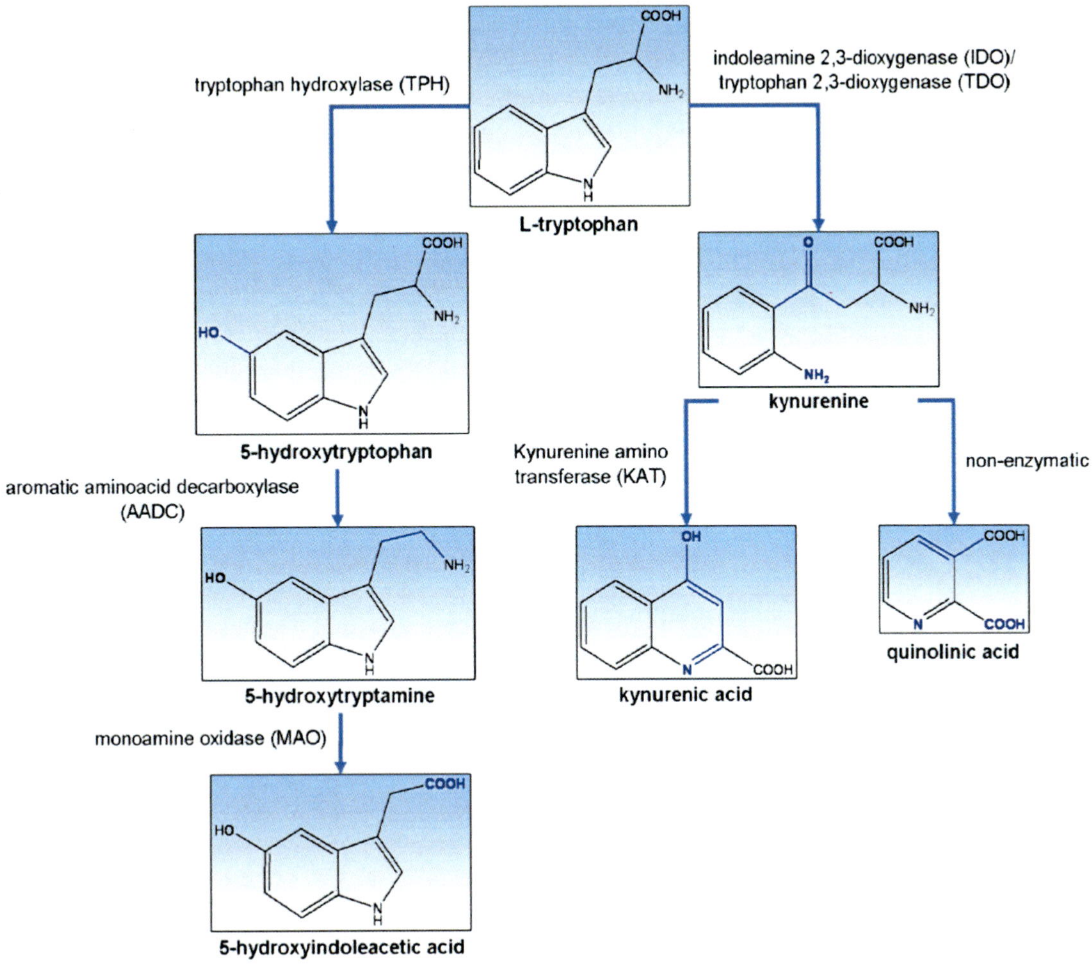

Figure 1: Tryptophan can either be metabolized in two different pathways or incorporated in proteins. The synthesis of 5-HT proceeds in two enzymatic steps: i) Conversion of Trp to 5-HTP by TPH ii) Catabolism of 5-HTP to 5-HT by AADC. Finally 5-HT is degraded to 5-HIAA by MAO.
The amount of Trp entering the kynurenine pathway is increased under inflammatory conditions. Kynurenine is formed by the enzymes IDO and TDO and is eventually degraded to quinolinic acid.

membrane and release 5-HT molecules into the synaptic cleft. Released 5-HT can bind to many different receptors, both postsynaptic and presynaptic or be taken up by the serotonergic reuptake transporter (SERT). There are at least fifteen different 5-HT receptors which are divided in seven distinct families (5-HT_{1-7}) [1]. An important role of 5-HT is the regulation of mood, and several 5-HT receptor subtypes are involved in the actions of antidepressants and antipsychotics. Serotonin synthesis may be of special interest because this process is controlled by 5-HT_{1A} receptors which are implied in the therapeutic efficacy of antidepressants [2].

It was observed that 5-HT influences many other neurotransmitter systems in an excitatory or inhibitory manner. One important key aspect that regulates serotonergic neurotransmission is the availability of the 5-HT precursor: the amino acid Trp.

In addition to conversion to serotonin, Trp is metabolized in the kynurenine-pathway and is being used for protein synthesis. The rate-limiting step in the kynurenine-pathway is the activity of indoleamine 2,3-dioxygenase (IDO) in the CNS and tryptophan 2,3-dioxygenase in peripheral organs.

Both enzymes convert Trp to kynurenine. Activation of IDO within the central nervous system takes place under the influence of proinflammatory cytokines, mainly within microglial cells. Increased cytokines and IDO activity have been linked to major depression in depressed subjects and in patients with inflammatory somatic disorders [3]. Increased IDO activity under inflammatory conditions may increase the amount of Trp used in the kynurenine pathway and consequently reduce the availability of Trp for 5-HT synthesis (see Fig. **1**).

All the above mentioned aspects of the serotonergic system may act in concert to enable the organism to function properly. The question is how we can obtain a reliable view of ongoing serotonergic processes in the living brain and what the contribution is of different receptor-subtypes and determinants of 5-HT release and its synthesis, considering the multitude of receptors, enzymatic activity and transport systems. The distribution of the different receptor subtypes contributes to the large variety of natural behaviours which involve the serotonergic system, and the different pathologies where 5-HT is implied to play a major role.

2. SEROTONERGIC FUNCTION IN AFFECTIVE DISORDERS

There have been many theories about the mechanisms leading to major depression. A depressive state is considered to result from a combination of genetic, neuronal and environmental determinants or a reaction to an environmental event and a failure to adapt [4]. However, the many neurobiological theories have not yet led to a comprehensive explanatory framework for the different categories of affective disorders proposed by classification systems such as the DSM-IV. Depression consists of multiple symptoms involving cognitive, affective and somatic symptoms and there appears to be a considerable heterogeneity among patients.

This heterogeneity is expressed in the wide range of symptoms like depressed mood and anhedonia, insomnia or hypersomnia, loss of appetite, decreased libido, concentration problems and activity disturbances. Expression of symptoms could be triggered by genotype or different environmental circumstances like upbringing, while eventually caused by disruptions of molecular signalling pathways and neurotransmission. The relation between the genetic aspects of susceptibility to mood disorders and possible defects at a neuronal level remains a topic of current research. 5-HT is the neurotransmitter most extensively associated with mood disorders such as depression.

Early studies revealed deficiencies in 5-HT concentrations and 5-HT turnover in depressive patients and relapse could partially be prevented by the administration of 5-HTP [5, 6]. Together with a large body of other studies, these data support the monoamine hypothesis of depression. In addition, several 5-HT receptor subtypes are related to the pathology of affective disorders and several of these receptors are involved in the actions of antidepressants and antipsychotics. Of most interest is the 5-HT_{1A} receptor, as it was hypothesized to be essential for antidepressant efficacy, and the 5-HT_{2A} receptor, which is a target of most antipsychotics. But also 5-HT_{2C} receptors seem to be able to augment the effects of antidepressants [7, 8]. These effects do probably not only involve the serotonergic system, but relate more to the interaction between 5-HT and, for example, the dopamine system. This implies that the modulatory effects of 5-HT may play an important role in the efficacy of antidepressants.

The development of different radioligands targeting different components of serotonergic neurotransmission could help to solve these questions. Positron Emission Tomography (PET) is a non-invasive technique that enables quantification of physiologic processes by measuring tracer kinetics. PET can reveal the dynamics of biological processes like 5-HT neurotransmission.

3. SEROTONERGIC RECEPTORS

Postsynaptic receptor binding can be either inhibitory or excitatory, depending on which subtype is stimulated. The presynaptic receptors (5-HT_{1A}, located on the somatodendrites and 5-HT_{1B}, located on axon terminals) are autoreceptors that inhibit serotonergic neurotransmission, while heteroreceptors influence the release of neurotransmitters other than 5-HT [9]. Almost all 5-HT receptors are G-protein coupled (metabotropic), with exception of the 5-HT_3 subtype which is a ligand-gated ion channel [1]. Different subtypes of the 5-HT receptor are diversely expressed across different brain regions and mediate distinct physiological and behavioural functions.

Much research has been focussing on the 5-HT_{1A} (auto)receptor, because of the early discovery of this subtype and the availability of its specific ligand 8-OH-DPAT. 5-HT_{1A} receptors are mainly located in the limbic forebrain, suggesting a role in the regulation of emotion [10]. This highly characterized receptor gained additional attention because of its association with antidepressant and anxiolytic drug efficacy. Since binding of 5-HT to 5-HT_{1A} receptors on cell bodies in the DRN putatively leads to regulating negative feedback of serotonergic neurotransmission (through neuronal hyperpolarisation), the therapeutic action of antidepressants such as the selective serotonin reuptake inhibitors (SSRIs) may be suppressed or delayed.

Another subtype of autoreceptors is the 5-HT_{1B} receptor. There was some confusion about the nomenclature of 5-HT_{1B} receptors because of species differences in the pharmacological characteristics of this subtype. Initially, the 5-HT_{1B} receptors were classified as 5-HT_{1D} receptors in some mammalian species including humans. 5-HT_{1B} receptors are autoreceptors located on the terminals of serotonergic neurons, particularly in the basal ganglia, and function as inhibitory heteroreceptors in several other brain areas like locus coeruleus and cingulate cortex [11, 12].

While the first receptor classified as 5-HT_{1D} actually turned out to be 5-HT_{1B}, another 5-HT_1 receptor with a similar pharmacological profile was discovered and named 5-HT_{1D} instead [13]. These receptors occur in very low quantities in the mammalian brain, but are most abundant in the basal ganglia, hippocampus and cortex [14]. Because of the strong homology in amino acid sequence, it is difficult to produce a ligand selective for either the 5-HT_{1B} or 5-HT_{1D} receptor. This makes it difficult to distinguish the pharmacological actions of both subtypes. Recently discovered selective antagonists have indicated that the autoreceptor function resides mainly in the 5-HT_{1B} receptor, whereas the 5-HT_{1D} subtype is probably a heteroreceptor.

The last members of the 5-HT_1 receptor family are the 5-HT_{1E} and 5-HT_{1F} subtypes which have a similar pharmacological profile, but with a different distribution pattern in the brain, with abundance of 5-HT_{1E} in cortex and caudate putamen and of 5-HT_{1F} receptor in hippocampus, DRN and cortex [14]. Little is known about their physiological role, although there are indications that potent 5-HT_{1F} agonists relieve migraine symptoms in an animal model and in clinical trials [15, 16].

Stimulation of 5-HT_2 receptors has a large variety of effects, *e.g.*, on conditioned responses, which correlates to their location in the forebrain. All 5-HT_2 receptor subtypes have low affinity for 5-HT. In contrast to 5-HT_1 receptors, upon their activation they increase the accumulation of Ca^{+2} and reduce potassium conductance, leading to neuronal excitation. The 5-HT_{2A} receptor is very well characterized and is present throughout the brain, especially in forebrain regions. This subtype is most abundant in cortical areas, caudate nucleus, nucleus accumbens, olfactory tubercle, amygdala and hippocampus [17]. The 5-HT_{2A} receptor is of special interest because of its putative role in regulating gene transcription of brain-derived neurotrophic factor, which is involved in antidepressant action [18]. Depressed patients have an increased expression of 5-HT_{2A} receptors in post-mortem tissue of the prefrontal cortex, while antidepressants can block $5\text{-}HT_{2A}$ binding [19]. Additionally, $5\text{-}HT_{2A}$ receptors are of interest because receptor stimulation can be hallucinogenic and therefore these receptors may be involved in regulating antipsychotic drug action [20-22].

Far less abundant is the $5\text{-}HT_{2B}$ receptor, which is particularly expressed in the dorsal hypothalamus, cerebellum, lateral septum and medial amygdala. There is evidence indicating a role for $5\text{-}HT_{2B}$ receptors in the regulation of anxiety, which corresponds to the location of this subtype in the medial amygdala [23].

The more widely distributed $5\text{-}HT_{2C}$ receptor is highly expressed in the choroid plexus and additionally present in cortex, limbic areas and basal ganglia [1]. Corresponding with its widespread distribution, this subtype is involved in the regulation of many aspects of behaviour like anxiety, food intake and sleep. Interestingly, besides a function in neuronal excitation $5\text{-}HT_{2C}$ receptors exert a tonic inhibitory effect on mesocorticolimbic dopamine and noradrenalin neurons, probably through stimulating GABA release, resulting in increased release of neurotransmitter after administration of a $5\text{-}HT_{2C}$ antagonist. Combined therapy of a $5\text{-}HT_{2C}$ antagonist and an SSRI could result in augmentation of antidepressant efficacy [24].

The $5\text{-}HT_3$ receptor is a ligand-gated ion channel. These receptors are most abundant in the dorsal vagal complex of the brainstem, where they are involved in the vomiting reflex which explains the antiemetic actions of $5\text{-}HT_3$ antagonists [25]. Other regions showing $5\text{-}HT_3$ expression are the hippocampus and amygdala, where the receptor is probably mostly expressed on GABAergic interneurons [26]. Because the $5\text{-}HT_3$ receptor influences many neurotransmitter systems like dopamine and acetylcholine, this subtype may be involved in the regulation of reward, anxiety and cognition.

$5\text{-}HT_4$ receptors are expressed throughout the brain with high levels in the nigrostriatal and mesolimbic system [27]. Stimulation of this receptor mainly increases neurotransmitter release by enhancing neuronal excitability and slowing down repolarisation. Its effects on the cholinergic system received most attention, but the $5\text{-}HT_4$ receptor is also present on dopaminergic neurons. However, the enhancing effect of $5\text{-}HT_4$ ligands on cognition seemed much more pronounced than effects on locomotion. Recently, also an antidepressant effect of the $5\text{-}HT_4$ partial agonist SL65.0155 has been reported [28].

Data on the $5\text{-}HT_5$ receptor family, which can be classified in two different subtypes $5\text{-}HT_{5A}$ and $5\text{-}HT_{5B}$, is very scarce. Both subtypes are distributed throughout the brain, but they are difficult to detect, especially the $5\text{-}HT_{5B}$ [29]. Little is known about the effects of receptor stimulation on behaviour [30].

High levels of $5\text{-}HT_6$ receptor binding have been detected in the striatum, olfactory tubercle, hippocampus and nucleus accumbens [31]. Like $5\text{-}HT_{1A}$ receptors, this subtype is associated with antidepressant and anxiolytic effects [32, 33] and it may be under inhibitory control by corticosteroids [34]. Therefore, the role of the $5\text{-}HT_6$ receptor in the physiological mechanisms of stress and depression deserves further attention. This receptor is also of interest because of its role in cognition, making it a possible drug target for Alzheimer's disease [35, 35, 36].

In addition to the expression of the $5\text{-}HT_{1A}$ and $5\text{-}HT_6$ genes, $5\text{-}HT_7$ receptor expression seems also to be regulated by corticosteroids [34, 37]. This subtype has a unique distribution with high levels in thalamus, hypothalamus and hippocampus and lower levels in other brain areas like cortex and amygdala [38]. Inactivation or blockade of $5\text{-}HT_7$ receptors results in an antidepressant-like effect in animal models of depression and this receptor is required for the antidepressant efficacy of some drugs [39, 40]. Its best described behavioural function is the induction of phase shifts in circadian rhythms [41]. Indeed, the mRNA for 5-HT_7 receptors is expressed in the suprachiasmatic nucleus, which is the main brain area involved in the regulation of circadian rhythms [42].

The distribution of the different 5-HT receptors and the projection areas of the 5-HT system are shown in Fig. **2**.

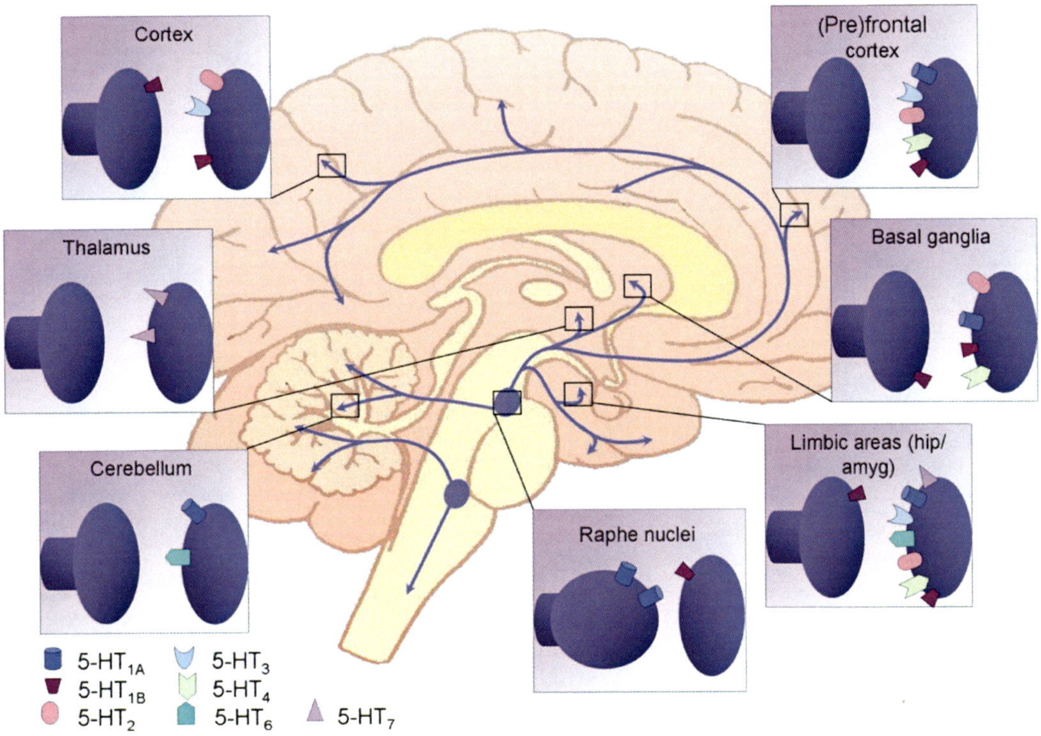

Figure 2: The serotonergic system.
The cell bodies of serotonergic neurons lay in the brainstem raphe nuclei. These neurons project to many brain areas like the cortex, basal ganglia, cerebellum, thalamus, limbic areas like hippocampus and amygdala, and spinal cord. Different 5-HT receptor subtypes have a specific distribution in the brain. In the figure autoreceptors in the raphe nuclei are depicted on neuronal cell bodies (5-HT_{1A}) or in terminal areas on the presynaps (5-HT_{1B}). The depiction of other 5-HT receptor subtypes in terminal areas can either represent heteroreceptors or postsynaptic receptors on 5-HT neurons.

4. THE USE OF POSITRON EMISSION TOMOGRAPHY IN PHARMACOLOGY

There are many applications of Positron Emission Tomography (PET) in pharmacology. The great advantage of PET is that in principle every physiological process in the body can be followed over time by labelling a compound with a radioactive isotope (tracer). These isotopes emit positrons that, when colliding with an electron in the surrounding tissue, emit 2 photons in exactly the opposite direction. This process is called annihilation. The PET scanner can detect these photons and it can calculate the position where the annihilation took place. Especially PET tracers for targets in the brain need extensive kinetic modelling in order to estimate the parameters that resemble the physiological process of interest. These kinetic models largely resemble the ones used in pharmacology for estimating drug kinetics, however, the essential properties of tracers and drugs are somewhat different. An example of a PET scan of a rat brain with the tracer [^{11}C]MDL 100907, which is able to measure 5-HT$_{2A}$ receptors in the brain, is given in Fig. **3**.

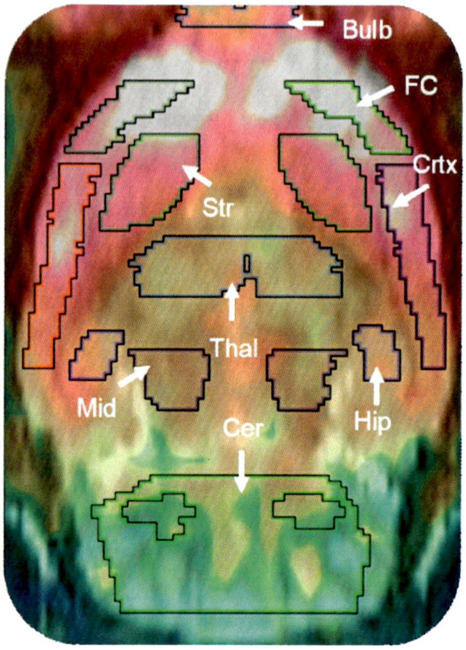

Figure 3: PET scan of rat brain with [^{11}C]MDL 100907
Example of a rat brain scanned with the 5-HT$_{2A}$ tracer [^{11}C] MDL 100907. The PET scan is transposed to an MRI image to delineate brain areas as shown in the figure. Bulb = bulbus olfactorius, Cer = cerebellum, Crtx = cortex, FC = frontal cortex, Hip = hippocampus, Mid = midbrain, Str = striatum, Thal = thalamus.

In general, there are three different kinds of tracers: the ones that only enter and exit the brain without binding to a target; the ones that bind to a receptor or a transporter; and the ones that are metabolized by enzymatic action. Data of such tracers need to be analyzed with a kinetic model that best suits their kinetic properties. An overview and more extensive explanation of pharmacokinetic models can be found in [43].

For PET tracers that only enter and exit the brain without binding, the 1-tissue compartment model (1TCM) can be used. In this model, the tissue concentration c_t can be described by the tracer concentration in plasma c_a, the influx constant K_1, and the efflux constant k_2. Tracers that are freely diffusible over the blood-brain barrier (BBB) and have a high permeability surface area product (meaning that they are easily extracted from plasma to tissue), are able to measure cerebral blood flow, like [^{15}O]water [44]. However, the kinetics of other tracers can also be analysed with a 1TCM, like [^{11}C]verapamil. This tracer is a substrate for the efflux transporter P-glycoprotein (P-gp), which actively pumps out [^{11}C]verapamil from the brain and [^{11}C]verapamil is therefore capable of measuring P-gp activity. As [^{11}C]verapamil uptake is sensitive to competition at the level of the transporter, it can be used to test if drugs are P-gp substrates. This is valuable information, because such drugs are less likely to accumulate in the brain or in tumours [45-47].

Kinetic data of tracers that enter the brain and bind to a target, like a receptor or transporter, can be analysed with a 2-tissue compartment model (2TCM), where the first compartment is the free concentration of the tracer c_f, and the second is the bound concentration of the tracer c_b. The model is usually simplified by ignoring the non-specific binding of the tracer, although such binding can contribute to the PET signal. Similar to the 1TCM, in the 2TCM K_1 and k_2 resemble influx and efflux of the tracer across the BBB. In addition, the constants k_3 and k_4 describe the exchange between free and specifically bound tracer (Fig. **4**). Binding potentials (BP), reflecting affinity of the tracer for its binding site and the amount of receptors, can be estimated according to an equation defined by Mintun *et al.* (1984) for *in vitro* binding studies [48]:

$$BP = \frac{B_{max}}{K_d}$$

Where B_{max} is the maximal amount of receptors available for binding, and the dissociation constant, K_d, is the concentration of free radioligand resulting in 50% of the maximal binding. The BP can generally also be expressed as k_3/k_4. For explanations about *in vitro* and *in vivo* differences and the generally excepted nomenclature of all the different parameters that can be measured with PET, see Innis *et al.* (2007) [49].

Every compound that has chemically favourable characteristics for labelling with a radioactive isotope could in principle be used as a tracer, although properties of the tracer should favour transport over the BBB and the labelled substrate should be specific for the target. On the other hand, the affinity for the target cannot be too high, as the parameters of the model (including k_4) have to be measured under equilibrium conditions within the time span of the PET scan of about 60-90 min. As k_4 resembles the k_{off} of the bound tracer from the target, high affinity of the tracer to the target prevents the measurement of BP within the time span of a PET scan.

Tracers that bind to targets in the brain can be used for a broad variety of applications, like measuring affinity, expression and occupancy of the targets. Also new chemical entities can be labelled with radioactive isotopes to investigate their distribution in the body and excretion route, although properties of the drug do not always favour its use as a tracer. Probably the most valuable asset of PET in pharmacology is the ability to calculate occupancy of certain drugs to, for example, a receptor. By applying different doses of a drug that potentially exerts its effect through occupancy of the target receptor, occupancy of the receptor by the test drug can be measured with PET in a non-invasive way.

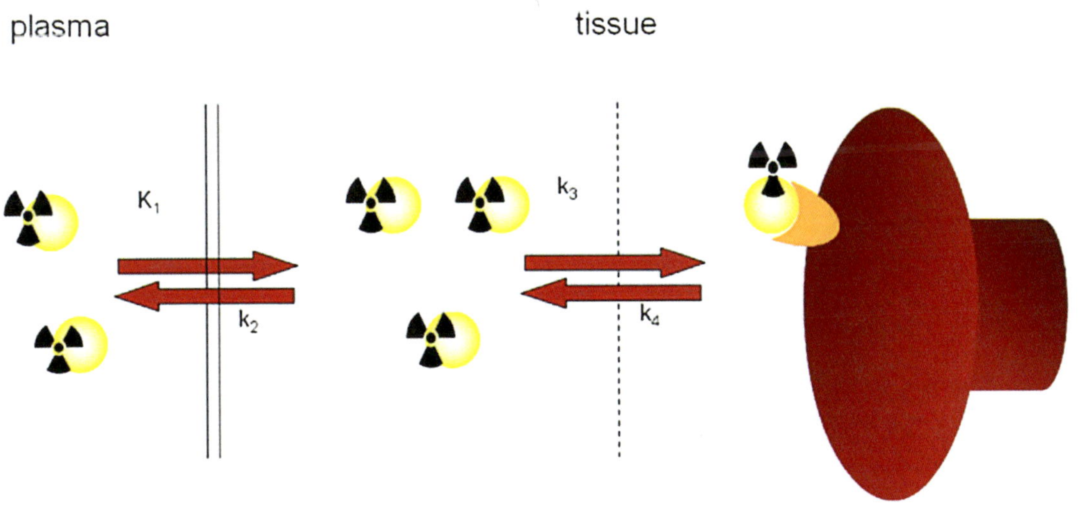

Figure 4: Kinetics of receptor tracers. Tracers are injected intravenously, where after they need to be transported over the BBB. Within tissue, there is a concentration of free (unbound) tracer and a concentration of bound tracer to the receptor. The tracer equilibrates between these stages with the constants depicted in the figure. K_1 and k_2 describe the kinetics between plasma and tissue and k_3 and k_4 describe the kinetics between free and specifically bound tracer.

Through this method, the minimum dose of the drug required to occupy sufficient receptors for a therapeutic effect can be measured [50, 51].

Tracers that are substrates for enzymes, and therefore are metabolized in a similar way as the endogenous substrate of the enzyme, can be used to measure the activity of that enzyme by analysis with a 2TCM with irreversible tracer trapping. The difference compared to the above mentioned 2TCM used for calculating BP, is that there is no k_4 in this model. Instead, a constant resembling a metabolic rate can be calculated from the formula:

$$K_i = \frac{k_3 * K_1}{k_3 + k_2}$$

The best known tracer in this category is [^{18}F]2-fluoro-2-deoxy-D-glucose (FDG), which is probably the most frequently used PET tracer at present (41959 hits in Pubmed search on "FDG PET"). FDG is an analogue of glucose and reflects energy consumption as it is metabolized by hexokinase to form FDG-6-PO_4. This radioactive labelled product is trapped in cells without any of the radiolabelled products leaving the brain (therefore $k_4 = 0$), so accumulation of radioactivity would reflect the metabolic rate of glucose consumption [52]. Especially brain, heart, lungs and tumours can be nicely visualised with FDG. In pharmacology, FDG is used to assess changes of glucose uptake after drug treatment, for example after cytostatic treatment to monitor treatment affectivity. In addition, the brain is a large consumer of glucose, and therefore the metabolic effects of CNS drugs can be measured with FDG.

Other PET tracers may have a less wide range of applications, but can still be very valuable to assess enzymatic activity or synthesis rates. Like [^{11}C]5-HTP, which is supposed to measure 5-HT synthesis rates [53] or [^{11}C]MP4A, which is a substrate for acetylcholinesterase and therefore measures acetylcholine breakdown [54]. Also here, compounds with chemically favourable characteristics for isotope labelling, which are a substrate for the enzyme of interest, could be labelled. Similar to tracers that bind to receptors, tracers that are a substrate for enzymes need to cross the BBB, and of course need to be specific for the target enzyme. In addition, the radioactive products should not leave the brain within the time frame of PET scanning, as this will lead to an underestimation of enzymatic activities.

The above mentioned models are the "golden standards", but these models can be simplified to make the measurement more robust and less prone to variability in individual rate constants. One way is by using the radioactivity from a reference region, devoid of specific binding of the tracer, instead of the plasma radioactivity to calculate the input function. This method has an additional advantage as no arterial blood sampling is needed, making the method less invasive.

There are several PET tracers available that can measure components of the serotonergic system. These tracers include receptor tracers and tracers that measure serotonin synthesis rates.

5. POSITRON EMISSION TOMOGRAPHY TRACERS FOR SEROTONIN RECEPTORS

In this section, we will first focus on radioligands for serotonin receptors or transporters (Table **1**). Such tracers are also reviewed elsewhere [55-57].

PET imaging with suitable radioligands gives a quantitative estimate of receptor distribution and density of the receptor in different brain areas. Kinetic analysis of tracer binding renders the BP as shown in equation 1. Unfortunately, radioligands are available for only a few of the 5-HT receptor subtypes mentioned above, but new radiotracers for the 5-HT system are constantly being developed. Fortunately, some of these radiotracers seem to be able to measure 5-HT release through competition with 5-HT at their binding site.

Many tracers have been developed for visualization of the 5-HT$_{1A}$ receptor, which resulted in increased insight regarding its function [58]. A reference tissue approach can be used for 5-HT$_{1A}$ receptor quantification as the 5-HT$_{1A}$ receptors are present at very low level in cerebellum. Most of the tracers are analogues of the agonist 8-OH-DPAT or the antagonist WAY-100635. Preclinical results in non-human primates have indicated a possible clinical use of the [^{11}C]robalzotan (or [^{11}C]NAD-299), an 8-OH-DPAT analogue [59]. The binding of [^{11}C]NAD-299 may be sensitive for competition of endogenous 5-HT and thus, [^{11}C]NAD-299 could be useful for measuring 5-HT release. Another agonist which shows high selectivity for 5-HT$_{1A}$ receptors in baboons is [^{11}C]CUMI-101 [60, 61]. Its usefulness in human was shown as kinetics were favourable in plasma and brain of healthy volunteers and test-retest variability was low [62].

A moderate-affinity ligand of which the binding may be sensitive for 5-HT competition is p-MPPF, although its sensitivity may be limited [63]. This compound is a silent antagonist at 5-HT$_{1A}$ receptors and [^{18}F]MPPF has shown specific binding in the brain [64]. However, it is a substrate of P-glycoprotein resulting in limited brain uptake. In humans, rapid metabolism of [^{18}F]MPPF causes low levels of the parent compound in plasma already after 10 minutes. A great advantage of this radioligand is that [^{18}F]MPPF can be distributed to other facilities, because of the longer half-life of fluorine-18 (109.8 min) as compared to carbon-11 (20 min).

The high-affinity radioligands [*carbonyl*-^{11}C]WAY-100635 (WAY) and [*carbonyl*-^{11}C]*desmethyl_* WAY-100635 (DWAY) are particularly suitable for imaging of the regional distribution of 5-HT$_{1A}$ receptors. Even the DRN is visible in the high contrast images. However, the binding of these potent tracers is not sensitive to competition by endogenous 5-HT. Despite the difficult production of WAY, many human studies have been performed with this tracer [57, 65]. A reduction of 5-HT$_{1A}$ receptor density was seen in unmedicated patients with major depression compared to healthy controls [66, 67]. Because DWAY shows greater signal intensity than WAY in human volunteers, this tracer may be preferred [68].

Recently, two radioligands were developed for 5-HT$_{1B}$ receptor imaging [69, 70]. Both [^{11}C] AZ10419369 and [^{11}C]P943 have been verified in humans or nonhuman primates and seem to be suitable for 5-HT$_{1B}$ receptor quantification. Both tracers have high affinity, particularly for the human receptor, and they show a regional distribution within the brain that is comparable to autoradiographic findings. As the cerebellum is virtually devoid of 5-HT$_{1B}$ receptors, a reference tissue model can be used for kinetic modelling. Interestingly, [^{11}C] AZ10419369 seems sensitive to endogenous 5-HT release induced by fenfluramine [71]. With the tracer [^{11}C]P943 a reduction in 5-HT$_{1B}$ heteroreceptor BP in ventral striatum / ventral pallidum of patients with a current major depressive episode was shown [72]. In this study they suggest that dysfunctional reward signalling in major depression may be attributed to abnormal 5-HT$_{1B}$ signalling in the striatum through interaction with other neurotransmitter systems, like dopamine, GABA or glutamate. These data indicate that both tracers are promising radioligands for human research in the future.

Another subtype that has been visualized with PET is the 5-HT$_{2A}$ receptor. The first selective radioligand that reached clinical application was [^{18}F]setoperone [73]. However, reliable measurements of 5-HT$_{2A}$ receptor density were only possible in cortex, because this tracer additionally labels dopamine D$_2$

receptors in the striatum. A more selective ligand which does not bind to D_2 receptors and may be more suitable for clinical assessment of 5-HT_{2A} receptor density is [^{18}F]altanserin [74]. However, a disadvantage of altanserin is that lipophilic metabolites pass the BBB and contribute to non-specific uptake of radioactivity within the brain, reducing signal to noise ratios. The most promising PET tracer for measuring 5-HT_{2A} receptor availability is [^{11}C]MDL-100907, a highly selective ligand with a high neocortex to cerebellum ratio [75]. Unfortunately, this tracer appears to be insensitive for competition by endogenous 5-HT and cannot detect changes in extracellular 5-HT [76]. Another disadvantage of [^{11}C]MDL-100907 is the rapid decay of carbon-11 (half-live of 20.4 min). Therefore Herth *et al* (2009) searched for MDL-100907 derivatives which can be labelled with fluorine-18 [77, 78]. They produced the promising radioligand [^{18}F]MH.MZ with comparable characteristics as MDL-100907. However, [^{18}F]MH.MZ binds with lower affinity to the 5-HT_{2A} receptor than [^{11}C]MDL-100907 and the washout from the brain is very slow, making it more difficult to obtain BP values. Clinical data for [^{18}F]MH.MZ have not been reported yet, but these are expected in the near future. Agonistic tracers may be more sensitive for competition with endogenous 5-HT, and development of these tracers, like [11C]Cimbi-36, is ongoing [79].

The 5-HT_4 receptor is of interest because of its putative role in cognition. To the best of our knowledge only one PET tracer has been developed for this subtype, [^{11}C]SB207145 [79]. The regional distribution of [^{11}C]SB207145 in the brain concurred with the distribution pattern of the 5-HT_4 receptor as known from autoradiography. This tracer appears suitable for clinical studies and the cerebellum can be used as a reference region, although this may result in underestimation of values in the striatum [80].

The latest identified and cloned subtype is the 5-HT_7 receptor. As this receptor has a typical distribution and seems to play not only a role in circadian rhythms, but is also implied in depression and the effect of antidepressants, there is recent interest in the development of radiotracers [39]. The first PET tracer was a carbon-11 labelled antagonist, DR4446. This tracer was evaluated in monkey and uptake of the tracer in different brain regions appeared to be decreased when cold (unlabelled) DR4446 was applied [81]. However, specificity to the 5-HT_7 receptor had yet to be tested and we could not find this study in literature. More recently, flurine-18 labelled analogues of the specific antagonist SB269970 were tested for their application as a 5-HT_7 PET tracer. From *in vivo* studies in rat, it appeared that the tracer [^{18}F]2FP3 is the most specific radiotracer and showed uptake distribution in accordance with the known distribution of 5-HT_7 receptors. Probably this tracer will subsequently be tested in humans [82].

Besides 5-HT receptors, SERT plays an important role in serotonergic neurotransmission and is involved in the therapeutic effect of SSRIs. Several PET tracers have been developed in order to depict SERT on the presynaptic terminals. Most tracers were SSRI derivatives labelled with carbon-11 and were not very successful because of a high level of nonspecific binding. A higher target to nontarget ratio was acquired with [^{11}C]McN5652 [83], although a long scanning time was required due to a relatively poor brain uptake of this compound. In cortex and midbrain, target-to-background ratios were still very low. For the midbrain this ratio can be improved by the use of [^{11}C]DASB, although in cortex target-to-background ratios remain low [84, 85]. [^{11}C]DASB is now the most frequently used SERT tracer, and in clinical studies a reduced binding of this ligand is observed after SSRI treatment. In addition, this tracer is used to measure occupancy of SERT by SSRIs at therapeutic doses [86]. Another tracer, [^{11}C]MADAM also seems to be promising to measure SERT BP [87], however, this tracer has been less applied in human studies. Although more studies are appearing and the tracer has good test-retest reproducibility [88] and occupancy studies have been performed as well to compare the SSRI's citalopram and escitalopram [89]. Most promising is the newly developed tracer [^{18}F]ADAM, which shows higher cortex-to-cerebellum ratios than [^{11}C]DASB in rat brain and has the benefits of fluorine-18 labelling [90]. However, the use of the cerebellum as a reference region is questionable, since standard uptake values in this brain area are reduced after treatment of animals with SSRIs.

The most commonly used radiotracers to measure aspects of the serotonin system are listed in Table **1**

Serotonergic component	Function	Radioligand	Literature
5-HT$_{1A}$	Autoreceptor on cell bodies in DRN/ inhibitory postsynaptic receptor	[^{11}C]NAD-195 [^{18}F]MPPF [*carbonyl*-^{11}C]WAY-100635 [*carbonyl*-^{11}C]*desmethyl*-WAY-100635 [^{18}F]FCWAY [^{18}F]MEFWAY [^{11}C]RWAY [^{11}C]CUMI-101	[59] [64] [65] [68] [92] [93] [94] [61]
5-HT$_{1B}$	Autoreceptor on nerve terminals/ inhibitory heteroreceptor	[^{11}C]AZ10419369 [^{11}C]P943	[69] [73]
5-HT$_{2A}$	Excitatory receptor (*e.g.*, regulation gene transcription)	[^{18}F]setoperone [^{18}F]altanserin [^{11}C]MDL-100907 [^{18}F]MH.MZ	[74] [75] [77] [79]
5-HT$_4$	Excitatory receptor	[^{11}C]SB207145	[81]
5-HT$_7$	Excitatory receptor	[^{11}C]DR4446 [^{18}F]2FP3	[82] [83]
SERT	Reuptake transporter (*e.g.*, target SSRI)	[^{11}C]McN5652 [^{11}C]DASB [^{11}C]MADAM [^{18}F]ADAM	[84] [85] [88] [91]
tryptophan	Precursor 5-HTP and substrate TPH	α-[^{11}C]methyl-tryptophan	[95]
5-HTP	Precursor 5-HT and substrate AADC	5-hydroxy-L-[β-^{11}C] tryptophan	[96]

Table 1: PET tracers used for research on serotonergic neurotransmission

6. MEASURING SEROTONIN SYNTHESIS RATES WITH POSITRON EMISSION TOMOGRPAHY

Recent technologies allow direct measurement of serotonin synthesis rates in living animals and humans. In the pathway for 5-HT synthesis, availability of Trp determines the rate of 5-HT formation, because the K_m values of TPH and AADC are greater than the physiological Trp concentrations, thus the enzymes are not saturated [97]. This means that analogues of Trp and 5-HTP can be used for measuring 5-HT synthesis rates. The first attempts at imaging 5-HT synthesis were conducted by labelling natural Trp with tritium. Some disadvantages were noted, like the incorporation of Trp into proteins, which reduces tracer availability [98, 99]. Therefore, other tracers have been developed with more favourable characteristics, such as α-[^{11}C]methyl-tryptophan ([^{11}C]AMT, Trp analogue) and 5-hydroxy-L-[β-^{11}C]tryptophan ([^{11}C]5-HTP, radiolabelled 5-HTP).

As Trp turned out to be unsuitable as a tracer, a radiolabelled analogue of Trp was introduced for measurement of 5-HT synthesis, α-methyltryptophan (AMT). This compound is a substrate of TPH and will eventually be converted to α-methylserotonin. Because α-methylserotonin is not degraded by MAO and cannot cross the BBB, it is trapped for a long period in the brain [100].

However, there are some contradictory results concerning the efficiency and reliability of radiolabelled AMT. The major problem is that labelled AMT can enter the kynurenine pathway, since it is an analogue of Trp and the activity of this pathway will increase the amount of radioactivity which is trapped in the brain [101]. Therefore, Chugani and colleagues refer to the constant reflecting the metabolic rate of 5-HT production, K_{acc}, as a reflection of the *capacity* of 5-HT synthesis, rather than the synthesis *rate* [102].

Tracer conversion to kynurenine can be prevented by labelling the direct precursor of 5-HT, which is only metabolized in the pathway for 5-HT synthesis. Injection of 5-HTP labelled in the β-position can provide insight in endogenously synthesized 5-HT, since 5-HTP is the substrate of the last enzyme involved in the production of 5-HT. [^{11}C]5-HTP will undergo the same conversions as 5-HTP and will eventually end up as [^{11}C]5-HIAA. Because of the difficulty of labelling 5-HTP in the β-position with carbon-11, a procedure which involves rapid enzymatic steps, this radiotracer has only been synthesized in a few imaging institutions [96, 103].

For both [^{11}C]AMT and [^{11}C]5-HTP a 3-compartment model, or 2TCM, with irreversible tracer trapping can be applied to fit the data and calculate the model parameters. The compartments described in the model are plasma, brain and irreversibly trapped tracer [95, 104]. Under steady-state conditions, the unidirectional trapping of the tracer is indicated by the constant K_{acc} or K^{α}. The K_{acc} describes an accumulation constant that takes all individual rate constants into account according to the formula:

$$K_{acc} = \frac{k_3 * K_1}{k_3 + k_2}$$

These constants all represent the speed of trapping of the radioactive compound in a certain region of interest. With a graphical method, called the Patlak plot, a similar constant (K_i) can be obtained, usually having a more robust outcome value. This graphical method is not constrained by individual rate constants, but is based on macro-system parameters, usually resulting in less variability. The slope of the Patlak plot, K_i, represents K_{acc}.

Both tracers have been used in preclinical and clinical research. From autoradiography studies with [^{14}C]AMT, it was shown that antidepressants had different effects after chronic and acute application, and changes in synthesis were also dependent on the brain region investigated [105, 106]. Possible explanations for the discrepancies between acute and chronic effects rely in the acute inhibiting effects on 5-HT synthesis of the autoreceptors 5-HT_{1A} and 5-HT_{1B}, and receptor desensitization after multiple stimulations. 5-HT_{1A} receptors decrease 5-HT synthesis after acute administration of the agonist buspirone, while chronic treatment abolished this effect [107]. In accordance, acute stimulation of 5-HT_{1B} receptors with compounds like CP-93,129, results in a decrease of 5-HT synthesis, while chronic administration abolishes this effect [108, 109].

In conclusion, both 5-HT_{1A} and 5-HT_{1B} autoreceptors can reduce 5-HT synthesis rates in the brain, but the receptors desensitize in response to chronic stimulation, so that their inhibitory effects are transient. The described studies with AMT are an excellent example of how PET tracers can provide novel insights regarding physiological processes.

Eventually a tracer should have the ability to visualize physiological processes in humans, in order to clarify the pathophysiology of disease and to be employed in clinical routine. Clinical studies with [^{11}C]AMT and [^{11}C]5-HTP provided insight on psychiatry-related pathologies (see reviews by [110, 111]).

Changes in Patlak K^{α} were detectable with [^{11}C]AMT PET in medication-free patients with major depression in the cingulate cortex. Surprisingly, K^{α} did not correlate with the severity of depression [112].

Treatment with the SSRI citalopram increased K^{α} in the cingulate cortex and this increase is associated with elevated mood as assessed by Hamilton rating scores [113]. It is known that blocking the 5-HT_{1A} receptor with pindolol can accelerate the therapeutic effects of antidepressants [114]. Indeed, at day 24 the increase in 5-HT synthesis rate induced by an SSRI was greater in patients who received pindolol at day 10, compared to placebo. Whether this increase in 5-HT synthesis is due to 5-HT_{1A} autoreceptor blocking remains questionable, because pindolol also excites dopaminergic and noradrenergic neurons [115]. Most probably the total blockage of central β-adrenoceptors by pindolol plays an important role [116].

In addition, the BP of [^{18}F]MPPF, a 5-HT_{1A} receptor ligand, could not be correlated to 5-HT synthesis rates as measured with [^{11}C]AMT in the raphe nuclei [117]. However, in terminal areas of serotonergic neurons (like hippocampus, anterior cingulate cortex and anterior insula) a negative correlation was found, indicating that decreased binding of [^{18}F]-MPPF to 5-HT_{1A} heteroreceptors increased 5-HT synthesis. These studies show that a combination of different tracers can lead to greater understanding of processes in the human brain.

While under healthy conditions [^{11}C]AMT may provide estimates of 5-HT synthesis, a recent human PET study confirmed that this tracer can actually enter the kynurenine pathway. It was shown that brain tumours show differences in IDO (the enzyme converting tryptophan to kynurenine) expression and that this expression was related to the amount of AMT taken up by the tumour [118].

To the best of our knowledge, the first PET study with [^{11}C]5-HTP in the human brain was performed in 1991 [119]. Patients suffering from major depression showed a reduced uptake of the tracer in their brains. A recent clinical study reported a relationship between [^{11}C]5-HTP trapping and mood states [120]. A clear negative correlation was observed between the cardinal symptoms of premenstrual dysphoria in women, like irritability and depressed mood, and changes in tracer trapping in the entire brain, prefrontal regions and some regions of the striatum. The opposite mood states, feelings of happiness and mental energy, showed a strong positive correlation with tracer trapping.

These studies indicate a prominent role for PET imaging in psychiatry, as this technique is able to reveal pathophysiological mechanisms, which can otherwise only be detected with invasive techniques.

7. CONCLUSIONS

The serotonergic system is complex, influencing many other neurotransmitter systems and behavioural functions. Monitoring 5-HT synthesis or other elements of serotonergic neurotransmission *in vivo* with PET gives insight into what is going on in the living brain. Research reviewed here shows the possibilities of this technique to elucidate processes otherwise not fully understood. However, refinement is necessary to increase resolution and increase target-to-background ratios. In addition, many elements of the 5-HT system have not yet been visualized, making the picture incomplete. The most elegant studies are studies where multiple tracers could be used, visualizing different aspects of serotonergic neurotransmission like receptor BP and 5-HT synthesis.

So far, PET imaging revealed the occupancy of different antidepressants on receptors and SERT, their effect on receptor expression and the differences between receptor expression in health and disease. In addition, effects of antidepressants on serotonin synthesis and differences of serotonin synthesis in health and disease were shown.

A unified theory of affective disorders can only be achieved if we consider different imaging methods and also take into account both animal and human histological data. In the future it may be worthwhile to develop tools to study both receptor density and 5-HT synthesis, and this will hopefully yield a better and more complete understanding of the processes involved in the pathophysiology of affective disorders. However, the studies discussed comprised only a small fraction of the affective disorders that exist and of course there is also much opportunity for application in neurodegenerative diseases.

REFERENCES

[1] Barnes NM, Sharp T. A review of central 5-HT receptors and their function. Neuropharmacology 1999, 38:1083-152.

[2] Richardson-Jones JW, Craige CP, Guiard BP, Stephen A, Metzger KL, Kung HF, Gardier AM, Dranovsky A, David DJ, Beck SG, Hen R, Leonardo ED. 5-HT_{1A} autoreceptor levels determine vulnerability to stress and response to antidepressants. Neuron 2010, 65:40-52.

[3] Dantzer R, O'Connor JC, Freund GG, Johnson RW, Kelley KW. From inflammation to sickness and depression: when the immune system subjugates the brain. Nat Rev Neurosci 2008, 9:46-56.

[4] aan het Rot M, Mathew SJ, Charney DS. Neurobiological mechanisms in major depressive disorder. CMAJ 2009, 180:305-13.

[5] van Praag HM, Korf J. Serotonin metabolism in depression: clinical application of the probenecid test. Int Pharmacopsychiatry 1974, 9:35-51.

[6] van Praag HM, de Haan S. Central serotonin metabolism and frequency of depression. Psychiatry Res 1979, 1:219-24.

[7] Jongsma ME, van der Hart MCG, Udo de Haes, Joanna I., Cremers TIFH, Westerink BHC, den Boer JA, Bosker FJ. Augmentation Strategies to Improve Treatment of Major Depression. Cent Nerv Syst Agents Med Chem 2006, 6:135-52.

[8] Dremencov E, Weizmann Y, Kinor N, Gispan-Herman I, Yadid G. Modulation of dopamine transmission by $5HT_{2C}$ and $5HT_3$ receptors: a role in the antidepressant response. Curr Drug Targets 2006, 7:165-75.

[9] Fink KB, Gothert M. 5-HT receptor regulation of neurotransmitter release. Pharmacol Rev 2007, 59:360-417.

[10] Pazos A, Probst A, Palacios JM. Serotonin receptors in the human brain--III. Autoradiographic mapping of serotonin-1 receptors. Neuroscience 1987, 21:97-122.

[11] Sari Y, Miquel MC, Brisorgueil MJ, Ruiz G, Doucet E, Hamon M, Verge D. Cellular and subcellular localization of 5-hydroxytryptamine1B receptors in the rat central nervous system: immunocytochemical, autoradiographic and lesion studies. Neuroscience 1999, 88:899-915.

[12] Verge D, Daval G, Marcinkiewicz M, Patey A, El Mestikawy S, Gozlan H, Hamon M. Quantitative autoradiography of multiple $5\text{-}HT_1$ receptor subtypes in the brain of control or 5,7-dihydroxytryptamine-treated rats. J Neurosci 1986, 6:3474-82.

[13] Hartig PR, Hoyer D, Humphrey PP, Martin GR. Alignment of receptor nomenclature with the human genome: classification of $5\text{-}HT_{1B}$ and $5\text{-}HT_{1D}$ receptor subtypes. Trends Pharmacol Sci 1996, 17:103-5.

[14] Bruinvels AT, Landwehrmeyer B, Gustafson EL, Durkin MM, Mengod G, Branchek TA, Hoyer D, Palacios JM. Localization of $5\text{-}HT_{1B}$, $5\text{-}HT_{1DA}$, $5\text{-}HT_{1E}$ and $5\text{-}HT_{1F}$ receptor messenger RNA in rodent and primate brain. Neuropharmacology 1994, 33:367-86.

[15] Ferrari MD, Farkkila M, Reuter U, Pilgrim A, Davis C, Krauss M, Diener HC, European COL-144 Investigators. Acute treatment of migraine with the selective $5\text{-}HT_{1F}$ receptor agonist lasmiditan--a randomised proof-of-concept trial. Cephalalgia 2010, 30:1170-8.

[16] Nelson DL, Phebus LA, Johnson KW, Wainscott DB, Cohen ML, Calligaro DO, Xu YC. Preclinical pharmacological profile of the selective $5\text{-}HT_{1F}$ receptor agonist lasmiditan. Cephalalgia 2010, 30:1159-69.

[17] Pazos A, Probst A, Palacios JM. Serotonin receptors in the human brain: IV. Autoradiographic mapping of serotonin-2 receptors. Neuroscience 1987, 21:123-39.

[18] Vaidya VA, Marek GJ, Aghajanian GK, Duman RS. $5\text{-}HT_{2A}$ receptor-mediated regulation of brain-derived neurotrophic factor mRNA in the hippocampus and the neocortex. J Neurosci 1997, 17:2785-95.

[19] Shelton RC, Sanders-Bush E, Manier DH, Lewis DA. Elevated $5\text{-}HT_{2A}$ receptors in postmortem prefrontal cortex in major depression is associated with reduced activity of protein kinase A. Neuroscience 2009, 158:1406-15.

[20] Di Pietro NC, Seamans JK. Dopamine and serotonin interactions in the prefrontal cortex: insights on antipsychotic drugs and their mechanism of action. Pharmacopsychiatry 2007, 40 Suppl 1:S27-33.

[21] Kometer M, Cahn BR, Andel D, Carter OL, Vollenweider FX. The 5-$HT_{2A/1A}$ agonist psilocybin disrupts modal object completion associated with visual hallucinations. Biol Psychiatry 2011, 69:399-406.

[22] Angelucci F, Bernardini S, Gravina P, Bellincampi L, Trequattrini A, Di Iulio F, Vanni D, Federici G, Caltagirone C, Bossu P, Spalletta G. Delusion symptoms and response to antipsychotic treatment are associated with the 5-HT_{2A} receptor polymorphism (102T/C) in Alzheimer's disease: a 3-year follow-up longitudinal study. J Alzheimers Dis 2009, 17:203-11.

[23] Duxon MS, Flanigan TP, Reavley AC, Baxter GS, Blackburn TP, Fone KC. Evidence for expression of the 5-hydroxytryptamine-2B receptor protein in the rat central nervous system. Neuroscience 1997, 76:323-9.

[24] Cremers TI, Giorgetti M, Bosker FJ, Hogg S, Arnt J, Mork A, Honig G, Bogeso KP, Westerink BH, den Boer H, Wikstrom HV, Tecott LH. Inactivation of 5-HT_{2C} receptors potentiates consequences of serotonin reuptake blockade. Neuropsychopharmacology 2004, 29:1782-9.

[25] Pratt GD, Bowery NG, Kilpatrick GJ, Leslie RA, Barnes NM, Naylor RJ, Jones BJ, Nelson DR, Palacids JM, Slater P, . Consensus meeting agrees distribution of 5-HT_3 receptors in mammalian hindbrain. Trends Pharmacol Sci 1990, 11:135-7.

[26] Morales M, Battenberg E, de Lecea L, Bloom FE. The type 3 serotonin receptor is expressed in a subpopulation of GABAergic neurons in the rat neocortex and hippocampus. Brain Res 1996, 731:199-202.

[27] Mengod G, Vilaro MT, Raurich A, Lopez-Gimenez JF, Cortes R, Palacios JM. 5-HT receptors in mammalian brain: receptor autoradiography and *in situ* hybridization studies of new ligands and newly identified receptors. Histochem J 1996, 28:747-58.

[28] Tamburella A, Micale V, Navarria A, Drago F. Antidepressant properties of the 5-HT_4 receptor partial agonist, SL65.0155: behavioral and neurochemical studies in rats. Prog Neuropsychopharmacol Biol Psychiatry 2009, 33:1205-10.

[29] Erlander MG, Lovenberg TW, Baron BM, de Lecea L, Danielson PE, Racke M, Slone AL, Siegel BW, Foye PE, Cannon K, . Two members of a distinct subfamily of 5-hydroxytryptamine receptors differentially expressed in rat brain. Proc Natl Acad Sci U S A 1993, 90:3452-6.

[30] Nelson DL. 5-HT_5 receptors. Curr Drug Targets CNS Neurol Disord 2004, 3:53-8.

[31] Kohen R, Metcalf MA, Khan N, Druck T, Huebner K, Lachowicz JE, Meltzer HY, Sibley DR, Roth BL, Hamblin MW. Cloning, characterization, and chromosomal localization of a human 5-HT_6 serotonin receptor. J Neurochem 1996, 66:47-56.

[32] Nikiforuk A, Kos T, Wesolowska A. The 5-HT_6 receptor agonist EMD 386088 produces antidepressant and anxiolytic effects in rats after intrahippocampal administration. Psychopharmacology (Berl) 2011, 217:411-8.

[33] Carr GV, Schechter LE, Lucki I. Antidepressant and anxiolytic effects of selective 5-HT_6 receptor agonists in rats. Psychopharmacology (Berl) 2011, 213:499-507.

[34] Yau JL, Noble J, Widdowson J, Seckl JR. Impact of adrenalectomy on 5-HT_6 and 5-HT_7 receptor gene expression in the rat hippocampus. Brain Res Mol Brain Res 1997, 45:182-6.

[35] King MV, Marsden CA, Fone KC. A role for the 5-HT_{1A}, 5-HT_4 and 5-HT_6 receptors in learning and memory. Trends Pharmacol Sci 2008, 29:482-92.

[36] Geldenhuys WJ, Van der Schyf CJ. The serotonin 5-HT_6 receptor: a viable drug target for treating cognitive deficits in Alzheimer's disease. Expert Rev Neurother 2009, 9:1073-85.

[37] Le Corre S, Sharp T, Young AH, Harrison PJ. Increase of 5-HT_7 (serotonin-7) and 5-HT_{1A} (serotonin-1A) receptor mRNA expression in rat hippocampus after adrenalectomy. Psychopharmacology (Berl) 1997, 130:368-74.

[38] Stowe RL, Barnes NM. Selective labelling of 5-HT_7 receptor recognition sites in rat brain using [3H]5-carboxamidotryptamine. Neuropharmacology 1998, 37:1611-9.

[39] Hedlund PB. The 5-HT_7 receptor and disorders of the nervous system: an overview. Psychopharmacology (Berl) 2009, 206:345-54.

[40] Sarkisyan G, Roberts AJ, Hedlund PB. The 5-HT_7 receptor as a mediator and modulator of antidepressant-like behavior. Behav Brain Res 2010.

[41] Ying SW, Rusak B. 5-HT_7 receptors mediate serotonergic effects on light-sensitive suprachiasmatic nucleus neurons. Brain Res 1997, 755:246-54.

[42] Colwell CS. Linking neural activity and molecular oscillations in the SCN. Nat Rev Neurosci 2011, 12:553-69.

[43] Maguire RP, Leenders KL. PET pharmacokinetic course. Japan: Kobe, 2007.

[44] Kety SS, Schmidt CF. The Nitrous Oxide Method for the Quantitative Determination of Cerebral Blood Flow in Man: Theory, Procedure and Normal Values. J Clin Invest 1948, 27:476-83.

[45] Luurtsema G, Molthoff CF, Schuit RC, Windhorst AD, Lammertsma AA, Franssen EJ. Evaluation of (R)-[11C]verapamil as PET tracer of P-glycoprotein function in the blood-brain barrier: kinetics and metabolism in the rat. Nucl Med Biol 2005, 32:87-93.

[46] de Klerk OL, Bosker FJ, Willemsen AT, Van Waarde A, Visser AK, de Jager T, Dagyte G, den Boer JA, Dierckx RA, Meerlo P. Chronic stress and antidepressant treatment have opposite effects on P-glycoprotein at the blood-brain barrier: an experimental PET study in rats. J Psychopharmacol 2010, 24:1237-42.

[47] Hendrikse NH, Franssen EJ, van der Graaf WT, Vaalburg W, de Vries EG. Visualization of multidrug resistance *in vivo*. Eur J Nucl Med 1999, 26:283-93.

[48] Mintun MA, Raichle ME, Kilbourn MR, Wooten GF, Welch MJ. A quantitative model for the *in vivo* assessment of drug binding sites with positron emission tomography. Ann Neurol 1984, 15:217-27.

[49] Innis RB, Cunningham VJ, Delforge J, Fujita M, Gjedde A, Gunn RN, Holden J, Houle S, Huang SC, Ichise M, Iida H, Ito H, Kimura Y, Koeppe RA, Knudsen GM, Knuuti J, Lammertsma AA, Laruelle M, Logan J, Maguire RP, Mintun MA, Morris ED, Parsey R, Price JC, Slifstein M, Sossi V, Suhara T, Votaw JR, Wong DF, Carson RE. Consensus nomenclature for *in vivo* imaging of reversibly binding radioligands. J Cereb Blood Flow Metab 2007, 27:1533-9.

[50] Lassen NA, Bartenstein PA, Lammertsma AA, Prevett MC, Turton DR, Luthra SK, Osman S, Bloomfield PM, Jones T, Patsalos PN. Benzodiazepine receptor quantification *in vivo* in humans using [11C]flumazenil and PET: application of the steady-state principle. J Cereb Blood Flow Metab 1995, 15:152-65.

[51] Cunningham VJ, Rabiner EA, Slifstein M, Laruelle M, Gunn RN. Measuring drug occupancy in the absence of a reference region: the Lassen plot re-visited. J Cereb Blood Flow Metab 2010, 30:46-50.

[52] Lucignani G, Schmidt KC, Moresco RM, Striano G, Colombo F, Sokoloff L, Fazio F. Measurement of regional cerebral glucose utilization with fluorine-18-FDG and PET in heterogeneous tissues: theoretical considerations and practical procedure. J Nucl Med 1993, 34:360-9.

[53] Visser AK, Van Waarde A, Willemsen AT, Bosker FJ, Luiten PG, Den Boer JA, Kema IP, Dierckx RA. Measuring serotonin synthesis: from conventional methods to PET tracers and their (pre)clinical implications. Eur J Nucl Med Mol Imaging 2010, 38:576-91.

[54] Irie T, Fukushi K, Namba H, Iyo M, Tamagami H, Nagatsuka S, Ikota N. Brain acetylcholinesterase activity: validation of a PET tracer in a rat model of Alzheimer's disease. J Nucl Med 1996, 37:649-55.

[55] Moresco RM, Matarrese M, Fazio F. PET and SPET molecular imaging: focus on serotonin system. Curr Top Med Chem 2006, 6:2027-34.

[56] Meltzer CC, Smith G, DeKosky ST, Pollock BG, Mathis CA, Moore RY, Kupfer DJ, Reynolds CF,III. Serotonin in aging, late-life depression, and Alzheimer's disease: the emerging role of functional imaging. Neuropsychopharmacology 1998, 18:407-30.

[57] Paterson LM, Kornum BR, Nutt DJ, Pike VW, Knudsen GM. 5-HT radioligands for human brain imaging with PET and SPECT. Med Res Rev 2011.

[58] Passchier J, Van Waarde A. Visualisation of serotonin-1A (5-HT_{1A}) receptors in the central nervous system. Eur J Nucl Med 2001, 28:113-29.

[59] Sandell J, Halldin C, Hall H, Thorberg SO, Werner T, Sohn D, Sedvall G, Farde L. Radiosynthesis and autoradiographic evaluation of [11C]NAD-299, a radioligand for visualization of the 5-HT_{1A} receptor. Nucl Med Biol 1999, 26:159-64.

[60] Milak MS, Severance AJ, Ogden RT, Prabhakaran J, Kumar JS, Majo VJ, Mann JJ, Parsey RV. Modeling considerations for 11C-CUMI-101, an agonist radiotracer for imaging serotonin-1A receptor *in vivo* with PET. J Nucl Med 2008, 49:587-96.

[61] Kumar JS, Prabhakaran J, Majo VJ, Milak MS, Hsiung SC, Tamir H, Simpson NR, Van Heertum RL, Mann JJ, Parsey RV. Synthesis and *in vivo* evaluation of a novel 5-HT_{1A} receptor agonist radioligand [O-methyl- 11C]2-(4-(4-(2-methoxyphenyl)piperazin-1-yl)butyl)-4-methyl-1,2,4-triazine -3,5(2H,4H)dione in nonhuman primates. Eur J Nucl Med Mol Imaging 2007, 34:1050-60.

[62] Milak MS, DeLorenzo C, Zanderigo F, Prabhakaran J, Kumar JS, Majo VJ, Mann JJ, Parsey RV. *In vivo* quantification of human serotonin 1A receptor using 11C-CUMI-101, an agonist PET radiotracer. J Nucl Med 2010, 51:1892-900.

[63] Udo de Haes JI, Bosker FJ, Van Waarde A, Pruim J, Willemsen AT, Vaalburg W, Den Boer JA. 5-HT_{1A} receptor imaging in the human brain: effect of tryptophan depletion and infusion on [(18)F] MPPF binding. Synapse 2002, 46:108-15.

[64] Shiue CY, Shiue GG, Mozley PD, Kung MP, Zhuang ZP, Kim HJ, Kung HF. P-[18F]-MPPF: a potential radioligand for PET studies of 5-HT_{1A} receptors in humans. Synapse 1997, 25:147-54.

[65] Pike VW, McCarron JA, Lammertsma AA, Osman S, Hume SP, Sargent PA, Bench CJ, Cliffe IA, Fletcher A, Grasby PM. Exquisite delineation of 5-HT_{1A} receptors in human brain with PET and [carbonyl-11 C]WAY-100635. Eur J Pharmacol 1996, 301:R5-7.

[66] Drevets WC, Frank E, Price JC, Kupfer DJ, Holt D, Greer PJ, Huang Y, Gautier C, Mathis C. PET imaging of serotonin 1A receptor binding in depression. Biol Psychiatry 1999, 46:1375-87.

[67] Drevets WC, Thase ME, Moses-Kolko EL, Price J, Frank E, Kupfer DJ, Mathis C. Serotonin-1A receptor imaging in recurrent depression: replication and literature review. Nucl Med Biol 2007, 34:865-77.

[68] Pike VW, Halldin C, McCarron JA, Lundkvist C, Hirani E, Olsson H, Hume SP, Karlsson P, Osman S, Swahn CG, Hall H, Wikstrom H, Mensonidas M, Poole KG, Farde L. [carbonyl-11C] Desmethyl-WAY-100635 (DWAY) is a potent and selective radioligand for central 5-HT_{1A} receptors *in vitro* and *in vivo*. Eur J Nucl Med 1998, 25:338-46.

[69] Pierson ME, Andersson J, Nyberg S, McCarthy DJ, Finnema SJ, Varnas K, Takano A, Karlsson P, Gulyas B, Medd AM, Lee CM, Powell ME, Heys JR, Potts W, Seneca N, Mrzljak L, Farde L, Halldin C. [11C]AZ10419369: a selective 5-HT_{1B} receptor radioligand suitable for positron emission tomography (PET). Characterization in the primate brain. Neuroimage 2008, 41:1075-85.

[70] Gallezot JD, Nabulsi N, Neumeister A, Planeta-Wilson B, Williams WA, Singhal T, Kim S, Maguire RP, McCarthy T, Frost JJ, Huang Y, Ding YS, Carson RE. Kinetic modeling of the serotonin 5-HT_{1B} receptor radioligand [(11)C]P943 in humans. J Cereb Blood Flow Metab 2009.

[71] Finnema SJ, Varrone A, Hwang TJ, Gulyas B, Pierson ME, Halldin C, Farde L. Fenfluramine-induced serotonin release decreases [11C]AZ10419369 binding to 5-HT_{1B}-receptors in the primate brain. Synapse 2010, 64:573-7.

[72] Murrough JW, Henry S, Hu J, Gallezot JD, Planeta-Wilson B, Neumaier JF, Neumeister A. Reduced ventral striatal/ventral pallidal serotonin1B receptor binding potential in major depressive disorder. Psychopharmacology (Berl) 2011, 213:547-53.

[73] Blin J, Pappata S, Kiyosawa M, Crouzel C, Baron JC. [18F]setoperone: a new high-affinity ligand for positron emission tomography study of the serotonin-2 receptors in baboon brain *in vivo*. Eur J Pharmacol 1988, 147:73-82.

[74] Lemaire C, Cantineau R, Guillaume M, Plenevaux A, Christiaens L. Fluorine-18-altanserin: a radioligand for the study of serotonin receptors with PET: radiolabeling and *in vivo* biologic behavior in rats. J Nucl Med 1991, 32:2266-72.

[75] Lundkvist C, Halldin C, Ginovart N, Nyberg S, Swahn CG, Carr AA, Brunner F, Farde L. [11C]MDL 100907, a radioligland for selective imaging of 5-HT_{2A} receptors with positron emission tomography. Life Sci 1996, 58:L-92.

[76] Hirani E, Sharp T, Sprakes M, Grasby P, Hume S. Fenfluramine evokes 5-HT_{2A} receptor-mediated responses but does not displace [11C]MDL 100907: small animal PET and gene expression studies. Synapse 2003, 50:251-60.

[77] Herth MM, Kramer V, Piel M, Palner M, Riss PJ, Knudsen GM, Rosch F. Synthesis and *in vitro* affinities of various MDL 100907 derivatives as potential 18F-radioligands for 5-HT_{2A} receptor imaging with PET. Bioorg Med Chem 2009, 17:2989-3002.

[78] Herth MM, Piel M, Debus F, Schmitt U, Luddens H, Rosch F. Preliminary *in vivo* and *ex vivo* evaluation of the 5-HT_{2A} imaging probe [(18)F]MH.MZ. Nucl Med Biol 2009, 36:447-54.

[79] Ettrup A, Hansen M, Santini MA, Paine J, Gillings N, Palner M, Lehel S, Herth MM, Madsen J, Kristensen J, Begtrup M, Knudsen GM. Radiosynthesis and *in vivo* evaluation of a series of substituted 11C-phenethylamines as 5-HT_{2A} agonist PET tracers. Eur J Nucl Med Mol Imaging 2011, 38:681-93.

[80] Marner L, Gillings N, Madsen K, Erritzoe D, Baare WF, Svarer C, Hasselbalch SG, Knudsen GM. Brain imaging of serotonin 4 receptors in humans with [(11)C]SB207145-PET. Neuroimage 2010.

[81] Marner L, Gillings N, Comley RA, Baare WF, Rabiner EA, Wilson AA, Houle S, Hasselbalch SG, Svarer C, Gunn RN, Laruelle M, Knudsen GM. Kinetic modeling of 11C-SB207145 binding to 5-HT4 receptors in the human brain *in vivo*. J Nucl Med 2009, 50:900-8.

[82] Zhang M, Haradahira T, Maeda J, Okauchi T, Kida T, Obayashi S, Suzuki K, Suhara T. Synthesis and preliminary PET study of the 5-HT_7 receptor antagonist [^{11}C]DR4446. J Label Compd Radiopharm 2002, 45:857-66.

[83] Lemoine L, Andries J, Le Bars D, Billard T, Zimmer L. Comparison of 4 Radiolabeled Antagonists for Serotonin 5-HT7 Receptor Neuroimaging: Toward the First PET Radiotracer. J Nucl Med 2011, 52:1811-8.

[84] Suehiro M, Scheffel U, Ravert HT, Dannals RF, Wagner HN,Jr. [11C](+)McN5652 as a radiotracer for imaging serotonin uptake sites with PET. Life Sci 1993, 53:883-92.

[85] Houle S, Ginovart N, Hussey D, Meyer JH, Wilson AA. Imaging the serotonin transporter with positron emission tomography: initial human studies with [11C]DAPP and [11C]DASB. Eur J Nucl Med 2000, 27:1719-22.

[86] Hinz R, Selvaraj S, Murthy NV, Bhagwagar Z, Taylor M, Cowen PJ, Grasby PM. Effects of citalopram infusion on the serotonin transporter binding of [11C]DASB in healthy controls. J Cereb Blood Flow Metab 2008, 28:1478-90.

[87] Voineskos AN, Wilson AA, Boovariwala A, Sagrati S, Houle S, Rusjan P, Sokolov S, Spencer EP, Ginovart N, Meyer JH. Serotonin transporter occupancy of high-dose selective serotonin reuptake inhibitors during major depressive disorder measured with [11C]DASB positron emission tomography. Psychopharmacology (Berl) 2007, 193:539-45.

[88] Halldin C, Lundberg J, Sovago J, Gulyas B, Guilloteau D, Vercouillie J, Emond P, Chalon S, Tarkiainen J, Hiltunen J, Farde L. [(11)C]MADAM, a new serotonin transporter radioligand characterized in the monkey brain by PET. Synapse 2005, 58:173-83.

[89] Lundberg J, Halldin C, Farde L. Measurement of serotonin transporter binding with PET and [11C]MADAM: a test-retest reproducibility study. Synapse 2006, 60:256-63.

[90] Lundberg J, Christophersen JS, Petersen KB, Loft H, Halldin C, Farde L. PET measurement of serotonin transporter occupancy: a comparison of escitalopram and citalopram. Int J Neuropsychopharmacol 2007, 10:777-85.

[91] Ma KH, Huang WS, Kuo YY, Peng CJ, Liou NH, Liu RS, Hwang JJ, Liu JC, Chen HJ, Shiue CY. Validation of 4-[18F]-ADAM as a SERT imaging agent using micro-PET and autoradiography. Neuroimage 2009, 45:687-93.

[92] Lang L, Jagoda E, Schmall B, Vuong BK, Adams HR, Nelson DL, Carson RE, Eckelman WC. Development of fluorine-18-labeled 5-HT_{1A} antagonists. J Med Chem 1999, 42:1576-86.

[93] Saigal N, Pichika R, Easwaramoorthy B, Collins D, Christian BT, Shi B, Narayanan TK, Potkin SG, Mukherjee J. Synthesis and biologic evaluation of a novel serotonin 5-HT_{1A} receptor radioligand, 18F-labeled mefway, in rodents and imaging by PET in a nonhuman primate. J Nucl Med 2006, 47:1697-706.

[94] Yasuno F, Zoghbi SS, McCarron JA, Hong J, Ichise M, Brown AK, Gladding RL, Bacher JD, Pike VW, Innis RB. Quantification of serotonin 5-HT1A receptors in monkey brain with [11C](R)-(-)-RWAY. Synapse 2006, 60:510-20.

[95] Diksic M, Nagahiro S, Sourkes TL, Yamamoto YL. A new method to measure brain serotonin synthesis *in vivo*. I. Theory and basic data for a biological model. J Cereb Blood Flow Metab 1990, 10:1-12.

[96] Bjurling P, Watanabe Y, Tokushige M, Oda T, Långström B. Syntheses of -^{11}C-labelled L-tryptophan and 5-hydroxy-L-tryptophan using a multi-enzymatic reaction route. J Chem Soc , Perkin Trans 1989:1331-4.

[97] Fernstrom JD, Wurtman RJ. Brain serotonin content: physiological dependence on plasma tryptophan levels. Science 1971, 173:149-52.

[98] Tracqui P, Morot-Gaudry Y, Staub JF, Brezillon P, Perault-Staub AM, Bourgoin S, Hamon M. Model of brain serotonin metabolism. II. Physiological interpretation. Am J Physiol 1983, 244:R206-15.

[99] Muzik O, Chugani DC, Chakraborty P, Mangner T, Chugani HT. Analysis of [C-11]alpha-methyl-tryptophan kinetics for the estimation of serotonin synthesis rate *in vivo*. J Cereb Blood Flow Metab 1997, 17:659-69.

[100] Roberge AG, Missala K, Sourkes TL. Alpha-methyltryptophan: effects on synthesis and degradation of serotonin in the brain. Neuropharmacology 1972, 11:197-209.

[101] Chugani DC. alpha-methyl-L-tryptophan: mechanisms for tracer localization of epileptogenic brain regions. Biomark Med 2011, 5:567-75.

[102] Chugani DC, Muzik O. Alpha[C-11]methyl-L-tryptophan PET maps brain serotonin synthesis and kynurenine pathway metabolism. J Cereb Blood Flow Metab 2000, 20:2-9.

[103] Hartvig P, Bergstrom M, Antoni G, Langstrom B. Positron emission tomography and brain monoamine neurotransmission -- entries for study of drug interactions. Curr Pharm Des 2002, 8:1417-34.

[104] Nagahiro S, Takada A, Diksic M, Sourkes TL, Missala K, Yamamoto YL. A new method to measure brain serotonin synthesis *in vivo*. II. A practical autoradiographic method tested in normal and lithium-treated rats. J Cereb Blood Flow Metab 1990, 10:13-21.

[105] Tsuiki K, Yamamoto YL, Diksic M. Effect of acute fluoxetine treatment on the brain serotonin synthesis as measured by the alpha-methyl-L-tryptophan autoradiographic method. J Neurochem 1995, 65:250-6.

[106] Muck-Seler D, Jevric-Causevic A, Diksic M. Influence of fluoxetine on regional serotonin synthesis in the rat brain. J Neurochem 1996, 67:2434-42.

[107] Okazawa H, Yamane F, Blier P, Diksic M. Effects of acute and chronic administration of the serotonin1A agonist buspirone on serotonin synthesis in the rat brain. J Neurochem 1999, 72:2022-31.

[108] Tohyama Y, Yamane F, Fikre Merid M, Blier P, Diksic M. Effects of serotine receptors agonists, TFMPP and CGS12066B, on regional serotonin synthesis in the rat brain: an autoradiographic study. J Neurochem 2002, 80:788-98.

[109] Hasegawa S, Watanabe A, Nishi K, Nguyen KQ, Diksic M. Selective 5-HT_{1B} receptor agonist reduces serotonin synthesis following acute, and not chronic, drug administration: results of an autoradiographic study. Neurochem Int 2005, 46:261-72.

[110] Diksic M, Young SN. Study of the brain serotonergic system with labeled alpha-methyl-L-tryptophan. J Neurochem 2001, 78:1185-200.

[111] Diksic M. Labelled alpha-methyl-L-tryptophan as a tracer for the study of the brain serotonergic system. J Psychiatry Neurosci 2001, 26:293-303.

[112] Rosa-Neto P, Diksic M, Okazawa H, Leyton M, Ghadirian N, Mzengeza S, Nakai A, Debonnel G, Blier P, Benkelfat C. Measurement of brain regional alpha-[11C]methyl-L-tryptophan trapping as a measure of serotonin synthesis in medication-free patients with major depression. Arch Gen Psychiatry 2004, 61:556-63.

[113] Berney A, Nishikawa M, Benkelfat C, Debonnel G, Gobbi G, Diksic M. An index of 5-HT synthesis changes during early antidepressant treatment: alpha-[11C]methyl-L-tryptophan PET study. Neurochem Int 2008, 52:701-8.

[114] Artigas F, Perez V, Alvarez E. Pindolol induces a rapid improvement of depressed patients treated with serotonin reuptake inhibitors. Arch Gen Psychiatry 1994, 51:248-51.

[115] Lejeune F, Millan MJ. Pindolol excites dopaminergic and adrenergic neurons, and inhibits serotonergic neurons, by activation of 5-HT_{1A} receptors. Eur J Neurosci 2000, 12:3265-75.

[116] Cremers TI, Wiersma LJ, Bosker FJ, Den Boer JA, Westerink BH, Wikstrom HV. Is the beneficial antidepressant effect of coadministration of pindolol really due to somatodendritic autoreceptor antagonism?. Biol Psychiatry 2001, 50:13-21.

[117] Frey BN, Rosa-Neto P, Lubarsky S, Diksic M. Correlation between serotonin synthesis and 5-HT_{1A} receptor binding in the living human brain: a combined alpha-[11C]MT and [18F]MPPF positron emission tomography study. Neuroimage 2008, 42:850-7.

[118] Batista CE, Juhasz C, Muzik O, Kupsky WJ, Barger G, Chugani HT, Mittal S, Sood S, Chakraborty PK, Chugani DC. Imaging correlates of differential expression of indoleamine 2,3-dioxygenase in human brain tumors. Mol Imaging Biol 2009, 11:460-6.

[119] Agren H, Reibring L, Hartvig P, Tedroff J, Bjurling P, Hornfeldt K, Andersson Y, Lundqvist H, Langstrom B. Low brain uptake of L-[11C]5-hydroxytryptophan in major depression: a positron emission tomography study on patients and healthy volunteers. Acta Psychiatr Scand 1991, 83:449-55.

[120] Eriksson O, Wall A, Marteinsdottir I, Agren H, Hartvig P, Blomqvist G, Langstrom B, Naessen T. Mood changes correlate to changes in brain serotonin precursor trapping in women with premenstrual dysphoria. Psychiatry Res 2006, 146:107-16.

Send Orders for Reprints to reprints@benthamscience.net

CHAPTER 4

PATHOPHYSIOLOGY OF MOOD DISORDERS: PHARMACOGENETIC ASPECTS

CHIARA FABBRI*, STEFANO PORCELLI, ALESSANDRO SERRETTI

Department of Biomedical and Neuromotor Sciences, University of Bologna, Bologna, Italy

Abstract: Major depressive disorder (MDD) is an emergent cause of personal and socio-economic burden, since its high lifetime prevalence (16.2%) and the unsatisfying response rate of the available antidepressant drugs. Among modulators of treatment outcome, genetic polymorphisms are thought to explain a significant share of the inter-individual variability, according to a complex multi-loci model.

Given the described scenario, the present chapter aims to summarize and compare the main pharmacogenetic findings regarding antidepressant treatment outcome, including both candidate gene studies and genome-wide association studies.

The literature provided replicated evidence of association between several genes (in particular, SLC6A4, HTR1A, HTR2A, COMT, MAOA, BDNF, GNB3, and MDR1) and antidepressant efficacy, but findings were mainly contradictory. Despite the inconsistent pharmacongetic results obtained so far, the increasing knowledge about MDD pathogenesis and antidepressant mechanisms of action, together with better awareness of the limitations of previous pharmacogenetic studies, may lead to the confirmations required to produce clinical applications. Technical improvement in genotyping procedures may help to translate the increasing theoretic knowledge into practical applications.

Keywords: Serotonin (5-HT), norepinephrine (NE), dopamine (DA), glutamate, Brain derived neurotrophic factor (BDNF), hypothalamic-pituitary-adrenal (HPA) axis, depression, antidepressant drugs, selective serotonin reuptake inhibitors (SSRIs), copy number variants (CNV), single nucleotide polymorphism (SNP), genome-wide association studies (GWAS)

1. INTRODUCTION

1.1. DEFINITIONS AND AIMS

Nowadays the choice of what antidepressant (AD) is suitable for each patient is based only on some general clinical principles, such as the presence of psychiatric co-morbidities, the personal or family history of response to a particular drug and the presence of medical diseases. Nevertheless, these clinical features do not allow to identify the ideal drug for each patient, thus, so far the effective drug is still found by trials and errors. Within this scenario, the 2-4 weeks lag before improvement during AD treatment is likely associated with the risk of clinical worsening, premature discontinuation and worse hopelessness feelings. Moreover, current remission rates of major depressive disorder are still low (30% of patients had not still attained remission after four carefully monitored interventions [1]). Clinical predictors of AD response have been extensively investigated, but with still controversial findings, and they cannot be translated into clinical practice [2]. Indeed, psychiatric disease phenotypes are very heterogeneous, and clinical features per se are not discriminative enough. On the other side, there is increasing evidence that genetic polymorphisms contribute substantially to the inter-individual variability in AD response [2]. It is well known that approximately 99,5% of the human

*Address correspondence to Chiara Fabbri: Department of Biomedical and Neuromotor Sciences, University of Bologna, Bologna, Italy; E-mail: chiara.fabbri@yahoo.it

Bruno P Guiard and Eliyahu Dremencov (Eds)

genome DNA sequence is identical among humans, so the 0,5% of the sequence is responsible of the different susceptibility to diseases and the other differences among humans. This difference consists in di, tri and tetra nucleotide repeats (satellite sequences); large variants > 1 kbp due to delections, insertions or duplications (copy number variants, CNV) and nucleotide substitutions [3]. We find 3 millions of substitution in each individual human genome and over the 80% of them is in form of single nucleotide polymorphism (SNP), so it is estimated that SNPs account for over 80% of the variability between humans, including disease predisposition [4]. Nowadays the HapMap project makes easier the research of SNPs and has currently mapped the location of over three million of SNPs (http://hapmap.ncbi.nlm.nih.gov/).

Pharmacogenetics is the research field dealing with the detection of genetic predictors of treatment response and side effects, with the aim of improving disease outcome. Pharmacogenetics deals with the investigation of single/few number of genetic polymorphisms, thus it provides a narrow potential in discovering the multiple loci involved in antidepressant effect. Thanks to technological improvement, pharmacogenomics is becoming the new horizon of research. Pharmacogenomics aims to broaden the coverage of genetic variants up to the whole genome and investigate also the relationships between genetic variants. Pharmacogenomics seems to be the best strategy to handle the genetic determinants of AD response, which result from the contribution of a high number of polymorphisms, each with a small effect size.

Through genotyping, in a more or less far future, the best drug for a patient could be selected a priori, overcoming the trial and error principle. The consequences would mark a turning point in the treatment of major depression, which has a life-time prevalence of 12.8% [5] and is responsible for the great burden attributable to non-fatal health outcomes [6].

1.2. PHARMACOGENETICS EVOLUTION OVER TIME AND OPEN ISSUES

A role of genetic polymorphisms in AD response arose from the observation that mood disorders and treatment response often show a familiar clustering. Indeed, mechanisms linked to the pathophysiology of mood disorders and mechanisms controlling drug response are supposed to be similar; for example the serotonin transporter gene is the most studied gene both as risk factor for mood disorders and predictor of AD response. Consistently, previous studies found that a proband's pharmacological response may allow the selection of sample of families which are homogeneous for mode of inheritance [7]. In the '90s', when pharmacogenetics moved its first steps, studies were based on the candidate gene method or functional candidate approach, *i.e.,* the analysis of genetic variants selected a priori on the basis of knowledge derived from biological/pharmacological studies and animal models. Genes selected through this method are mainly the ones coding for key molecular components of the serotoninergic, noradrenergic and dopaminergic systems. Indeed, the pathophysiology of depression involves functional abnormalities of these systems and their restoration might be related to the AD efficacy [8]. In principle, the candidate-gene method is useful to test founded candidates, even if it has produced mainly inconsistent findings. Indeed, it shows a fundamental limitation: the multiple loci with small effect size involved in treatment response are not detectable through this approach in realistic sample sizes. Thanks to technical improvements, in the last years a new approach is spreading in order to overcome this issue: the genome-wide association method. Genome-wide association studies (GWAS), through the use of micro-array technology, have at disposal information about hundreds of thousands of polymorphic loci, allowing to cover the greatest part of the genetic variability associated to a phenotype. They overcome the need of any a priori hypothesis, a very useful tool since AD mechanisms of action are not fully understood. Moreover, biological plausibility is not an initial requirement for a convincing statistical association, as there are many examples in human genetics of previously unsuspected candidate genes nonetheless showing highly compelling associations [9]. GWAS have already produced promising results in the study of other complex diseases, such as coronary artery disease, type 1 and 2 diabetes and rheumatoid arthritis [10], showing to be a powerful method for the identification of genes involved in common human diseases. With regard to AD pharmacogenetics, three independent studies performed as far as now [11] did not find loci which reached the genome-wide threshold of significance. Indeed, the multitude of comparisons made in a GWAS result in a huge increase of the risk of type I error, since the probability of making at least one type I error in a study is: 1-(1-alpha)n (where n is the number of independent comparisons made). Therefore, the standard genome-wide threshold of significance has been set to p < 10-7 and p < 10-8, which correspond to an alpha error = 0.05 and 0.01, respectively. This standard is based on a Bonferroni's correction for an assumed million independent variants in the human genome [12]. The lack of genome-wide significant results as well as the poor replication of findings are probably due to some still unsolved limitations of GWAS. Firstly, the inadequate sample size, since our current knowledge suggests that future GWAS will need samples of tens of thousands rather than the thousands traditionally used [13]. Another issue is placed on a technical level. Indeed, reliable genotyping should be extended to polymorphisms present in < 5% of the population and also rare variants (< 1% of the population), which the current GWAS technology is not able to detect. Moreover, the available genotyping platforms are able to provide only a relative narrow genomic coverage (*e.g.*, less of 50% in the larger GWAS which has been performed till now [11]). A third but not less important issue pertains to phenotype definition. As a matter of fact, mood disorders show a wide range of clinical presentations and standard diagnostic criteria (DSM-IV or ICD-10) could not completely reflect them. Thus, the effect of a number of stratification factors might be a source of bias [14]. Given these matters, there are aldready emerging strategies to solve them. Indeed, the use of large replication samples is nowadays possible thanks to the growth of controlled-access data repositories *via* the NIMH Human Genetics Initiative (http://nimhgenetics.org). Moreover, an increasing number of studies provide a detailed collection of clinical and environmental information other than genotyping, allowing their inclusion in statistical models. This is expected to increase the specificity of genetic information, by the definition of genetic profiles of response which are associated to specific clinical characteristics. The improvement in genotyping procedures probably will make the rest.

2. PHARMACOGENETIC FINDINGS

Before entering into the details of pharmacogenetic findings, some preliminary remarks are required. We collected and compared available pharmacogenetic studies focused on antidepressant drugs, following a functional criteria, *i.e.*, grouping genes pertaining to the same neurotransmitter system, the same biological pathway (*e.g.*, the hypothalamic-pituitary-adrenal axis) or carrying out similar biological functions. We discussed the biological/molecular rationale of findings in the view of MDD pathophysiology and antidepressant mechanisms of action. Main replicated genes (i.e., almost six positive findings) were deeply discussed, but also less replicated results (i.e., between six and three positive findings) and preliminary findings (i.e., less than three positive findings) were mentioned (see Table **1**). GWAS results were discussed in a separate paragraph (2.8), since their particular methodology showed specific strengths and limits and provided different findings compared to candidate gene studies.

2.1. SEROTONINERGIC SYSTEM

Genes pertaining to the serotoninergic system are probably the most investigated, since the first theory of depression pathophysiology ascribed the main mechanism of the disease to a depletion of monoamines in the central nervous system (CNS). The so called monoaminergic theory of depression arose from the observation that some compounds, such as iproniazide and reserpine, shared the property of influencing the monoamines balance in the CNS and showed unexpected AD effect. Ever

Serotoninergic system						
Main replicated genes						
Gene	**Polymorphism**	**Drug class**	**Therapeutic effects**		**Side effects**	
			Positive results	**Negative results**	**Positive results**	**Negative results**
SLC6A4	HTTLPR	SSRIs	[21-27, 29-33, 35, 42, 44-46, 48-50, 61, 300-306]	[37, 39, 41, 54, 67, 81, 307, 308]	[37, 43, 67, 69, 71]	[50, 74, 130, 306, 309]
		Other/ Mixed	[28, 40, 47, 51, 52, 310]	[36, 53, 59, 117, 307]	[28, 68]	[72, 83, 311]
		augm.	[43, 312]		[43]	
	STin2 VNTR	SSRIs	[31, 33, 44, 46, 51, 81]	[39, 49, 82]	[68]	[69]
		Other/ Mixed	[40, 46, 51]	[32]		[83]
	rs25531	SSRIs	[61]	[33, 37, 38, 41, 303]	[37]	
		Other/ Mixed		[42, 59]		
HTR1A	rs6295 (-1019C/G)	SSRIs	[49, 102-105, 107, 109]	[81, 92, 108, 111, 230]		[74]
		Other/ Mixed	[101]	[230]		
	rs1800042 (Gly272Asp)	SSRIs	[110]	[102, 111]		
	rs10042486 and rs1364043	Other/ Mixed				
HTR2A	rs6311 (1438G/A)	SSRIs	[50, 118]	[92, 120]	[50, 71, 121, 313]	[314]
		Other/ Mixed	[315]	[53]		[83]
	rs6313 (102T/C) (LD with rs6311)	SSRIs		[49, 92, 119]		[74, 130]
		Other/ Mixed	[117]		[316]	

HTR2A	rs6314 (452His/Tyr)	SSRIs	[40]	[126]		[74]
	rs7997012	SSRIs	[122, 126]	[92]		
		Other/Mixed	[239]	[128, 149]		
	rs1928040	SSRIs	[317]			
		Other/Mixed		[128, 149]		
Less replicated genes						
TPH1	rs1800532 (A218C)	SSRIs	[84-86, 93]	[30, 49, 81, 89-92]		[91, 309]
TPH2	1463G/A	SSRIs	[81, 318]			
		Other/Mixed				[319]
	rs1843809, rs1386494 and rs1487276	SSRIs	[81]			
	rs10897346 and rs1487278	SSRIs	[95]			
		Other		[95]		
	rs2171363		[96]			
Preliminary findings						
HTR1B	rs6298	SSRIs	[107]			
	rs130058	SSRIs	[107]	[320]		
HTR2C	rs3813929	SSRIs				[74]
		Other/Mixed				[72]
HTR3A	rs1062613 (178C/T)	SSRIs	[50]		[130]	[50, 74, 121, 131]
HTR3B	rs1176744 (A27373G)	SSRIs			[131]	[74, 121, 130]
	-100 -102 AAG delection	SSRIs			[130]	
	rs35312182	SSRIs				[74]
HTR6	rs1805054 (C267T)	SSRIs		[92, 127]		
		Other/Mixed	[137]	[40, 138]		

Noradrenergic system						
Main replicated genes						
COMT	rs4680 (Val108/158Met)	SSRIs	[140, 143, 145]	[147, 321]		
		Other/Mixed	[142, 144, 146]		[72]	
MAO-A	VNTR 1.2 kb upstream the coding sequence	SSRIs	[322]	[81, 89, 119, 323]	[314]	
		Other/Mixed	[156, 324]	[154]		[83]
	rs1465108	SSRIs	[81]			
	rs6323	SSRIs	[81, 155]			
	rs1799835	Other/Mixed	[155]			
SLC6A2	rs2242446 (T-182C)	Other/Mixed	[53]	[42, 51]		[83]
	rs5569 (G1287A)	Other/Mixed	[46, 53]	[51]		
	rs1362621	SSRIs	[152]			
	rs5564	Other/Mixed	[152]			
	rs58532686	Other/Mixed	[42]			
	rs60329 and rs1532701	Other/Mixed	[125]			
	rs35915, rs28386840, rs168924, rs36017, rs47958 and rs171798	Other/Mixed		[42]		
Preliminary findings						
ADRB1	rs180253 (G1165C)	SSRIs		[160]		
		Other/Mixed	[159]			
	rs1801252	SSRIs		[160]		
ADRA2A	rs1800544 (-1291C/G)	Other/Mixed	[161]	[162]	[162]	
Dopaminergic system						
Preliminary findings						
SLC6A3	3' UTR 40-bp VNTR	Other/Mixed	[36, 171]			
DRD4	3rd exon 48 bp VNTR	SSRIs		[174]		
		Other/Mixed	[178]			
DRD2	rs1801028	SSRIs		[174, 176]		
DRD3	rs167770, rs6280 and rs2134655	augm.	[177]			

Hypothalamic-pituitary-adrenal (HPA) axis						
Main replicated genes						
FKBP5	rs1360780	SSRIs	[195, 205]	[325, 326]		
		Other/Mixed	[203, 204]	[125, 327]		
	rs3800373	Other/Mixed	[204]	[149, 203, 327]		
	rs4713916	SSRIs	[205]			
		Other/Mixed		[149]		
Less replicated genes						
CRHR1	rs1876828, rs242939 and rs242941 (haplotype)	SSRIs	[194]			
		Other/Mixed	[193]			
	rs12942300	SSRIs	[196]			
Preliminary findings						
CRHBP	rs10473984	SSRIs	[196]			
CRHR2	rs2270007	SSRIs	[195]			
NR3C1	ER22/23EK	Other/mixed	[198]			
	rs852977, rs10482633 and rs10052957	Other/mixed		[125]		
	BclI	SSRIs		[202]		
Signal transduction pathways and growth factors						
Main replicated genes						
BDNF	rs6265 (196G/A)	SSRIs	[328-331]	[220, 332]	[220]	
		Other/Mixed	[218, 223, 333, 334]	[222, 229, 335]		
	rs90887	Other/Mixed	[221]			
	rs61888800	Other/Mixed	[222]			
	rs7124442	Other/Mixed	[222, 223]			
	rs11030104	Other/Mixed	[218, 222]			
GNB3	rs5443 (C825T)	SSRIs	[227]	[49, 231]		[231, 313]
		Other/Mixed	[27, 226, 228-230, 336]	[232]	[336]	

Preliminary findings						
CREB1	C deletion in intron 8	Other/Mixed		[229]		
	18 SNPs within the gene	Other/Mixed		[152]		
	rs2253206-rs7569963, rs7569963-rs4675690 and rs7569963	Other/Mixed	[234]			
NTRK2	NT_023935.17_16651920, rs1624327	SSRIs	[152]			
	NT_023935.17_16593339, NT_023935.17_16593340, rs2289658, rs2289657	Other/Mixed	[152]			
Enzymes						
Less replicated genes						
ACE	insertion (I)/deletion (D)	Other/Mixed	[337-340]	[341]		
GSK3B	rs334558 (-50 T/C)	SSRIs	[342]			
		Lithium Aug.	[343]			
Preliminary findings						
PDE1A	rs1549870	SSRIs		[344]		
		Other/Mixed	[345]			
PDE11A	rs1880916	SSRIs	[346]	[344]		
		Other/Mixed	[345]			
Glutamatergic system						
Preliminary findings						
GRIK4	rs1954787	SSRIs	[238]			
		Other/Mixed	[239]	[123, 240]		
GRIK2	rs9404130, rs2518302 and rs513216	SSRIs			[124]	
GRIA1	rs1994862 rs10515697 and rs1864205	SSRIs			[124]	
GRIA3	rs2285127 rs2269551 and rs550640	SSRIs			[124]	
GRIN3A	rs1323427, rs1323423 and rs2050641	SSRIs			[124]	
GRM3	rs6465084	SSRIs		[241]		
GRM2	rs3821829, rs12487957 and rs4687771	SSRIs		[241]		

Pharmacokinetic genes*						
Main replicated genes						
MDR1	rs2032582 (G2677T/A)	SSRIs	[250, 251]	[254-256]		[256]
		Other/Mixed		[257]		[257]
	rs1045642 (C3435T)	SSRIs	[250]	[254-256]		[256]
		Other/Mixed		[259]	[258]	[259]
	11 SNPs	Other/Mixed	[253]			
	rs2032583 and rs2235040	SSRIs	[252]			
	rs2214103 and rs3842	Other/Mixed	[152]			
Other genes						
Preliminary findings						
CLOCK	rs1801260 (3111 T/C)	SSRIs	[347]	[323]		
	rs3736544 and rs3749474	SSRIs	[348]			
IL-1β	rs16944 (C-511T)	SSRIs	[349, 350]			
		Other/Mixed	[351]			
DTNBP1	rs760761	SSRIs	[352, 353]			
		Other/Mixed		[354]		
TREK1	rs2841616, rs2841608, rs12136349, rs10494996, rs7549184 and rs10779646	SSRIs	[355]			
	rs6686529	SSRIs	[356]			
OPRM1	rs540825	SSRIs	[357]			
		Other/Mixed		[240]		

Table 1: Pharmacogenetic findings in relation to antidepressant response and side effects (treatment emergent suicidal ideation was not included). Results of GWAS (paragraph 2.8) were not reported here for lack of comparability with results of candidate gene studies.

Main replicated genes: almost six positive findings

Less replicated genes: almost three positive findings

Preliminary findings: less than three positive findings

augm. = augmentation

* Results pertaining to CYP450 genes are not reported here, for a review see [263].

since, the most part of AD drugs were engineered upon this observation, like the selective serotonin re-uptake inhibitors (SSRIs), which represent the most used AD class nowadays.

2.1.1. Serotonin transporter (SLC6A4)

Taking into account the previously reported issues, it is understandable the reason why the serotonin transporter gene (SLC6A4) is a priori excellent candidate. Its product (SERT) regulates brain serotonin neurotransmission by transporting the neurotransmitter serotonin from synaptic cleft to pre-synaptic neurons. The interest toward it arose also from its involvement in depression pathophysiology: SERT KO mice showed a behavioral phenotype that is reminding of some symptoms of depressive episodes, such as inhibited exploratory locomotion, increased anxiety, together with a reduction in aggressive behavior and home cage activity [15, 16]. The most studied polymorphism within the SLC6A4 gene is without doubt the 5-HTTLPR, a 44bp insertion/deletion involving two units in a sequence of sixteen repeated elements in the promoter. This polymorphism shows a functional effect: the long (l) 5-HTTLPR allele is associated with a twice basal SERT expression compared to the short (s) allele [17]. Despite evidence of a functional effect of this polymorphism *in vitro*, *in vivo* studies did not provide consistent findings. Indeed, more than one recent positron emission tomography (PET) study reported that the expression of the serotonin transporter was not regulated by 5-HTTLPR l/s and rs25531 variants [18, 19]. These inconsistent findings may result from small participant numbers, the use of sub-optimal radiotracer for measuring the SERT activity, the effect of other polymorphisms influencing the expression of the gene (*e.g.,* rs16965628 [20]). Moreover, 5-HTTLPR and rs25531 could impact on aspects of brain function only in specific areas and/or as a result of particular internal or external stimuli or pathological conditions. About that, one the most confirmed finding is a greater amygdala activation in response to negative emotional stimuli in s carriers, which was demonstrated by functional magnetic resonance imaging (fMRI) [18]. Moving from molecular findings to pharmacogenetics, several studies reported an association between this polymorphism and AD response. Particularly, the most part of them found that the l allele is a predictor of higher AD efficacy in Caucasian populations [21-35] although negative findings have been reported as well [36-43]. On the other side, in Asians results were more contradictory. Indeed, several studies associated the s allele or the s/s genotype to better antidepressant response [44-48], while other found opposite [49-52] or negative results [53, 54]. It is important to underline that the ethnic origin of the sample is of particular relevance in pharmacogenetic studies, since polymorphisms can show very different frequencies in relation to the ethnic group. This is just the case of 5-HTTLPR: the l/l genotype is present in 29-43% of Caucasians, but in 1-13% of East Asians [55]. In order to better understand the 5-HTTLPR effect on AD efficacy and try to dissect the role of ethnicity, also meta-analyses have been performed, unfortunately without reaching any conclusive result. Indeed, a first meta-analysis reported an association between the l/l genotype and l allele and both remission and response rates [56], without evidence of rough differences between Caucasian and Asian samples. On the other hand, a more recent meta-analysis failed to replicate this result [57], but Caucasian and Asian samples were not analyzed also separately, possibly explaining the different findings. Moreover, the latter meta-analysis included also the results of the Sequenced Treatment Alternatives to Relieve Depression (STAR*D) study, the largest antidepressant trial performing a GWAS so far. The STAR*D study included a multiethnic sample, and no evidence of association between 5-HTTLPR and antidepressant response was found in the whole sample [37]. In spite of the great impact of STAR*D results within the scientific community, the pharmacogenetic study did not show so a careful design. Indeed, blood sample for DNA analysis (available for 1953 subjects from the whole 4041 sample) was not collected prior to the initiation of drug therapy. This may introduce a selection bias, since most patients with drug-related adverse events or poor response are at risk of dropping out of treatment early on and they would not be included in the pharmacogenetic analysis. Besides ethnicity and deficit in study design, other stratification factors have been suggested, for example a possible interaction between 5-HTTLPR and environmental factors as stressful life events [34, 58, 59](although this topic is still controversial [60]), or the mechanism of AD action [28]. Moreover, other genetic variants within SLC6A4 gene or other related genes may interact with 5-HTTLPR, modulating its effects on AD efficacy. For example, rs25531, located just upstream of the 5-HTTLPR, was found to impact the AD response [33, 61-63], maybe affecting the expression of the gene [64]. Nevertheless, the role of rs25531 in relation to AD response [38, 41, 42] and its functional effects are still unclear [65]. Finally, another complication arises from the observation that 5-HTTLPR may influence not only AD response but also antidepressant induced side effects: the s/s genotype seems to be a predictor of higher side effect risk [28, 37, 43, 66-69], possibly reducing the compliance in this group. Anyway, some opposite [70, 71] or negative [72-74] findings exist and results may depend on the mechanism of AD action [28].

Another polymorphism influencing SERT expression, is a 17bp VNTR (Variable Number of Tandem Repeats) polymorphism within intron 2 (STin2). Some evidences suggested this polymorphism as a risk factor for depressive disorder [75-77] and suicide behavior [78, 79], maybe with a synergistic effect with 5-HTTLPR [80]. Furthermore, several studies showed an effect of STin2 on AD response [31, 33, 40, 44, 46, 51, 81], even without univocal results [32, 39, 82]. Also STin2 has been associated with the risk of side effects during AD treatment (SSRIs, SNRIs, TCAs, mirtazapine, IMAO) [68], although other Authors failed to replicated this result during SSRI [69] and milnacipram [83] treatment.

2.1.2. Tryptophan hydroxylase

Tryptophan hydroxylase (TPH) is a key enzyme for the synthesis of serotonin, since it catalyzes the limiting step of the process. There are two distinct TPH genes that encode two different homologous enzymes: TPH1 and TPH2. TPH1 is mostly expressed in peripheral tissues like the skin, the gut and the pineal gland but it is also expressed in the CNS. TPH2 is exclusively expressed in neuronal cells and it is the predominant isoform in the CNS. For these reasons TPH genes have been considered among the of the most promising genes concerning the genetic modulation of AD response.

Several studies reported an association between TPH1 polymorphisms and SSRI response [84-86]. Unfortunately following studies found controversial results [30, 49, 81, 87-92]. Nevertheless, recent studies reported consistently results about rs1800532 (or A218C), which is the most investigated SNP of TPH1 and might modulate AD effects, concerning both clinical response [93] and side effect profile [72]. These recent data suggest that the role of TPH1 polymorphisms is not yet deeply understood and needs further investigation. In particular, it could be interesting the investigation of possible interactions among TPH1 polymorphisms and other polymorphisms within correlated genes (like 5-HT_{2A}, GNB3 and COMT) [72, 94].

Also TPH2 polymorphisms have been associated with AD response: rs1843809, rs1386494 and rs1487276 [81], rs10897346 and rs1487278 [95], rs2171363 [96]. Although these results need to be replicated, overall these data suggest a role for TPH2 gene in AD pharmacogenetics as well.

2.1.3. Serotonin (5-hydroxytryptamine)-1A (5-HT1A) receptor

Serotonin-1A receptor is a G protein-coupled receptor located both pre- and post-synaptically and widely distributed in regions that receive serotonergic input from the raphe nuclei: the frontal cortex, septum, amygdala, hippocampus and hypothalamus [97]. It also modulates the serotonergic activity of these areas by reducing the firing rate of raphe nuclei neurons, the amount of serotonin released per action potential, and the synthesis of the neurotransmitter. The 5-HT_{1A} receptor is coded by the 5-hydroxytryptamine receptor 1A gene (HTR1A). An involvement of this gene in AD response was suggested because several ADs desensitize raphe 5-HT_{1A} autoreceptors, leading to an enhancement of the serotonergic neurotransmission that could be responsible, at least partially, of the AD effect. Moreover, it has been reported that the block of the 5-HT_{1A} autoreceptors may accelerate AD action [98].

In pharmacogenetics, the most investigated HTR1A variants are C(-1019)G (rs6295) and Gly272Asp (rs1800042). Among these, the most promising one concerning AD response is rs6295, which is located in the promoter region of the gene and seems to influence the expression of the receptor [99, 100]. Particularly, the G allele was associated with higher risk of depression, suicidal behavior and AD resistance [49, 99, 101-107]. Nonetheless, conflicting results were reported as well [81, 108]. Interestingly, some Authors found an association between rs6295 and AD response only in particular subgroups of patients, like females [102] and patients with melancholic depression [109], suggesting the importance to take into consideration demographic and clinical modulators in pharmacogenetic studies. The same SNP, together with rs1800042, was studied also in relation to paroxetine discontinuation syndrome, a common side effect after paroxetine sudden suspension, but they did not show any predictive value [74]. On the other hand, as well as rs6295, also rs1800042 seems to be a promising SNP as predictor of AD response [110], although following studies did not confirm the result [102, 111]. For other two SNPs (rs10042486 and rs1364043), preliminary data suggest a possible role [103].

Thus, taking into account the scarcity and inconsistency of available data, further studies are needed in order to clarify the role of the gene, by the investigation also of other variants within it [112]. Also studies investigating HTR1A variants in relation to AD side effects are particularly required.

2.1.4. Serotonin (5-hydroxytryptamine)-2A (5-HT2A) receptor

Serotonin-2A receptor is a G protein-coupled receptor coded by the HTR2A gene. It is expressed widely throughout the CNS, near most of the serotoninergic terminal rich areas, including neocortex (mainly prefrontal, parietal, and somatosensory cortex) and the olfactory tubercle. An increasing body of evidence suggest that 5-HTR2A levels and activity are altered in psychiatric disorders like major depression [113-116]. The most investigated polymorphisms within HTR2A are: A-1438G (rs6311), C102T (rs6313) and His452Tyr (rs6314). rs6313 was associated with AD response [117], but mainly to the risk of side-effects (Table **1**), as well as rs6311 [50, 118], a SNP in high linkage disequilibrium with the previous one. Unfortunately, other studies failed to replicate these positive findings [49, 53, 81, 92, 119-121]. Nonetheless, a relevant role for this gene in AD pharmacogenetics has suggested by several positive findings concerning other variants within it [40, 81, 119, 122-128]. Overall data suggested a role for the HTR2A gene in AD response, although a wider knowledge of this gene is needed in order to better disentangle this issue [129].

2.1.5. Serotonin (5-hydroxytryptamine)-3A/3B (5-HT3A/3B) receptors

Serotonin-3 receptors are expressed throughout the central and peripheral nervous systems and mediates a variety of physiological functions; it is the only ion channel subtype in the serotonin family. Five different subunits (A–E) of the 5-HT_3 receptor have been identified. In the AD pharmacogenetics field, these genes have been investigated mainly concerning the side effect profile rather than the treatment response. In particular, HTR3A rs1062613 (C178T) and two polymorphisms in HTR3B (-100 -102 AAG delection variant and rs1176744) have been associated with vomiting and nausea due to paroxetine treatment [50, 130, 131]. On the other side, studies on gastrointestinal side effects during SSRIs treatment alone showed no association with HTR3B rs1176744 [121, 130] and HTR3A rs1062613 (C195T) [131]. Furthermore, no association was detected between HTR3A (rs1062613) and HTR3B (rs35312182 and rs1176744) polymorphisms and paroxetine discontinuation syndrome [74].

2.1.6. Serotonin (5-hydroxytryptamine)-6 (5-HT6) receptor

The 5-HT_6 receptor is a G protein-coupled receptor which is expressed almost exclusively in the brain. Genetic variants within this gene likely have an effect on brain and several studies investigated the possible association between HTR6 variants and brain-related features, like behavior traits, finding positive results [132, 133]. Furthermore, it seems to be involved in AD mechanisms of action [134, 135]. Consistently, the C267T variant (rs1805054) seems to modulate the AD response [136, 137]. Anyway, also negative findings were reported in literature [40, 92, 138] and further investigation is required.

2.2. NORADRENERGIC SYSTEM

Noradrenergic system has been deeply investigated in the field of AD pharmacogenetics in the light of the monoaminergic theory of depression and because it is one of the main target of tricyclic AD. Among the key genes within this system, the most investigated are catechol-O-methyltransferase (COMT), monoamine oxidase A (MAO-A) (both clearly involved also in other systems, such as the dopaminergic one) and norepinephrine transporter (SLC6A2) genes, which code for the main enzymes responsible for the amine metabolism.

2.2.1. Catechol-O-methyltransferase (COMT)

Within the COMT gene, the most investigated SNP was without doubt the functional rs4680 (Val158Met), firstly described by Weinshilboum and colleagues [139]. It has been hypothesized that rs4680 may affect SSRI response through the modulation of the dopamine bioavailability in the pre-frontal cortex [140]. Indeed, the clinical effect of serotonergic antidepressants might be related to an optimization of the dopaminergic activity [141]. Consistently, several studies reported an association between rs4680 and AD response [140, 142-146], although it is still unclear which the favourable genotype is. Nonetheless, the fact that only one study did not find any association between this SNP and AD response [147] suggests it likely plays a role in AD response. On the other side, there are also some preliminary findings about a possible effect of rs4680 on the risk to gain weight during treatment with various antidepressants [72]. Consistently, the same genotype was found to be a predictor of weight gain during buproprion treatment for smoking cessation, although only in association with the dopamine receptor type 2 Taq1 locus polymorphism [148].

Recently, two studies investigated other SNPs within the COMT gene, finding associations with response to various AD [149, 150]. Although these results clearly needed further validation, they further support the role of COMT gene variants in AD response.

2.2.2. Norepinephrine transporter (SLC6A2)

The norepinephrine transporter or NET is encoded by the SLC6A2 gene. It is a monoamine transporter that reuptakes the neurotransmitters norepinephrine (NE) from the synapse back to cytosol, hence other transporters VMAT (vesicular monoamine transporter) sequester NE into vesicles for later storage and release.

Several functional polymorphisms within the SLC6A2 gene have been associated with AD response [46, 53, 151]. Particularly, rs5569 (G1287A) was associated to nortryptiline response [46] and to the onset of milnacipran response [53]. On the other hand, no effect of this SNP on SSRIs and venlafaxine response was detected [46, 51] and it seems not to modulate the final milnacipran response [53]. The rs2242446 (T182C) was associated to milnacipran response instead [53], although this result was not replicated by a further study with SSRIs and venlafaxine [51].

Recently, some studies investigated other genetic variants within the SLC6A2 gene finding interesting results. Particularly, Uher *et al.* showed an association among two SNPs (rs60329 and rs1532701) and nortritpyline response [125], and Dong *et al.* found that rs5564 and rs1362621 were associated with remission with desipramine and fluoxetine treatment [152]. Nevertheless, a more recent study failed to find any association among seven polymorphisms (rs35915, rs28386840, rs168924, rs2242446, rs36017, rs47958, rs171798) within the SLC6A2 gene and AD response [42].

These data taken together suggest the need of further studies in order to better elucidate the role of this gene in the field of AD pharmacogenetics.

2.2.3. Monoamine Oxidase A (MAO-A)

Monoamine oxidases (MAO) are a family of enzymes that catalyze the oxidation of monoamines. There are two types of MAO in humans: MAO-A and MAO-B, both expressed in the CNS, particularly in neurons and astroglia. The MAO-A isoform, coded by the homonym gene, metabolizes several important amines and catecholamines including dopamine, serotonin, and norepinephrine (NE). The most investigated polymorphism within this gene is a VNTR located in the promoter region (1.2 Kb upstream of the MAO-A gene), which regulates the transcriptional level of the gene and has been linked to variations in the enzyme activity [153]. Taking into account that this variant might influence the neurotransmitter concentrations, it was considered a good candidate for AD pharmacogenetic analyses. Despite the good assumptions, several studies did not find any association between this polymorphism and AD response [81, 89, 119, 154]. Nonetheless these discouraging initial results, two more recent studies reported an association between this variant and mirtazapine response [155, 156], supporting the need of further investigation on this issue.

Some other polymorphisms within this gene were investigated concerning AD response, although with less replicated results. Particularly, positive associations were reported between rs1465108, rs6323 and fluoxetine response [81], rs1799835 and mirtazapine response (only in females) [155] and rs6323 and placebo response [157].

2.2.4. Adrenoreceptor beta-1 (ADRB1) and Adrenoreceptor alpha2 (ADRA2A)

The ADRB1 and ADRA2A are G-protein associated receptors: ADRB1 stimulates adenylate cyclase while ADRA2A inactivates adenylate cyclase and seems to be related to pretreatment HPA axis hyperactivity and increased adrenocorticotropin levels in male depressed patients [158].

Recently, an interesting functional polymorphism within the ADRB1 gene (rs180253 or G1165C) was described. It was associated with an enhanced coupling to the stimulatory Gs protein and increased adenylyl cyclase activation, resulting in a better and faster response to AD treatment [159]. Unfortunately, a further study failed to replicate this result in a sample of depressed patients treated with citalopram [160].

Concerning the ADRA2A gene, preliminary evidence of an effect on response to SNRI but not to SSRI response was provided [161]. Following studies did not confirm a role in antidepressant response but they found that ADRA2A may predict the risk of body weight gain during treatment with mirtazapine [162] and suicidal ideation among nortriptyline treated patients [163].

2.3. DOPAMINERGIC SYSTEM

Despite both pre-clinical [164] and clinical data [165] showed an involvement of the dopaminergic system in the pathogenesis of major depression, this system was less investigated in the field of AD pharmacogenetics compared to the previous ones. Indeed, a specific role for dopaminergic impairment was proposed in melancholic depression [166], although an excessive dopaminergic stimulation might be even detrimental for depressed patients [167]. Finally, several studies support dopamine receptor 2 (DRD2) involvement in AD pharmacodynamics, leading to the hypothesis that dopaminergic-mesolimbic pathway may represent a final common pathway in AD action [168, 169].

2.3.1. Dopamine transporter (SLC6A3)

The dopamine transporter (or DAT) is responsible for the dopamine reuptake from the synaptic cleft into presynaptic neurons, causing the end of the dopaminergic signal. Thus, it might modulate also AD clinical effects, as exposed above. Interestingly, it has been reported that AD drugs, particularly SSRIs, modulate the availability of DAT, supporting the relevant role of the dopaminergic system in AD mechanisms of action [169, 170].

The relatively most investigated polymorphism within the SLC6A3 gene is a VNTR located at the 3' end. Particularly, one study reported an association among the 9/10 and 9/9 genotypes and a higher risk of poorer and slower response to various AD drugs [36], while the 10/10 genotype was associated with an endophenotype of late-life depression that responds preferentially to methylphenidate added to a SSRI [171].

2.3.2. Dopamine receptors

Dopamine receptors are divided into the D_1-like family (D_1 and D_5, which are coupled to a Gs protein and activate adenylate cyclase), and D_2-like family (D_2, D_3 and D_4, which are coupled to a G_I protein and inhibit adenylate cyclase). Only the D_2-like family was associated to depressive disorders.

Concerning the AD pharmacogenetics, some data suggested a role of the D_2 receptor gene (DRD2) [169, 172, 173]. On the other side, several studies failed to find any association between this gene and AD response. Particularly, a functional polymorphism (rs1801028) has been repeatedly investigated with negative findings [174-176]. On the other hand, a recent study showed an association between the DRD2 rs4245147 and lamotrigine response in a sample of bipolar depressed patients [177], suggesting a possible role of this gene in the AD response of this group of patients. In the same study also an association among three DRD3 SNPs (rs167770, rs6280 and rs2134655) and olanzapine/fluoxetine combination response was shown.

Finally, several studies investigated the VNTR polymorphism in the third exon of the DRD4 gene in relation to AD response, unfortunately with negative results [174], except for Garriock *et al.* who found a significant modulating effect on various AD medications [178].

2.4. HYPOTHALAMIC-PITUITARY-ADRENAL (HPA) AXIS

A growing body of evidence suggested an involvement of the hypothalamic-pituitary-adrenal (HPA) axis in the pathogenesis of mood disorders, particularly major depression, since HPA axis dysfunctions were detected up to 70% of depressed patients [179]. HPA axis hyperactivity was hypothesized to be linked to the pathogenesis, treatment and course of depression [180]. Consistently, the most part of AD treatments seem to attenuate or normalize HPA axis activity [181-184]. The main neuroendocrine regulator of the HPA axis is the corticotrophin releasing hormone (CRH), and in the CNS corticotrophin releasing hormone receptors 1 and 2 (CRHR1 and CRHR2) are the two fundamental sub-types of CRH receptors. Several studies suggested a key role for CHR in depression [185-191], as well as for the CRHR1 gene, which seems to mediate the CRH elicited effects in depression and anxiety [192].

2.4.1. CRH receptors (CRHR1 and CRHR2)

Some polymorphisms within the CRHR1 gene (rs242941 and one haplotype including two other SNPs, *i.e.,* rs1876828 and rs242939) were found related to fluoxetine response [193, 194]. Interestingly, the association was more robust for a cluster of patients with anxious depression, although a further study failed to replicate this result [195].

Concerning the CRHR2 gene, Papiol *et al.* found an association between rs2270007 and citalopram response [195].

Recently, confirmations for both these genes were provided, with also positive findings for the CRH-binding protein (CRHBP) gene [196].

2.4.2. Glucocorticoid receptor (GR)

Hyperactivity of HPA axis might be caused also by impaired glucocorticoid signaling. Glucocorticoids act through the glucocorticoid receptor (GR, coded by the NR3C1 gene), a ligand-activated transcription factor. Thus, genetic variants occurring within the NR3C1 gene may affect significantly the sensitivity to glucocorticoids. Consistently, several NR3C1 polymorphisms were associated to depression as well as to AD response. Particularly, the ER22/23EK polymorphism, which consists of two linked point mutations in codons 22 and 23 [197], was associated with a faster clinical response [198]. Also the BclI polymorphism, that identified two alleles with fragment lengths of 4.5 and 2.3 kb, gained attention, since several clinical investigations suggested it is linked to altered GR function [199-201]. It was associated with baseline ACTH values in depressed patients as well as to AD response (even if only a trend) [202]. Finally, a recent GWAS gave rise to the hypothesis of a role of some SNPs (rs852977, rs10482633, rs10052957) within this gene in AD response, although none of them survived after correction for hypothesis-wide effective number of comparisons [125].

Another possible level of modulation in the glucocorticoid signalling pathway is FKBP5, a protein that interacts functionally with mature corticoid receptor hetero-complexes. Thus, several polymorphisms within the FKBP5 gene have been investigated in the AD pharmacogenetic field, with promising results. Particularly, rs1360780, rs3800373 and rs4713916 were associated to AD response [195, 203-205]. Furthermore, Horstmann *et al.* reported an interaction between rs1360780 (FKBP5) and rs12800734 (GRIK4) on remission prediction [123]. Nevertheless, in literature negative findings exist as well (Table **1**).

2.5. SIGNAL TRANSDUCTION PATHWAYS AND GROWTH FACTORS

In depressed subjects hippocampal and prefrontal atrophy, together with the hypertrophy of other regions like amygdale [206], suggest an imbalance in neurogenesis and neuroplasticity processes. Indeed, in adults neurogenesis persists at a given level and the growth factors expressed during brain development control neuroplasticity [207, 208]. Consistently, the acute synaptic increase in monoamine levels brought about by antidepressants probably acts through changes of brain plasticity in the long term. This is thought to happen thanks to molecular changes in transcription and translation processes [209, 210].

2.5.1. Brain derived neurotrophic factor (BDNF)

The researchers' attention has been especially turned to BDNF, member of the nerve growth factor (NGF)-superfamily. The reasons are the key role played by neurotrophins in neuronal growth and plasticity, other than the under-expression of the BDNF gene during depressive states [211]. Consistently, it has been hypothesized that antidepressant treatments may work through the re-establishing of BDNF balance, modifying its expression in different brain areas [212-216]. Particularly, chronic SSRIs or electroconvulsive seizure (ECT) administration was associated to increased BDNF expression in the hippocampus of adult rats [217].

Given it is an excellent candidate gene, BDNF polymorphisms were extensively studied, especially a valine to methionine (V66M) substitution in position 196 (rs6265). Its role in AD response is supported by an increasing body of evidence (Table **1**), although it is still controversial whether allele or genotype has to be considered the risk factor [2].

As stated above for 5-HTTLPR, this mismatch may be partially linked to ethnic stratification of the examined samples [218], since considerable BDNF allele and haplotype diversity among global populations were reported [219]. Some evidence about the involvement of this SNP also in the risk of side effects was found [220], but confirmations are needed.

Some other polymorphisms within the gene were associated to AD response. Among them, rs90887 [221], rs61888800 [222], rs7124442 [222, 223] and rs11030104 [218, 222]. The last one was found to interact with temperamental trait harm avoidance in predicting AD response [218], remembering us the complex network of interactions which leads to a certain response to AD treatments (Figure **1**). Not only gene x environment interactions are nowadays more often recognized, but also gene x gene interactions. Indeed, recently the NTRK2 gene (that codes for the BDNF receptor) received attention since its possible interaction with the BDNF gene [163].

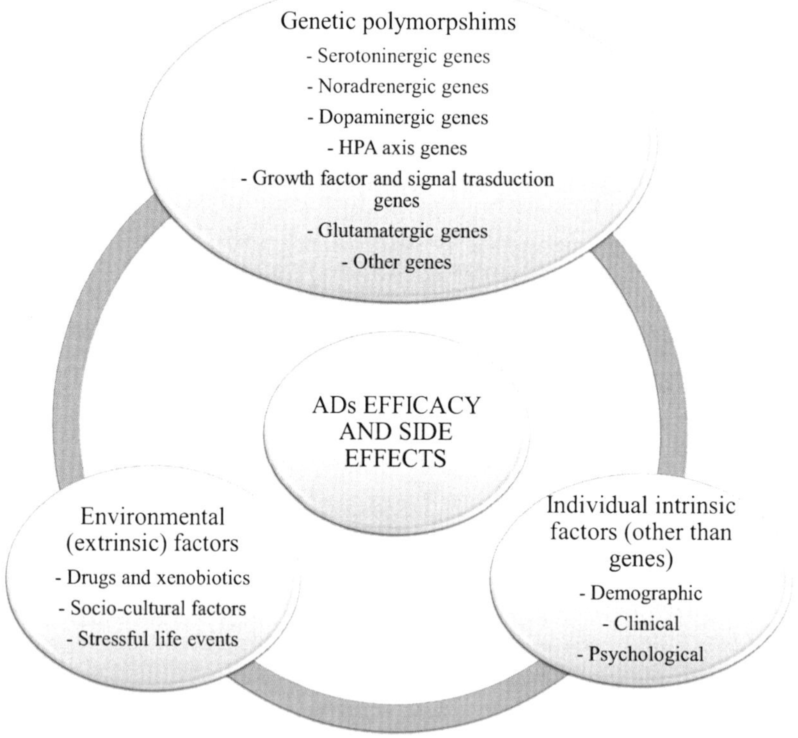

Figure 1: The determinants of antidepressant (ADs) response. The three groups of determinants are not independent, but interactions act both within and among them.

2.5.2. Beta polypeptide of guanine nucleotide binding protein (GNB3)

Among signal transduction proteins, previous studies mainly focused on the GNB3 gene, which codes for the beta3 subunit of the G protein complex. Given the high complexity of G protein signal transduction cascades and their high diffusion, they are thought to be involved in the neuronal plasticity [224] as well as to play a role in AD response. Indeed, they have a key role in the downstream signalling cascade following monoamine receptors activation.

Within the GNB3 gene, the most promising variant is rs5443 (C825T), because it was associated to the occurrence of a splice variant which showed an altered activity. Indeed, the splice variant, called Gbeta3s, seems to be less active than the wild form in terms of modulation of ion channels and formation of heterodymers with other proteins [225]. The larger part of studies published until now found that the T variant predict better AD response [27, 226-229], while only one opposite result exists [230]. Nevertheless, some other Authors did not find any association [49, 231, 232].

2.5.3. c-AMP response-element binding (CREB)

CREB encodes a transcription factor which binds to the cAMP-responsive element and induces transcription of genes in response to stimulation of the cAMP pathway. Alternate splicing of this gene results in two transcript variants encoding different isoforms, of which only CREB1 has been studied in relation to AD pharmacogenetics. CREB is a good candidate, since it seems to play a role both in the aetiology and pharmacotherapy of major depression [233], but its polymorphisms are still poorly investigated in the field and as far as now, with negative findings [152, 229]. Recently, it was proposed that some alleles or haplotypes within CREB1 could be related to treatment resistance rather than to response [234]. Finally, the gene may have a role in suicidal behaviours in patients with major depression and in treatment-emergent suicidal ideation [235].

2.6. GLUTAMATERGIC SYSTEM

Glutamate is the principal excitatory neurotransmitter in the CNS and acts both on metabotropic and ionotropic receptors. By the last ones, it plays a key role in the plasticity of synapses and is involved in long-term potentiation, an activity-dependent increase in the efficiency of synaptic transmission which is thought to underlie certain kinds of memory and learning. The glutamatergic system seems to have a relevant role in the pathogenesis of depression, since glutamate levels are increased in patients with major depressive disorder [236], suggesting enhanced glutamatergic transmission. On the other side, chronic SSRI treatment has been reported to attenuate glutamatergic transmission in the rat cerebral cortex [237]. To test the role of glutamatergic genetic variants in depressed patients during citalopram treatment, Paddock *et al.* studied the GRIK4 (glutamate receptor, ionotropic, kainate 4) gene, finding that the rs1954787 polymorphism was a predictor of response [238]. This preliminary finding was confirmed by a following report [239] although more recent studies did not replicate the result [123, 240]. In regard to genes coding for metabotropic receptors, preliminary negative results have been reported both for GRM2 (glutamate receptor, metabotropic 2) and GRM3 (glutamate receptor, metabotropic 3) [241]. Other genes (GRIK2 and GRIA3 (glutamate receptor, ionotrophic, AMPA 3)) were associated to treatment-emergent suicidal ideation [242, 243] and antidepressant induced sexual dysfunction (GRIK2, GRIA1, GRIA3 and GRIN3A (glutamate receptor, ionotropic, N-methyl-D-aspartate 3A)) [124]. Nevertheless, these positive findings need confirmations, which were not found in the case of treatment-emergent suicidal ideation [244].

2.7. PHARMACOKINETIC FINDINGS

Differences in AD metabolism may affect AD plasma concentration and consequently treatment efficacy and safety. AD pharmacokinetics may be modified by enzyme inhibitors/enhancers [245], aging [246], pregnancy [247], but also genetic polymorphisms within P glycoprotein and 450 isoenzymes genes.

2.7.1. P glycoprotein

P-glycoprotein, a member of the superfamily of ATP-binding cassette (ABC) and MDR/TAP subfamily transporter proteins, is a coded by the ABCB1 gene. It is an ATP-dependent drug efflux pump for xenobiotic compounds which is expressed widely in the body, mainly in organs involved in the catabolism and the elimination of drugs. Its localization in the endothelial cells of the blood–brain barrier [248] regulates xenobiotics intake in the brain and may play a role in psychotropic drugs efficacy and side effects. So far, several SNPs within the ABCB1 gene have been studied for their possible effect on AD treatment outcome. The most studied ones are at positions 2677 (rs2032582) and 3435 (rs1045642), because they have been associated with alteration of P glycoprotein expression and/or function [249]. Positive associations were found between rs2032582 [250, 251] and rs1045642 (as well as the haplotype rs2032582/rs1128503) [250] and SSRI response. Two associations with rs2032583 and rs2235040 have been already replicated [252, 253], although not in patients treated with mirtazapine (which is though not to be a substrate of P glycoprotein) [252]. The potential role of other SNPs (rs17064, rs2214103, rs3842) was proposed [152]. Despite these encouraging results, other studies failed to find any effect of rs2032582 and rs1045642 [254-257], rs10280101, rs7787082, rs2032583 and rs2235040 [240]. Regarding side effect risk, evidence supporting the involvement of the ABCB1 gene is still poor [258], while several negative findings exist [256, 257, 259].

2.7.2. Cytochrome P450 (CYP450)

The cytochrome P450 superfamily is a class of proteins mainly expressed in the liver and represent the major enzymes responsible for the phase I oxidative reactions of both drugs and endogenous compounds. The genes coding for these enzymes are very polymorphic, particularly those involved in AD metabolism (mainly CYP2D6, CYP2C19, CYP2B6, CYP2C9 and CYP3A4). The known alleles show normal, reduced/absent or increased activity (http://www.cypalleles.ki.se/), allowing to distinguish some metabolizing groups. Anyway, this classification does not exactly reflect the metabolic status, because it does not take into account that some alleles are only partially active and some alleles show different activity depending on the drug metabolized [260]. According to this classification, the wild type genotype is defined as extensive metabolizer (EM), which is characterized by the presence of two active alleles, while intermediate metabolizer (IM) is characterized by the presence of one wild type allele plus a partially or totally defective allele and it is expected to be between the EMs and the poor metabolizers (PMs). PM shows a combination of two partially or totally defective alleles. Finally, the ultrarapid metabolizer (UM) category exists only for CYP2D6 and it is usually linked to multiple allele copies. In this paragraph only the CYP2D6 and CYP2C19 genes are discussed, since their polymorphisms were associated with the metabolism of a wide group of AD drugs [261, 262]. For a global review see [263].

The CYP2D6 gene received particular attention in the field. There is good evidence for a linear relationship between CYP2D6 gene copy number and metabolism of several ADs (*e.g.*, amitriptyline and nortriptyline [264, 265], imipramine [266], paroxetine [267-269] and venlafaxine [270, 271]), even if some negative results exist [254, 272-274]. These controversial results may be explained by the contribution of different CYP isoenzymes to the metabolism of a drug, a common event for ADs, and different allele distribution among populations [263]. Despite the good relation found between CYP2D6 genotype and AD plasma levels, the same cannot be reported for AD efficacy and safety. Indeed, some Authors reported positive association with therapeutic effects [275, 276] or side effects [121, 275, 277], but several others found lack of association [74, 256, 265, 278, 279]. Concerning this, a direct correlation between AD plasma concentrations and AD clinical outcomes was not found for most ADs, with the exception of tricyclic ADs [263].

After the CYP2D6 gene, the CYP2C19 one is the most studied in the field. The available studies are mainly focused on pharmacokinetic parameters, showing that the CYP2C19 genotype affects the metabolism and plasma levels of several ADs, particularly citalopram [280-282], escitalopram [246, 276, 283, 284] and amitriptyline [264, 274, 285].

The described picture brings out that there is not yet evidence to support the recommendation of CYP genotyping in the clinical practice, since the effect of CYP variants on clinical outcomes is still not totally clear also for the most studied isoenzymes. Besides the approval of the AmpliChipTM test, which allows to classify subjects on CYP2D6 and CYP2C19 phenotypes by DNA micro-array technology [286], guidelines has not yet recommended it for lacking of cost/benefit evidence [287]. Thus, even if genotyping technologies and dose adjustments based on pharmacokinetic findings [288] are already available, further investigation is expected to clarify the usefulness and applicability in the clinical practice. The current knowledge suggests that genotyping might be important when the parent drug or its metabolites are critical for drug safety and polymorphic drug metabolism might affect the risk for side effects. For example this might be the case for antidepressant drug therapy with tricyclic ADs (largely affected by the CYP2D6 polymorphisms).

2.8. FOCUS ON GENOME-WIDE ASSOCIATION STUDIES (GWAS)

In the last years the shift from the study of single genes to wide-genome studies has progressively become a need, since increasing evidence suggests that the candidate gene method was not enough powerful to investigate the genetic complexity of mood disorders and AD response.

As far as now, three large trials implemented the genome-wide approach to detect genetic variants associated to AD response: the Sequenced Treatment Alternatives to Relieve Depression study (STAR*D) (n=1953) [289], the Genome-based Therapeutic Drugs for Depression study (GENDEP) (n=706) [290] and the Munich Antidepressant Response Study (MARS) (n=339) [291]. In spite of the lack of results which reached the genome-wide significance threshold, these studies brought out top markers which should further investigated in order to clarify their role. The strongest findings include rs1126757 (IL11 gene) and rs2500535 (UST gene) [290], rs6966038 (UBE3C gene), rs6127921 (BMP7 gene) and rs809736 (RORA gene) [289], rs6989467 (CDH17 gene) and rs1502174 (EPHB1 gene) [291]. Also genetic predictors of treatment-emergent suicidal ideation were investigated on genome-wide data. Two studies on the GENDEP sample led to the replication of NTRK2 gene association to suicidal risk [163, 292]. On the other side, in the STAR*D different markers emerged (top markers in the PAPLN and IL28RA genes) [244].

Besides the low number of GWAS performed in the field until now and the poor replication of results, the technical improvement in genotyping platforms and computation procedures, other than the increasing knowledge of gene x gene and gene x environment interactions, are expected to fully realize the potentiality of GWAS in the field.

3. CONCLUSION

As we have traced in the previous paragraphs, a high number of pharmacokinetic and pharmacodynamic genes may contribute to the clinical outcomes of AD treatments, but results are poorly replicated and often contradictory. For this reason, the clinical impact of AD pharmacogenetics is still poor. Nonetheless, as it often happens for a novel field of research, a more or less long period of development is needed to obtain practical applications. The opportunities are bright, since clinical applications of pharmacogenetic research have already produced relevant effects in other fields of medicine, especially oncology [293, 294] and in psychiatry the number of replicated findings increases every day. In the psychiatric field, the available evidence suggest that several strong candidate genes are involved in AD response, but replication is thought to be a need, since the high risk of false positive findings [295]. A number of factors are probably responsible for poor replication of results. Among these, differences in inclusion criteria, medication, outcome and side effect measures, ethnicity and genetic coverage. The lack of standardized study design makes meta-analyses as well as comparisons across studies difficult. Another point is the difficulty to cover the complexity of AD response, which results from the interaction of different type of determinants (Figure **1**). Indeed, genetic factors are thought to explain about the 50% of the variance in AD response [141], while the other part results from extrinsic environmental and intrinsic non-genetic (clinical, demographic, psychological) modulators. Obviously, interactions among these determinants may occur both intra- and inter-them. *E.g.*, the so-called flip-flop phenomenon, *i.e.*, the interaction of multiple loci and environmental effects in determining susceptibility to complex diseases, may lead to ambiguous results. Flip-flop associations are seen particularly when the risk allele at the target locus is a relatively common allele. Additionally, for loci with a minor-allele frequency <5%, it may be more likely that flip-flop phenomena indicates spurious results than confirmatory ones confounded by the multilocus effect. Flip-flop associations can also be due to investigation of a non-causal variant in LD (linkage disequilibrium) with a genuine causal variant. Indeed notable difference in LD across populations were found (*e.g.*, for COMT gene) and, less obviously, sampling variation can lead to variation in observed LD patterns. For this reason, markers in weak LD with each other (*e.g.*, $r2<0.3$) may need to be considered carefully [296]. In order to overcome this phenomenon, the analysis of multiple variant interactions is needed. Actually, one of the most promising approach to achieve this objective is pathway analysis, *i.e.*, the analysis of several genetic variants within genes involved in the same biological pathway. So far, the usefulness of this approach in the AD pharmacogenomics has been shown [291, 297] as well as its potential for better understanding the AD mechanisms of action.

Concerning clinical-demographic determinants instead, ambiguous findings may result from studies including both bipolar and unipolar patients or patients with multiple and a single episode of major depression, who seem to have a lower genetic load [298], without correct analysis for these discrepancies. Indeed, there is increasing evidence that some genetic variants may affect AD response only in certain subgroups of patients, *e.g.*, the s allele of the 5-HTTLPR polymorphism was found to predict poor AD response only in a subgroup of patients with anxious depression [42]. Also psychological modulators may define subgroups of patients with more homogeneous genetic determinants, *e.g.*, harm avoidance (a personality dimension defined by the Temperament and Character Inventory or TCI [299]) was found to predict treatment response in interaction with rs11030104 (BDNF gene) [218]. For these reasons, growing importance is given to the identification of peculiar and homogeneous subgroup of patients, the so-called endophenotypes (*e.g.*, early onset, psychotic symptoms). Under this point of view, the use of the HAM-D as a whole to measure the outcome does not allow to value if a patient reach remission of some symptoms with persistence of others. Thus, in order to define endophenotypes and recognize stratification factors, the assessment of psycho-social characteristics and the use of HAM-D symptom clusters should become a standard in pharmacogenetic studies.

Regarding studies performed on pharmacokinetic genes, other specific limitations have to be considered. Firstly, a single drug is metabolized by specific enzymes, but the result of this reaction may be an active molecule that can be metabolized by different enzyme/s. Secondly, drug interactions may deeply impact the activity of the cytochromes in a way that may be dependent on the genetics, but to an extent that is still difficult to define. *E.g.,* the enzyme activity of a genetic PM cannot be affected by inducers or inhibitors. On the other hand, EMs or UMs can be converted to the PM phenotype by strong enzyme inhibitors. Finally, drugs can be metabolized by a set of cytocromes: they should all be investigated by a single test in order to infer sufficient predictive information about the drug blood levels. In order to overcome this problematic issue in the pharmacokinetic field, further studies considering these confounding factors are clearly required to provide definitive results. Future studies on this topic should also solve some methodological deficits of past studies [263].

The increasing knowledge of the limits which have affected AD pharmacogenetic studies until now, together with technological improvement, are gradually expected to allow their overcoming. Given this assumption, there is great hope that pharmacogenomics will offer personalized treatments based on genetic profiles of response/side effects, thus leading to a radical improvement of major depression prognosis, as well as for other common and disabling psychiatric diseases.

REFERENCES

[1] Warden D, Rush AJ, Trivedi MH, Fava M, Wisniewski SR. The STAR*D Project results: a comprehensive review of findings. Current psychiatry reports 2007, 9:449-59.

[2] Porcelli S, Drago A, Fabbri C, Gibiino S, Calati R, Serretti A. Pharmacogenetics of antidepressant response. J Psychiatry Neurosci 2011, 36:87-113.

[3] McCarroll SA. Extending genome-wide association studies to copy-number variation. Human molecular genetics 2008, 17(R2):R135-42.

[4] Roberts R, Wells GA, Stewart AF, Dandona S, Chen L. The genome-wide association study--a new era for common polygenic disorders. Journal of cardiovascular translational research 2010, 3:173-82.

[5] Alonso J, Angermeyer MC, Bernert S, Bruffaerts R, Brugha TS, Bryson H, *et al.* Disability and quality of life impact of mental disorders in Europe: results from the European Study of the Epidemiology of Mental Disorders (ESEMeD) project. Acta psychiatrica Scandinavica 2004(420):38-46.

[6] WHO. Ten statistical highlights in global public health. World Health statistics 2007 [cited 2011 6 March]; Available from: http://www.who.int/whosis/whostat2007_10highlights.pdf

[7] Serretti A, Franchini L, Gasperini M, Rampoldi R, Smeraldi E. Mode of inheritance in mood disorders families according to fluvoxamine response. Acta psychiatrica Scandinavica 1998, 98:443-50.

[8] Nutt DJ, Baldwin DS, Clayton AH, Elgie R, Lecrubier Y, Montejo AL, *et al.* Consensus statement and research needs: the role of dopamine and norepinephrine in depression and antidepressant treatment. The Journal of clinical psychiatry 2006, 67 Suppl 6:46-9.

[9] Psychiatric GWAS Consortium Steering Committee. A framework for interpreting genome-wide association studies of psychiatric disorders. Molecular psychiatry 2009, 14:10-7.

[10] Wellcome Trust Case Control Consortium. Genome-wide association study of 14,000 cases of seven common diseases and 3,000 shared controls. Nature 2007, 447:661-78.

[11] Laje G, McMahon FJ. Genome-wide association studies of antidepressant outcome: A brief review. Progress in neuro-psychopharmacology & biological psychiatry 2010, 27.

[12] Johnson RC, Nelson GW, Troyer JL, Lautenberger JA, Kessing BD, Winkler CA, *et al.* Accounting for multiple comparisons in a genome-wide association study (GWAS). BMC genomics 2010, 11:724.

[13] O'Donovan MC, Craddock NJ, Owen MJ. Genetics of psychosis; insights from views across the genome. Human genetics 2009, 126:3-12.

[14] Serretti A, Kato M, Kennedy JL. Pharmacogenetic studies in depression: a proposal for methodologic guidelines. The pharmacogenomics journal 2008, 8:90-100.

[15] Holmes A, Murphy DL, Crawley JN. Abnormal behavioral phenotypes of serotonin transporter knockout mice: parallels with human anxiety and depression. Biological psychiatry 2003, 54:953-9.

[16] Holmes A, Yang RJ, Lesch KP, Crawley JN, Murphy DL. Mice lacking the serotonin transporter exhibit 5-HT_{1A} receptor-mediated abnormalities in tests for anxiety-like behavior. Neuropsychopharmacology 2003, 28:2077-88.

[17] Heils A, Teufel A, Petri S, Stöber G, Riederer P, Bengel D, *et al.* Allelic variation of human serotonin trasporter gene expression. Journal of neurochemistry 1996, 66:2621-4.

[18] Murthy NV, Selvaraj S, Cowen PJ, Bhagwagar Z, Riedel WJ, Peers P, *et al.* Serotonin transporter polymorphisms (SLC6A4 insertion/deletion and rs25531) do not affect the availability of 5-HTT to [11C] DASB binding in the living human brain. NeuroImage 2010, 52:50-4.

[19] Shioe K, Ichimiya T, Suhara T, Takano A, Sudo Y, Yasuno F, *et al.* No association between genotype of the promoter region of serotonin transporter gene and serotonin transporter binding in human brain measured by PET. Synapse New York, NY. 2003, 48:184-8.

[20] Martin J, Cleak J, Willis-Owen SA, Flint J, Shifman S. Mapping regulatory variants for the serotonin transporter gene based on allelic expression imbalance. Molecular psychiatry 2007, 12:421-2.

[21] Smeraldi E, Zanardi R, Benedetti F, Dibella D, Perez J, Catalano M. Polymorphism Within the Promoter of the Serotonin Transporter Gene and Antidepressant Efficacy of Fluvoxamine. Molecular psychiatry 1998, 3:508-11.

[22] Zanardi R, Benedetti F, DiBella D, Catalano M, Smeraldi E. Efficacy of paroxetine in depression is influenced by a functional polymorphism within the promoter of serotonin transporter gene. Journal of clinical psychopharmacology 2000, 20:105-7.

[23] Zanardi R, Serretti A, Rossini D, Franchini L, Cusin C, Lattuada E, *et al.* Factors affecting fluvoxamine antidepressant activity: influence of pindolol and 5-HTTLPR in delusional and nondelusional depression. Biological psychiatry 2001, 50:323-30.

[24] Pollock BG, Ferrell RE, Mulsant BH, Mazumdar S, Miller M, Sweet RA, *et al.* Allelic Variation in the Serotonin Transporter Promoter Affects Onset of Paroxetine Treatment Response in Late-Life Depression. Neuropsychopharmacology 2000, 23:587-90.

[25] Rausch JL, Johnson ME, Fei Y-J, Li JQ, Shendarkar N, Mac Hobby H, *et al.* Initial conditions of serotonin transporter kinetics and genotype: influence on ssri treatment trial outcome. Biological psychiatry 2002 5/1, 51:723-32.

[26] Arias B, Catalan R, Gasto C, Gutierrez B, Fananas L. 5-HTTLPR polymorphism of the serotonin transporter gene predicts non-remission in major depression patients treated with citalopram in a 12-weeks follow up study. Journal of clinical psychopharmacology 2003, 23:563-7.

[27] Joyce PR, Mulder RT, Luty SE, McKenzie JM, Miller AL, Rogers GR, *et al.* Age-dependent antidepressant pharmacogenomics: polymorphisms of the serotonin transporter and G protein beta3 subunit as predictors of response to fluoxetine and nortriptyline. The international journal of neuropsychopharmacology / official scientific journal of the Collegium Internationale Neuropsychopharmacologicum (CINP) 2003, 6:339-46.

[28] Murphy GM, Jr., Hollander SB, Rodrigues HE, Kremer C, Schatzberg AF. Effects of the serotonin transporter gene promoter polymorphism on mirtazapine and paroxetine efficacy and adverse events in geriatric major depression. Archives of general psychiatry 2004, 61:1163-9.

[29] Durham LK, Webb SM, Milos PM, Clary CM, Seymour AB. The serotonin transporter polymorphism, 5HTTLPR, is associated with a faster response time to sertraline in an elderly population with major depressive disorder. Psychopharmacology 2004, 174:525-9.

[30] Serretti A, Cusin C, Rossini D, Artioli P, Dotoli D, Zanardi R. Further evidence of a combined effect of SERTPR and TPH on SSRIs response in mood disorders. Am J Med Genet B Neuropsychiatr Genet 2004, 129:36-40.

[31] Bozina N, Peles AM, Sagud M, Bilusic H, Jakovljevic M. Association study of paroxetine therapeutic response with SERT gene polymorphisms in patients with major depressive disorder. World J Biol Psychiatry 2008, 9:190-7.

[32] Huezo-Diaz P, Uher R, Smith R, Rietschel M, Henigsberg N, Marusic A, *et al.* Moderation of antidepressant response by the serotonin transporter gene. Br J Psychiatry 2009, 195:30-8.

[33] Mrazek DA, Rush AJ, Biernacka JM, O'Kane DJ, Cunningham JM, Wieben ED, *et al.* SLC6A4 variation and citalopram response. Am J Med Genet B Neuropsychiatr Genet 2009, 150B:341-51.

[34] Mandelli L, Marino E, Pirovano A, Calati R, Zanardi R, Colombo C, *et al.* Interaction between SERTPR and stressful life events on response to antidepressant treatment. Eur Neuropsychopharmacol 2009, 19:64-7.

[35] Illi A, Poutanen O, Setala-Soikkeli E, Kampman O, Viikki M, Huhtala H, *et al.* Is 5-HTTLPR linked to the response of selective serotonin reuptake inhibitors in MDD? European archives of psychiatry and clinical neuroscience 2010.

[36] Kirchheiner J, Nickchen K, Sasse J, Bauer M, Roots I, Brockmoller J. A 40-basepair VNTR polymorphism in the dopamine transporter (DAT1) gene and the rapid response to antidepressant treatment. The pharmacogenomics journal 2006.

[37] Hu XZ, Rush AJ, Charney D, Wilson AF, Sorant AJ, Papanicolaou GJ, *et al.* Association between a functional serotonin transporter promoter polymorphism and citalopram treatment in adult outpatients with major depression. Archives of general psychiatry 2007, 64:783-92.

[38] Kraft JB, Peters EJ, Slager SL, Jenkins GD, Reinalda MS, McGrath PJ, *et al.* Analysis of association between the serotonin transporter and antidepressant response in a large clinical sample. Biological psychiatry 2007, 61:734-42.

[39] Dogan O, Yuksel N, Ergun MA, Yilmaz A, Ilhan MN, Karslioglu HE, *et al.* Serotonin transporter gene polymorphisms and sertraline response in major depression patients. Genet Test 2008, 12:225-31.

[40] Wilkie MJ, Smith G, Day RK, Matthews K, Smith D, Blackwood D, *et al.* Polymorphisms in the SLC6A4 and HTR2A genes influence treatment outcome following antidepressant therapy. The pharmacogenomics journal 2009, 9:61-70.

[41] Maron E, Tammiste A, Kallassalu K, Eller T, Vasar V, Nutt DJ, *et al.* Serotonin transporter promoter region polymorphisms do not influence treatment response to escitalopram in patients with major depression. Eur Neuropsychopharmacol 2009, 19:451-6.

[42] Baffa A, Hohoff C, Baune BT, Muller-Tidow C, Tidow N, Freitag C, *et al.* Norepinephrine and serotonin transporter genes: impact on treatment response in depression. Neuropsychobiology 2010, 62:121-31.

[43] Reimherr F, Amsterdam J, Dunner D, Adler L, Zhang S, Williams D, *et al.* Genetic polymorphisms in the treatment of depression: speculations from an augmentation study using atomoxetine. Psychiatry research 2010, 175:67-73.

[44] Kim DK, Lim SW, Lee S, Sohn SE, Kim S, Hahn CG, *et al.* Serotonin transporter gene polymorphism and antidepressant response. Neuroreport 2000, 11:215-9.

[45] Yoshida K, Ito K, Sato K, Takahashi H, Kamata M, Higuchi H, *et al.* Influence of the serotonin transporter gene-linked polymorphic region on the antidepressant response to fluvoxamine in Japanese depressed patients. Progress in neuro-psychopharmacology & biological psychiatry. 2002, 26:383-6.

[46] Kim H, Lim SW, Kim S, Kim JW, Chang YH, Carroll BJ, *et al.* Monoamine transporter gene polymorphisms and antidepressant response in koreans with late-life depression. Jama 2006, 296:1609-18.

[47] Kang R-H, Wong M-L, Choi M-J, Paik J-W, Lee M-S. Association study of the serotonin transporter promoter polymorphism and mirtazapine antidepressant response in major depressive disorder. Progress in Neuro-Psychopharmacology and Biological Psychiatry. 2007 2007/8/15, 31:1317-21.

[48] Umene-Nakano W, Yoshimura R, Ueda N, Suzuki A, Ikenouchi-Sugita A, Hori H, *et al.* Predictive factors for responding to sertraline treatment: views from plasma catecholamine metabolites and serotonin transporter polymorphism. Journal of psychopharmacology (Oxford, England) 2009.

[49] Hong CJ, Chen TJ, Yu YW, Tsai SJ. Response to fluoxetine and serotonin 1A receptor (C-1019G) polymorphism in Taiwan Chinese major depressive disorder. The pharmacogenomics journal 2006, 6:27-33.

[50] Kato M, Fukuda T, Wakeno M, Fukuda K, Okugawa G, Ikenaga Y, *et al.* Effects of the serotonin type 2A, 3A and 3B receptor and the serotonin transporter genes on paroxetine and fluvoxamine efficacy and adverse drug reactions in depressed Japanese patients. Neuropsychobiology 2006, 53:186-95.

[51] Min W, Li T, Ma X, Li Z, Yu T, Gao D, *et al.* Monoamine transporter gene polymorphisms affect susceptibility to depression and predict antidepressant response. Psychopharmacology 2009, 205:409-17.

[52] Lee SH, Choi TK, Lee E, Seok JH, Lee SH, Lee HS, *et al.* Serotonin transporter gene polymorphism associated with short-term treatment response to venlafaxine. Neuropsychobiology 2010, 62:198-206.

[53] Yoshida K, Takahashi H, Higuchi H, Kamata M, Ito K, Sato K, *et al.* Prediction of antidepressant response to milnacipran by norepinephrine transporter gene polymorphisms. The American journal of psychiatry 2004, 161:1575-80.

[54] Yoshimura R, Umene-Nakano W, Suzuki A, Ueda N, Miyamoto K, Ikenouchi-Sugita A, *et al.* Rapid response to paroxetine is associated with plasma paroxetine levels at 4 but not 8 weeks of treatment, and is independent of serotonin transporter promoter polymorphism in Japanese depressed patients. Human psychopharmacology 2009, 24:489-94.

[55] Goldman N, Glei DA, Lin YH, Weinstein M. The serotonin transporter polymorphism (5-HTTLPR): allelic variation and links with depressive symptoms. Depression and anxiety 2010, 27:260-9.

[56] Serretti A, Kato M, De Ronchi D, Kinoshita T. Meta-analysis of serotonin transporter gene promoter polymorphism (5-HTTLPR) association with selective serotonin reuptake inhibitor efficacy in depressed patients. Molecular psychiatry 2007, 12:247-57.

[57] Taylor MJ, Sen S, Bhagwagar Z. Antidepressant Response and the Serotonin Transporter Gene-Linked Polymorphic Region. Biological psychiatry 2010.

[58] Keers R, Uher R, Huezo-Diaz P, Smith R, Jaffee S, Rietschel M, *et al.* Interaction between serotonin transporter gene variants and life events predicts response to antidepressants in the GENDEP project. The pharmacogenomics journal 2010.

[59] Bukh JD, Bock C, Vinberg M, Werge T, Gether U, Vedel Kessing L. Interaction between genetic polymorphisms and stressful life events in first episode depression. Journal of affective disorders 2009, 119:107-15.

[60] Coventry WL, James MR, Eaves LJ, Gordon SD, Gillespie NA, Ryan L, *et al.* Do 5HTTLPR and stress interact in risk for depression and suicidality? Item response analyses of a large sample. Am J Med Genet B Neuropsychiatr Genet 2010, 153B:757-65.

[61] Kraft J, Slager S, McGrath P, Hamilton S. Sequence analysis of the serotonin transporter and associations with antidepressant response. Biological psychiatry 2005, 58(374-381).

[62] Smeraldi E, Serretti A, Artioli P, Lorenzi C, Catalano M. Serotonin transporter gene-linked polymorphic region: possible pharmacogenetic implications of rare variants. Psychiatric genetics 2006, 16:153-8.

[63] Bonvicini C, Minelli A, Scassellati C, Bortolomasi M, Segala M, Sartori R, *et al.* Serotonin transporter gene polymorphisms and treatment-resistant depression. Progress in neuro-psychopharmacology & biological psychiatry 2010.

[64] Hu XZ, Lipsky RH, Zhu G, Akhtar LA, Taubman J, Greenberg BD, *et al.* Serotonin transporter promoter gain-of-function genotypes are linked to obsessive-compulsive disorder. American journal of human genetics 2006, 78:815-26.

[65] Perroud N, Salzmann A, Saiz PA, Baca-Garcia E, Sarchiapone M, Garcia-Portilla MP, *et al.* Rare genotype combination of the serotonin transporter gene associated with treatment response in severe personality disorder. Am J Med Genet B Neuropsychiatr Genet 2010, 153B:1494-7.

[66] Kato M, Serretti A. Review and meta-analysis of antidepressant pharmacogenetic findings in major depressive disorder. Molecular psychiatry 2010, 15:473-500.

[67] Perlis RH, Mischoulon D, Smoller JW, Wan YJ, Lamon-Fava S, Lin KM, *et al.* Serotonin transporter polymorphisms and adverse effects with fluoxetine treatment. Biological psychiatry 2003, 54:879-83.

[68] Popp J, Leucht S, Heres S, Steimer W. Serotonin transporter polymorphisms and side effects in antidepressant therapy--a pilot study. Pharmacogenomics 2006, 7:159-66.

[69] Smits K, Smits L, Peeters F, Schouten J, Janssen R, Smeets H, *et al.* Serotonin transporter polymorphisms and the occurrence of adverse events during treatment with selective serotonin reuptake inhibitors. International clinical psychopharmacology 2007, 22:137-43.

[70] Lanctot KL, Rapoport MJ, Chan F, Rajaram RD, Strauss J, Sicard T, *et al.* Genetic predictors of response to treatment with citalopram in depression secondary to traumatic brain injury. Brain Inj 2010, 24:959-69.

[71] Bishop JR, Ellingrod VL, Akroush M, Moline J. The association of serotonin transporter genotypes and selective serotonin reuptake inhibitor (SSRI)-associated sexual side effects: possible relationship to oral contraceptives. Human psychopharmacology 2009, 24:207-15.

[72] Secher A, Bukh J, Bock C, Koefoed P, Rasmussen HB, Werge T, *et al.* Antidepressive-drug-induced bodyweight gain is associated with polymorphisms in genes coding for COMT and TPH1. International clinical psychopharmacology 2009, 24:199-203.

[73] Higuchi H. [Prediction of antidepressant response to milnacipran and fluvoxamine using pharmacogenetical methods]. Nihon shinkei seishin yakurigaku zasshi = Japanese journal of psychopharmacology 2010, 30:71-6.

[74] Murata Y, Kobayashi D, Imuta N, Haraguchi K, Ieiri I, Nishimura R, *et al.* Effects of the serotonin 1A, 2A, 2C, 3A, and 3B and serotonin transporter gene polymorphisms on the occurrence of paroxetine discontinuation syndrome. Journal of clinical psychopharmacology 2010, 30:11-7.

[75] MacKenzie A, Quinn J. A serotonin transporter gene intron 2 polymorphic region, correlated with affective disorders, has allele-dependent differential enhancer-like properties in the mouse embryo. Proceedings of the National Academy of Sciences of the United States of America 1999, 96:15251-5.

[76] Ogilvie AD, Battersby S, Bubb VJ, Fink G, Harmar AJ, Goodwin GM, *et al.* Polymorphism in serotonin transporter gene associated with susceptibility to major depression. Lancet 1996, 347:731-3.

[77] Gutierrez B, Pintor L, Gasto C, Rosa A, Bertranpetit J, Vieta E, *et al.* Variability in the serotonin transporter gene and increased risk for major depression with melancholia. Hum Gen 1998, 103:319-22.

[78] Gaysina D, Zainullina A, Gabdulhakov R, Khusnutdinova E. The serotonin transporter gene: polymorphism and haplotype analysis in Russian suicide attempters. Neuropsychobiology 2006, 54:70-4.

[79] Lopez de Lara C, Dumais A, Rouleau G, Lesage A, Dumont M, Chawky N, *et al.* STin2 variant and family history of suicide as significant predictors of suicide completion in major depression. Biological psychiatry 2006, 59:114-20.

[80] Hranilovic D, Stefulj J, Schwab S, Borrmann-Hassenbach M, Albus M, Jernej B, *et al.* Serotonin transporter promoter and intron 2 polymorphisms: relationship between allelic variants and gene expression. Biological psychiatry 2004, 55:1090-4.

[81] Peters EJ, Slager SL, McGrath PJ, Knowles JA, Hamilton SP. Investigation of serotonin-related genes in antidepressant response. Molecular psychiatry 2004, 9:879-89.

[82] Ito K, Yoshida K, Sato K, Takahashi H, Kamata M, Higuchi H, *et al.* A variable number of tandem repeats in the serotonin transporter gene does not affect the antidepressant response to fluvoxamine. Psychiatry research 2002, 111:235-9.

[83] Higuchi H, Takahashi H, Kamata M, Yoshida K. Influence of serotonergic/noradrenergic gene polymorphisms on nausea and sweating induced by milnacipran in the treatment of depression. Neuropsychiatric disease and treatment 2009, 5:393-8.

[84] Serretti A, Zanardi R, Cusin C, Rossini D, Lorenzi C, Smeraldi E. Tryptophan hydroxylase gene associated with paroxetine antidepressant activity. European Neuropsychopharmacology 2001, 11:375-80.

[85] Serretti A, Zanardi R, Rossini D, Cusin C, Lilli R, Smeraldi E. Influence of tryptophan hydroxylase and serotonin transporter genes on fluvoxamine antidepressant activity. Molecular psychiatry 2001, 6:586-92.

[86] Ham BJ, Lee BC, Paik JW, Kang RH, Choi MJ, Choi IG, *et al.* Association between the tryptophan hydroxylase-1 gene A218C polymorphism and citalopram antidepressant response in a Korean population. Progress in neuro-psychopharmacology & biological psychiatry 2007, 31:104-7.

[87] Rujescu D, Giegling I, Sato T, Hartmann A, Moller H. Genetic variations in tryptophan hydroxylase in suicidal behavior: analysis and meta-analysis. Biological psychiatry 2003, 54:465-73.

[88] Bellivier F, Chaste P, Malafosse A. Association between the TPH gene A218C polymorphism and suicidal behavior: a meta-analysis. Am J Med Genet B Neuropsychiatr Genet 2004, 124:87-91.

[89] Yoshida K, Naito S, Takahashi H, Sato K, Ito K, Kamata M, *et al.* Monoamine oxidase: A gene polymorphism, tryptophan hydroxylase gene polymorphism and antidepressant response to fluvoxamine

in Japanese patients with major depressive disorder. Progress in neuro-psychopharmacology & biological psychiatry 2002, 26:1279-83.

[90] Ham B, Lee M, Lee H, Kang R, Han C, Choi M, *et al.* No association between the tryptophan hydroxylase gene polymorphism and major depressive disorders and antidepressant response in a Korean population. Psychiatric genetics 2005, 15:229-301.

[91] Kato M, Wakeno M, Okugawa G, Fukuda T, Azuma J, Kinoshita T, *et al.* No association of TPH1 218A/C polymorphism with treatment response and intolerance to SSRIs in Japanese patients with major depression. Neuropsychobiology 2007, 56:167-71.

[92] Illi A, Setala-Soikkeli E, Viikki M, Poutanen O, Huhtala H, Mononen N, *et al.* 5-HTR1A, 5-HTR2A, 5-HTR6, TPH1 and TPH2 polymorphisms and major depression. Neuroreport 2009 5, 20:1125-8.

[93] Viikki M, Kampman, O, Illi, A, Setala-Soikkeli, E, Anttila, S, Huuhka, M. TPH1 218A/C polymorphism is associated with major depressive disorder and its treatment response. Neuroscience letters 2010, 468:80-4.

[94] Anttila S, Huuhka K, Huuhka M, Rontu R, Mattila KM, Leinonen E, *et al.* Interaction between TPH1 and GNB3 genotypes and electroconvulsive therapy in major depression. Journal of neural transmission 2007, 114:461-8.

[95] Tzvetkov MV, Brockmoller J, Roots I, Kirchheiner J. Common genetic variations in human brain-specific tryptophan hydroxylase-2 and response to antidepressant treatment. Pharmacogenetics and genomics 2008, 18:495-506.

[96] Tsai SJ, Hong CJ, Liou YJ, Yu YW, Chen TJ, Hou SJ, *et al.* Tryptophan hydroxylase 2 gene is associated with major depression and antidepressant treatment response. Progress in neuro-psychopharmacology & biological psychiatry 2009 , 33:637-41.

[97] Lesch KP, Gutknecht L. Focus on the 5-HT_{1A}receptor: emerging role of a gene regulatory variant in psychopathology and pharmacogenetics. The international journal of neuropsychopharmacology / official scientific journal of the Collegium Internationale Neuropsychopharmacologicum (CINP) 2004, 7:381-5.

[98] Perez V, Gilaberte I, Faries D, Alvarez E, Artigas F. Randomised, double-blind, placebo-controlled trial of pindolol in combination with fluoxetine antidepressant treatment. Lancet 1997, 349:1594-7.

[99] Lemonde S, Turecki G, Bakish D, Du L, Hrdina P, Bown C, *et al.* Impaired trans-repression at a 5-HT_{1A} receptor gene polimorphism associated with major depression and suicide. J Neurosci 2003 2003, 23:8788-99.

[100] Albert PR, Lemonde S. 5-HT_{1A} receptors, gene repression, and depression: guilt by association. Neuroscientist 2004, 10:575-93.

[101] Lemonde S, Du L, Bakish D, Hrdina P, Albert PR. Association of the C(1019)G 5-HT_{1A} functional promoter polymorphism with antidepressant response. The international journal of neuropsychopharmacology / official scientific journal of the Collegium Internationale Neuropsychopharmacologicum (CINP) 2004, 7:501-6.

[102] Yu YW, Tsai SJ, Liou YJ, Hong CJ, Chen TJ. Association study of two serotonin 1A receptor gene polymorphisms and fluoxetine treatment response in Chinese major depressive disorders. Eur Neuropsychopharmacol 2006, 16:498-503.

[103] Kato M, Fukuda T, Wakeno M, Okugawa G, Takekita Y, Watanabe S, *et al.* Effect of 5-HT_{1A} gene polymorphisms on antidepressant response in major depressive disorder. Am J Med Genet B Neuropsychiatr Genet 2009, 150B:115-23.

[104] Serretti A, Artioli P, Lorenzi C, Pirovano A, Tubazio V, Zanardi R. The C(-1019)G polymorphism of the 5-HT_{1A} gene promoter and antidepressant response in mood disorders: preliminary findings. The international journal of neuropsychopharmacology / official scientific journal of the Collegium Internationale Neuropsychopharmacologicum (CINP) 2004, 7:453-60.

[105] Arias B, Catalan R, Gasto C, Gutierrez B, Fananas L. Evidence for a combined genetic effect of the 5-HT_{1A} receptor and serotonin transporter genes in the clinical outcome of major depressive patients treated with citalopram. Journal of psychopharmacology (Oxford, England) 2005, 19:166-72.

[106] Parsey RV, Olvet DM, Oquendo MA, Huang YY, Ogden RT, Mann JJ. Higher 5-HT_{1A} receptor binding potential during a major depressive episode predicts poor treatment response: preliminary data from a naturalistic study. Neuropsychopharmacology 2006, 31:1745-9.

[107] Villafuerte SM, Vallabhaneni K, Sliwerska E, McMahon FJ, Young EA, Burmeister M. SSRI response in depression may be influenced by SNPs in HTR1B and HTR1A. Psychiatric genetics 2009, 19:281-91.

[108] Noro M, Antonijevic I, Forray C, Kasper S, Kocabas NA, Lecrubier Y, *et al.* $5HT_{1A}$ and $5HT_{2A}$ receptor genes in treatment response phenotypes in major depressive disorder. International clinical psychopharmacology 2010, 25:228-31.

[109] Baune BT, Hohoff C, Roehrs T, Deckert J, Arolt V, Domschke K. Serotonin receptor 1A -1019C/G variant: Impact on antidepressant pharmacoresponse in melancholic depression? Neuroscience letters 2008, 436:111-5.

[110] Suzuki Y, Sawamura K, Someya T. The effects of a 5-hydroxytryptamine 1A receptor gene polymorphism on the clinical response to fluvoxamine in depressed patients. Pharmacoeconomics J 2004, 4:283-6.

[111] Levin GM, Bowles TM, Ehret MJ, Langaee T, Tan JY, Johnson JA, *et al.* Assessment of human serotonin 1A receptor polymorphisms and SSRI responsiveness. Molecular diagnosis & therapy 2007, 11:155-60.

[112] Drago A, De Ronchi D, Serretti A. Incomplete Coverage of Candidate Genes: A Poorly Considered Bias. Current Genomics 2008, ahead of print.

[113] Bhagwagar Z, Hinz R, Taylor M, Fancy S, Cowen P, Grasby P. Increased 5-HT_{2A} receptor binding in euthymic, medication-free patients recovered from depression: a positron emission study with [(11)C]MDL 100,907. The American journal of psychiatry 2006, 163:1580-7.

[114] Yatham LN, Liddle PF, Dennie J, Shiah IS, Adam MJ, Lane CJ, *et al.* Decrease in brain serotonin-2 receptor binding in patients with major depression following desipramine treatment-A

positron emission tomography study with fluorine-18-labeled setoperone. Archives of general psychiatry 1999, 56:705-11.

[115] Meyer JH, Kapur S, Eisfeld B, Brown GM, Houle S, DaSilva J, *et al.* The Effect of Paroxetine on 5-HT_{2A} Receptors in Depression: An [18F]Setoperone PET Imaging Study. The American journal of psychiatry 2001, 158:78–85.

[116] Yamauchi M, Takako M, Tetsuya M, Imanishi T. Desensitization of 5-HT_{2A} receptor function by chronic administration of selective serotonin reuptake inhibitors. Brain Res 2005:164-9.

[117] Minov C, Baghai TC, Schule C, Zwanzger P, Schwarz MJ, Zill P, *et al.* Serotonin-2A-receptor and -transporter polymorphisms: lack of association in patients with major depression. Neuroscience letters 2001, 303:119-22.

[118] Choi M, Kang R, Ham B, Jeong H, Lee M. Serotonin receptor 2A gene polymorphism (-1438A/G) and short-term treatment response to citalopram. Neuropsychobiology 2005, 52:155-62.

[119] Cusin C, Serretti A, Zanardi R, Lattuada E, Rossini D, Lilli R, *et al.* Influence of monoamine oxydase A and serotonin receptor 2A polymorphisms in SSRIs antidepressant activity. International Journal of Neuropsychopharmacology 2002, 5:27-35.

[120] Sato K, Yoshida K, Takahashi H, Ito K, Kamata M, Higuchi H, *et al.* Association between -1438G/A promoter polymorphism in the 5-HT_{2A} receptor gene and fluvoxamine response in Japanese patients with major depressive disorder. Neuropsychobiology 2002, 46:136-40.

[121] Suzuki Y, Sawamura K, Someya T. Polymorphisms in the 5-hydroxytryptamine 2A receptor and CytochromeP4502D6 genes synergistically predict fluvoxamine-induced side effects in japanese depressed patients. Neuropsychopharmacology 2006, 31:825-31.

[122] McMahon FJ, Buervenich S, Charney D, Lipsky R, Rush AJ, Wilson AF, *et al.* Variation in the gene encoding the serotonin 2A receptor is associated with outcome of antidepressant treatment. American journal of human genetics 2006, 78:804-14.

[123] Horstmann S, Lucae S, Menke A, Hennings JM, Ising M, Roeske D, *et al.* Polymorphisms in GRIK4, HTR2A, and FKBP5 show interactive effects in predicting remission to antidepressant treatment. Neuropsychopharmacology 2010, 35:727-40.

[124] Perlis RH, Laje G, Smoller JW, Fava M, Rush AJ, McMahon FJ. Genetic and clinical predictors of sexual dysfunction in citalopram-treated depressed patients. Neuropsychopharmacology 2009, 34:1819-28.

[125] Uher R, Huezo-Diaz P, Perroud N, Smith R, Rietschel M, Mors O, *et al.* Genetic predictors of response to antidepressants in the GENDEP project. The pharmacogenomics journal 2009, 9:225-33.

[126] Peters EJ, Slager SL, Jenkins GD, Reinalda MS, Garriock HA, Shyn SI, *et al.* Resequencing of serotonin-related genes and association of tagging SNPs to citalopram response. Pharmacogenetics and genomics 2009, 19:1-10.

[127] Kishi T, Fukuo Y, Yoshimura R, Okochi T, Kitajima T, Naitoh H, *et al.* Pharmacogenetic study of serotonin 6 receptor gene with antidepressant response in major depressive disorder in the Japanese population. Human psychopharmacology 2010, 25:481-6.

[128] Lucae S, Ising M, Horstmann S, Baune BT, Arolt V, Muller-Myhsok B, *et al.* HTR2A gene variation is involved in antidepressant treatment response. Eur Neuropsychopharmacol 2010, 20:65-8.

[129] Serretti A, Calati R, Giegling I, Hartmann AM, Moller HJ, Colombo C, *et al.* 5-HT_{2A} SNPs and the Temperament and Character Inventory. Progress in neuro-psychopharmacology & biological psychiatry 2007, 31:1275-81.

[130] Tanaka M, Kobayashi D, Murakami Y, Ozaki N, Suzuki T, Iwata N, *et al.* Genetic polymorphisms in the 5-hydroxytryptamine type 3B receptor gene and paroxetine-induced nausea. The international journal of neuropsychopharmacology / official scientific journal of the Collegium Internationale Neuropsychopharmacologicum (CINP) 2008, 11:261-7.

[131] Sugai T, Suzuki Y, Sawamura K, Fukui N, Inoue Y, Someya T. The effect of 5-hydroxytryptamine 3A and 3B receptor genes on nausea induced by paroxetine. The pharmacogenomics journal 2006, 6:351-6.

[132] Ballaz SJ, Akil H, Watson SJ. Analysis of 5-HT_6 and 5-HT_7 receptor gene expression in rats showing differences in novelty-seeking behavior. Neuroscience 2007, 147:428-38.

[133] Mitchell ES, Sexton T, Neumaier JF. Increased expression of 5-HT_6 receptors in the rat dorsomedial striatum impairs instrumental learning. Neuropsychopharmacology 2007, 32:1520-30.

[134] Svenningsson P, Tzavara ET, Qi H, Carruthers R, Witkin JM, Nomikos GG, *et al.* Biochemical and behavioral evidence for antidepressant-like effects of 5-HT_6 receptor stimulation. J Neurosci. 2007, 27:4201-9.

[135] Wesolowska A, Nikiforuk A. Effects of the brain-penetrant and selective 5-HT_6 receptor antagonist SB-399885 in animal models of anxiety and depression. Neuropharmacology 2007, 52:1274-83.

[136] Kohen R, Metcalf MA, Khan N, Druck T, Huebner K, Lachowicz JE, *et al.* Cloning, characterization, and chromosomal localization of a human 5-HT_6 serotonin receptor. Journal of neurochemistry 1996, 66:47-56.

[137] Lee S, Lee K, Lee H, Ham B, Ryu S, Lee M. Association between the 5-HT_6 receptor C267T polymorphism and response to antidepressant treatment in major depressive disorder. Psychiatry Clin Neurosci 2005, 59:140-5.

[138] Wu WH, Huo SJ, Cheng CY, Hong CJ, Tsai SJ. Association Study of the 5-HT_6 Receptor Polymorphism (C267T) and Symptomatology and Antidepressant Response in Major Depressive Disorders. Neuropsychobiology 2001, 44:172-5.

[139] Weinshilboum RM, Otterness DM, Szumlanski CL. Methylation pharmacogenetics: catechol O-methyltransferase, thiopurine methyltransferase, and histamine N-methyltransferase. Annu Rev Pharmacol Toxicol 1999, 39:19-52.

[140] Arias B, Serretti A, Lorenzi C, Gasto C, Catalan R, Fananas L. Analysis of COMT gene (Val 158 Met polymorphism) in the clinical response to SSRIs in depressive patients of European origin. Journal of affective disorders 2006, 90:251-6.

[141] Porcelli S, Fabbri C, Drago A, Gibiino S, De Ronchi D, Serretti A Genetics and antidepressants: where we are. Clin Neuropsych. 2011, 8,2:99-150.

[142] Baune BT, Hohoff C, Berger K, Neumann A, Mortensen S, Roehrs T, *et al.* Association of the COMT val158met variant with antidepressant treatment response in major depression. Neuropsychopharmacology 2008, 33:924-32.

[143] Benedetti F, Colombo C, Pirovano A, Marino E, Smeraldi E. The catechol-O-methyltransferase Val(108/158)Met polymorphism affects antidepressant response to paroxetine in a naturalistic setting. Psychopharmacology 2009, 203:155-60.

[144] Yoshida K, Higuchi H, Takahashi H, Kamata M, Sato K, Inoue K, *et al.* Influence of the tyrosine hydroxylase val81met polymorphism and catechol-O-methyltransferase val158met polymorphism on the antidepressant effect of milnacipran. Human psychopharmacology 2008, 23:121-8.

[145] Tsai SJ, Gau YT, Hong CJ, Liou YJ, Yu YW, Chen TJ. Sexually dimorphic effect of catechol-O-methyltransferase val158met polymorphism on clinical response to fluoxetine in major depressive patients. Journal of affective disorders 2009, 113:183-7.

[146] Szegedi A, Rujescu D, Tadic A, Muller MJ, Kohnen R, Stassen HH, *et al.* The catechol-O-methyltransferase Val108/158Met polymorphism affects short-term treatment response to mirtazapine, but not to paroxetine in major depression. The pharmacogenomics journal 2005, 5:49-53.

[147] Illi A, Setala-Soikkeli E, Kampman O, Viikki M, Nuolivirta T, Poutanen O, *et al.* Catechol-O-methyltransferase val108/158met genotype, major depressive disorder and response to selective serotonin reuptake inhibitors in major depressive disorder. Psychiatry research 2010, 176:85-7.

[148] Hu J, Redden DT, Berrettini WH, Shields PG, Restine SL, Pinto A, *et al.* No evidence for a major role of polymorphisms during bupropion treatment. Obesity (Silver Spring) 2006, 14:1863-7.

[149] Perlis RH, Fijal B, Adams DH, Sutton VK, Trivedi MH, Houston JP. Variation in catechol-O-methyltransferase is associated with duloxetine response in a clinical trial for major depressive disorder. Biological psychiatry 2009, 65:785-91.

[150] Kocabas NA, Antonijevic I, Faghel C, Forray C, Kasper S, Lecrubier Y, *et al.* Dysbindin gene (DTNBP1) in major depressive disorder (MDD) patients: lack of association with clinical phenotypes. World J Biol Psychiatry 2010, 11:985-90.

[151] Hahn MK, Mazei-Robison MS, Blakely RD. Single nucleotide polymorphisms in the human norepinephrine transporter gene affect expression, trafficking, antidepressant interaction, and protein kinase C regulation. Mol Pharmacol 2005, 68:457-66.

[152] Dong C, Wong ML, Licinio J. Sequence variations of ABCB1, SLC6A2, SLC6A3, SLC6A4, CREB1, CRHR1 and NTRK2: association with major depression and antidepressant response in Mexican-Americans. Molecular psychiatry 2009, 14:1105-18.

[153] Sabol SZ, Hu S, Hamer D. A functional polymorphism in the monoamine oxidase A gene promoter. Human Genetic 1998, 103:273-9.

[154] Muller DJ, Schulze TG, Macciardi F, Ohlraun S, Gross MM, Scherk H, *et al.* Moclobemide

response in depressed patients: association study with a functional polymorphism in the monoamine oxidase A promoter. Pharmacopsychiatry 2002, 35:157-8.

[155] Tadic A, Muller MJ, Rujescu D, Kohnen R, Stassen HH, Dahmen N, *et al.* The MAOA T941G polymorphism and short-term treatment response to mirtazapine and paroxetine in major depression. Am J Med Genet B Neuropsychiatr Genet 2007, 144:325-31.

[156] Tzeng DS, Chien CC, Lung FW, Yang CY. MAOA gene polymorphisms and response to mirtazapine in major depression. Human psychopharmacology 2009, 24:293-300.

[157] Leuchter AF, McCracken JT, Hunter AM, Cook IA, Alpert JE. Monoamine oxidase a and catechol-o-methyltransferase functional polymorphisms and the placebo response in major depressive disorder. Journal of clinical psychopharmacology 2009, 29:372-7.

[158] Haefner S, Baghai TC, Schule C, Eser D, Spraul M, Zill P, *et al.* Impact of gene-gender effects of adrenergic polymorphisms on hypothalamic-pituitary-adrenal axis activity in depressed patients. Neuropsychobiology 2008, 58:154-62.

[159] Zill P, Baghai TC, Engel R, Zwanzger P, Schule C, Minov C, *et al.* Beta-1-adrenergic receptor gene in major depression: Influence on antidepressant treatment response. Am J Med Genet 2003, 120B:85-9.

[160] Crowley JJ, Lipsky RH, Lucki I, Berrettini WH. Variation in the genes encoding vesicular monoamine transporter 2 and beta-1 adrenergic receptor and antidepressant treatment outcome. Psychiatric genetics 2008, 18:248-51.

[161] Wakeno M, Kato M, Okugawa G, Fukuda T, Hosoi Y, Takekita Y, *et al.* The alpha 2A-adrenergic receptor gene polymorphism modifies antidepressant responses to milnacipran. Journal of clinical psychopharmacology 2008, 28:518-24.

[162] Lee HY, Kang RH, Paik JW, Jeong YJ, Chang HS, Han SW, *et al.* Association of the adrenergic alpha 2a receptor--1291C/G polymorphism with weight change and treatment response to mirtazapine in patients with major depressive disorder. Brain Res 2009, 1262:1-6.

[163] Perroud N, Aitchison KJ, Uher R, Smith R, Huezo-Diaz P, Marusic A, *et al.* Genetic predictors of increase in suicidal ideation during antidepressant treatment in the GENDEP project. Neuropsychopharmacology 2009, 34:2517-28.

[164] McClure DJ. The role of dopamine in depression. Canadian Psychiatric Association journal 1973, 18:309012.

[165] Willner P. Dopamine and depression: a review of recent evidence. I. Empirical studies. Brain Res 1983, 287:211-24.

[166] Malhi GS, Berk M. Does dopamine dysfunction drive depression? Acta psychiatrica Scandinavica 2007:116-24.

[167] Dailly E, Chenu F, Renard CE, Bourin M. Dopamine, depression and antidepressants. Fundamental & clinical pharmacology 2004, 18:601-7.

[168] Porcelli S, Drago A, Fabbri C, Serretti A. Mechanisms of antidepressant action: An integrated dopaminergic perspective. Progress in neuro-psychopharmacology & biological psychiatry. 2011.

[169] Willner P, Hale AS, Argyropoulos S. Dopaminergic mechanism of antidepressant action in depressed patients. Journal of affective disorders 2005, 86:37-45.

[170] Zhou Z, Roy A, Lipsky R, Kuchipudi K, Zhu G, Taubman J, *et al.* Haplotype-based linkage of tryptophan hydroxylase 2 to suicide attempt, major depression, and cerebrospinal fluid 5-hydroxyindoleacetic acid in 4 populations. Archives of general psychiatry 2005, 62:1109-18.

[171] Lavretsky H, Siddarth P, Kumar A, Reynolds CF, 3rd. The effects of the dopamine and serotonin transporter polymorphisms on clinical features and treatment response in geriatric depression: a pilot study. International journal of geriatric psychiatry 2008, 23:55-9.

[172] Dziedzicka-Wasylewska M, Solich J. Neuronal cell lines transfected with the dopamine D2 receptor gene promoter as a model for studying the effects of antidepressant drugs. Brain research 2004, 128:75-82.

[173] Maj J, Papp M, Skuza G, Bigajska K, Zazula M. The influence of repeated treatment with imipramine, (+)- and (-)-oxaprotiline on behavioural effects of dopamine D-1 and D-2 agonists. Journal of neural transmission 1989, 76:29-38.

[174] Serretti A, Zanardi R, Cusin C, Rossini D, Lilli R, Lorenzi C, *et al.* No association between dopamine D2 and D4 receptor gene variants and antidepressant activity of two selective serotonin reuptake inhibitors. Psychiatry research 2001, 104:195-203.

[175] Benedetti F, Serretti A, Colombo C, Lilli R, Lorenzi C, Smeraldi E. Dopamine receptor D2 and D3 gene variants are not associated with the antidepressant effect of total sleep deprivation in bipolar depression. Psychiatry research 2003, 118:241-7.

[176] Serretti A, Artioli P, Zanardi R, Lorenzi C, Rossini D, Cusin C, *et al.* Genetic features of antidepressant induced mania and hypo-mania in bipolar disorder. Psychopharmacology 2004, 174:504-11.

[177] Perlis RH, Adams DH, Fijal B, Sutton VK, Farmen M, Breier A, *et al.* Genetic association study of treatment response with olanzapine/fluoxetine combination or lamotrigine in bipolar I depression. The Journal of clinical psychiatry 2010, 71:599-605.

[178] Garriock HA, Delgado P, Kling MA, Carpenter LL, Burke M, Burke WJ, *et al.* Number of risk genotypes is a risk factor for major depressive disorder: a case control study. Behav Brain Funct. 2006, 2:24.

[179] Holsboer F. The corticosteroid receptor hypothesis of depression. Neuropsychopharmacology 2000, 23:477-501.

[180] Nemeroff CB, Owens MJ. Treatment of mood disorders. Nature neuroscience 2002, 5 Suppl:1068-70.

[181] De Bellis MD, Gold PW, Geracioti TD, Jr., Listwak SJ, Kling MA. Association of fluoxetine treatment with reductions in CSF concentrations of corticotropin-releasing hormone and arginine vasopressin in patients with major depression. The American journal of psychiatry 1993, 150:656-7.

[182] Ising M, Kunzel HE, Binder EB, Nickel T, Modell S, Holsboer F. The combined dexamethasone/CRH test as a potential surrogate marker in depression. Progress in neuro-psychopharmacology & biological psychiatry 2005, 29:1085-93.

[183] Ising M, Horstmann S, Kloiber S, Lucae S, Binder EB, Kern N, *et al.* Combined dexamethasone/corticotropin releasing hormone test predicts treatment response in major depression - a potential biomarker? Biological psychiatry 2007, 62:47-54.

[184] Schule C, Baghai TC, Eser D, Hafner S, Born C, Herrmann S, *et al.* The combined dexamethasone/CRH Test (DEX/CRH test) and prediction of acute treatment response in major depression. PloS one 2009, 4:e4324.

[185] Liu ZC, Luo XN, Wang GH. Corticotropin-releasing factor andmajor depression. Foreign Medical Sci (Section Of Psychiatry) 2 2002:156–8.

[186] Nemeroff CB, Widerlov E, Bissette G, Walleus H, Karlsson I, Eklund K, *et al.* Elevated concentrations of CSF corticotropin-releasing factor-like immunoreactivity in depressed patients. Science New York, NY, 1984, 226:1342-4.

[187] Nemeroff CB, Owens MJ, Bissette G, Andorn AC, Stanley M. Reduced corticotropin releasing factor binding sites in the frontal cortex of suicide victims. Archives of general psychiatry 1988, 45:577-9.

[188] Raadsheer FC, Hoogendijk WJ, Stam FC, Tilders FJ, Swaab DF. Increased numbers of corticotropin-releasing hormone expressing neurons in the hypothalamic paraventricular nucleus of depressed patients. Neuroendocrinology 1994, 60:436-44.

[189] Brady LS, Gold PW, Herkenham M, Lynn AB, Whitfield HJ, Jr. The antidepressants fluoxetine, idazoxan and phenelzine alter corticotropin-releasing hormone and tyrosine hydroxylase mRNA levels in rat brain: therapeutic implications. Brain Res 1992, 572:117-25.

[190] Gold PW, Chrousos GP. Organization of the stress system and its dysregulation in melancholic and atypical depression: high vs low CRH/NE states. Molecular psychiatry 2002, 7:254-75.

[191] Michelson D, Galliven E, Hill L, Demitrack M, Chrousos G, Gold P. Chronic imipramine is associated with diminished hypothalamic-pituitary-adrenal axis responsivity in healthy humans. The Journal of clinical endocrinology and metabolism 1997, 82:2601-6.

[192] Van Pett K, Viau V, Bittencourt JC, Chan RK, Li HY, Arias C, *et al.* Distribution of mRNAs encoding CRF receptors in brain and pituitary of rat and mouse. J Comp Neurol 2000, 428:191-212.

[193] Licinio J, O'Kirwan F, Irizarry K, Merriman B, Thakur S, Jepson R, *et al.* Association of a corticotropin-releasing hormone receptor 1 haplotype and antidepressant treatment response in Mexican-Americans. Molecular psychiatry 2004, 9:1075-82.

[194] Liu Z, Zhu F, Wang G, Xiao Z, Tang J, Liu W, *et al.* Association study of corticotropin-releasing hormone receptor1 gene polymorphisms and antidepressant response in major depressive disorders. Neuroscience letters 2007, 414:155-8.

[195] Papiol S, Arias B, Gasto C, Gutierrez B, Catalan R, Fananas L. Genetic variability at HPA axis in major depression and clinical response to antidepressant treatment. Journal of affective disorders 2007, 104:83-90.

[196] Binder EB, Owens MJ, Liu W, Deveau TC, Rush AJ, Trivedi MH, *et al.* Association of polymorphisms in genes regulating the corticotropin-releasing factor system with antidepressant treatment response. Archives of general psychiatry 2010, 67:369-79.

[197] van Rossum EF, Voorhoeve PG, te Velde SJ, Koper JW, Delemarre-van de Waal HA, Kemper HC, *et al.* The ER22/23EK polymorphism in the glucocorticoid receptor gene is associated with a beneficial body composition and muscle strength in young adults. The Journal of clinical endocrinology and metabolism 2004, 89:4004-9.

[198] van Rossum EF, Binder EB, Majer M, Koper JW, Ising M, Modell S, *et al.* Polymorphisms of the glucocorticoid receptor gene and major depression. Biological psychiatry 2006, 59:681-8.

[199] Rosmond R, Chagnon YC, Holm G, Chagnon M, Perusse L, Lindell K, *et al.* A glucocorticoid receptor gene marker is associated with abdominal obesity, leptin, and dysregulation of the hypothalamic-pituitary-adrenal axis. Obesity research 2000, 8:211-8.

[200] Panarelli M, Holloway CD, Fraser R, Connell JM, Ingram MC, Anderson NH, *et al.* Glucocorticoid receptor polymorphism, skin vasoconstriction, and other metabolic intermediate phenotypes in normal human subjects. The Journal of clinical endocrinology and metabolism 1998, 83:1846-52.

[201] Ukkola O, Rosmond R, Tremblay A, Bouchard C. Glucocorticoid receptor Bcl I variant is associated with an increased atherogenic profile in response to long-term overfeeding. Atherosclerosis 2001, 157:221-4.

[202] Brouwer JP, Appelhof BC, van Rossum EF, Koper JW, Fliers E, Huyser J, *et al.* Prediction of treatment response by HPA-axis and glucocorticoid receptor polymorphisms in major depression. Psychoneuroendocrinology 2006, 31:1154-63.

[203] Binder EB, Salyakina D, Lichtner P, Wochnik GM, Ising M, Putz B, *et al.* Polymorphisms in FKBP5 are associated with increased recurrence of depressive episodes and rapid response to antidepressant treatment. Nature genetics 2004, 36:1319-25.

[204] Kirchheiner J, Lorch R, Lebedeva E, Seeringer A, Roots I, Sasse J, *et al.* Genetic variants in FKBP5 affecting response to antidepressant drug treatment. Pharmacogenomics 2008, 9:841-6.

[205] Lekman M, Laje G, Charney D, Rush AJ, Wilson AF, Sorant AJ, *et al.* The FKBP5-gene in depression and treatment response--an association study in the Sequenced Treatment Alternatives to Relieve Depression (STAR*D) Cohort. Biological psychiatry 2008, 63:1103-10.

[206] Sapolsky RM. Stress and plasticity in the limbic system. Neurochemical research 2003, 28:1735-42.

[207] Duman RS, Monteggia LM. A neurotrophic model for stress-related mood disorders. Biological psychiatry 2006, 59:1116-27.

[208] Monteggia LM, Barrot M, Powell CM, Berton O, Galanis V, Gemelli T, *et al.* Essential role of brain-derived neurotrophic factor in adult hippocampal function. Proceedings of the National Academy of Sciences of the United States of America 2004, 101:10827-32.

[209] Nestler EJ, Barrot M, DiLeone RJ, Eisch AJ, Gold SJ, Monteggia LM. Neurobiology of depression. Neuron 2002, 34:13-25.

[210] Pittenger C, Duman RS. Stress, depression, and neuroplasticity: a convergence of mechanisms. Neuropsychopharmacology 2008, 33:88-109.

[211] Brunoni AR, Lopes M, Fregni F. A systematic review and meta-analysis of clinical studies on major depression and BDNF levels: implications for the role of neuroplasticity in depression. The international journal of neuropsychopharmacology / official scientific journal of the Collegium Internationale Neuropsychopharmacologicum (CINP) 2008, 11:1169-80.

[212] Follesa P, Biggio F, Gorini G, Caria S, Talani G, Dazzi L, *et al.* Vagus nerve stimulation increases norepinephrine concentration and the gene expression of BDNF and bFGF in the rat brain. Brain Res 2007, 1179:28-34.

[213] Rogoz Z, Skuza G, Legutko B. Repeated co-treatment with imipramine and amantadine induces hippocampal brain-derived neurotrophic factor gene expression in rats. J Physiol Pharmacol 2007, 58:219-34.

[214] Reagan LP, Hendry RM, Reznikov LR, Piroli GG, Wood GE, McEwen BS, *et al.* Tianeptine increases brain-derived neurotrophic factor expression in the rat amygdala. European journal of pharmacology 2007, 565:68-75.

[215] Calabrese F, Molteni R, Maj PF, Cattaneo A, Gennarelli M, Racagni G, *et al.* Chronic duloxetine treatment induces specific changes in the expression of BDNF transcripts and in the subcellular localization of the neurotrophin protein. Neuropsychopharmacology 2007, 32:2351-9.

[216] Conti B, Maier R, Barr AM, Morale MC, Lu X, Sanna PP, *et al.* Region-specific transcriptional changes following the three antidepressant treatments electro convulsive therapy, sleep deprivation and fluoxetine. Molecular psychiatry 2007, 12:167-89.

[217] Nibuya M, Morinobu S, Duman RS. Regulation of BDNF and trkB mRNA in rat brain by chronic electroconvulsive seizure and antidepressant drug treatments. J Neurosci 1995, 15:7539-47.

[218] Mandelli L, Mazza M, Martinotti G, Tavian D, Colombo E, Missaglia S, *et al.* Further evidence supporting the influence of brain-derived neurotrophic factor on the outcome of bipolar depression: independent effect of brain-derived neurotrophic factor and harm avoidance. Journal of psychopharmacology (Oxford, England) 2010.

[219] Petryshen TL, Sabeti PC, Aldinger KA, Fry B, Fan JB, Schaffner SF, *et al.* Population genetic study of the brain-derived neurotrophic factor (BDNF) gene. Molecular psychiatry 2010, 15:810-5.

[220] Zou YF, Wang Y, Liu P, Feng XL, Wang BY, Zang TH, *et al.* Association of brain-derived neurotrophic factor genetic Val66Met polymorphism with severity of depression, efficacy of fluoxetine and its side effects in Chinese major depressive patients. Neuropsychobiology 2010, 61:71-8.

[221] Gratacos M, Soria V, Urretavizcaya M, Gonzalez JR, Crespo JM, Bayes M, *et al.* A brain-derived neurotrophic factor (BDNF) haplotype is associated with antidepressant treatment outcome in mood disorders. The pharmacogenomics journal 2008, 8:101-12.

[222] Licinio J, Dong C, Wong ML. Novel sequence variations in the brain-derived neurotrophic factor gene and association with major depression and antidepressant treatment response. Archives of general psychiatry 2009, 66:488-97.

[223] Domschke K, Lawford B, Laje G, Berger K, Young R, Morris P, *et al.* Brain-derived neurotrophic factor (BDNF) gene: no major impact on antidepressant treatment response. The international journal of neuropsychopharmacology / official scientific journal of the Collegium Internationale Neuropsychopharmacologicum (CINP) 2010, 13:93-101.

[224] Chen G, Hasanat KA, Bebchuk JM, Moore GJ, Glitz D, Manji HK. Regulation of signal transduction pathways and gene expression by mood stabilizers and antidepressants. Psychosom Med 1999, 61:599-617.

[225] Ruiz-Velasco V, Ikeda SR. A splice variant of the G protein beta 3-subunit implicated in disease states does not modulate ion channels. Physiological genomics 2003, 13:85-95.

[226] Zill P, Baghai TC, Zwanzger P, Schule C, Minov C, Riedel M, *et al.* Evidence for an association between a G-protein beta3-gene variant with depression and response to antidepressant treatment. Neuroreport 2000, 11:1893-7.

[227] Serretti A, Lorenzi C, Cusin C, Zanardi R, Lattuada E, Rossini D, *et al.* SSRIs antidepressant activity is influenced by Gbeta3 variants. Eur Neuropsychopharmacol 2003, 13:117-22.

[228] Lee HJ, Cha JH, Ham BJ, Han CS, Kim YK, Lee SH, *et al.* Association between a G-protein beta3 subunit gene polymorphism and the symptomatology and treatment responses of major depressive disorders. The pharmacogenomics journal 2004, 4:29-33.

[229] Wilkie MJ, Smith D, Reid IC, Day RK, Matthews K, Wolf CR, *et al.* A splice site polymorphism in the G-protein beta subunit influences antidepressant efficacy in depression. Pharmacogenetics and genomics 2007, 17:207-15.

[230] Lin E, Chen PS, Chang HH, Gean PW, Tsai HC, Yang YK, *et al.* Interaction of serotonin-related genes affects short-term antidepressant response in major depressive disorder. Progress in neuro-psychopharmacology & biological psychiatry 2009, 33:1167-72.

[231] Kato M, Wakeno M, Okugawa G, Fukuda T, Takekita Y, Hosoi Y, *et al.* Antidepressant response and intolerance to SSRI is not influenced by G-protein beta3 subunit gene C825T polymorphism in Japanese major depressive patients. Progress in neuro-psychopharmacology & biological psychiatry 2008, 32:1041-4.

[232] Kang RH, Hahn SW, Choi MJ, Lee MS. Relationship between G-protein beta-3 subunit C825T polymorphism and mirtazapine responses in Korean patients with major depression. Neuropsychobiology 2007, 56:1-5.

[233] Blendy JA. The role of CREB in depression and antidepressant treatment. Biological psychiatry 2006, 59:1144-50.

[234] Serretti A, Chiesa A, Calati R, Massat I, Linotte S, Kasper S, *et al.* A preliminary investigation of the influence of CREB1 gene on treatment resistance in major depression. Journal of affective disorders 2011, 128:56-63.

[235] Perlis RH, Purcell S, Fava M, Fagerness J, Rush AJ, Trivedi MH, *et al.* Association between treatment-emergent suicidal ideation with citalopram and polymorphisms near cyclic adenosine monophosphate response element binding protein in the STAR*D study. Archives of general psychiatry 2007, 64:689-97.

[236] Sanacora G, Mason GF, Rothman DL, Behar KL, Hyder F, Petroff OA, *et al.* Reduced cortical gamma-aminobutyric acid levels in depressed patients determined by proton magnetic resonance spectroscopy. Archives of general psychiatry 1999, 56:1043-7.

[237] Boyer PA, Skolnick P, Fossom LH. Chronic administration of imipramine and citalopram alters the expression of NMDA receptor subunit mRNAs in mouse brain. A quantitative *in situ* hybridization study. J Mol Neurosci 1998, 10:219-33.

[238] Paddock S, Laje G, Charney D, Rush AJ, Wilson AF, Sorant AJ, *et al.* Association of GRIK4 with outcome of antidepressant treatment in the STAR*D cohort. The American journal of psychiatry 2007, 164:1181-8.

[239] Horstmann S, Lucae S, Menke A, Ising M, Muller-Myhsok B, Holsboer F, *et al.* Association of GRIK4 and HTR2A genes with antidepressant treatment in the MARS cohort of depressed inpatients. European Neuropsychopharmacology 2008, 18:S214-S5.

[240] Perlis RH, Fijal B, Dharia S, Heinloth AN, Houston JP. Failure to replicate genetic associations with antidepressant treatment response in duloxetine-treated patients. Biological psychiatry 2010, 67:1110-3.

[241] Tsunoka T, Kishi T, Ikeda M, Kitajima T, Yamanouchi Y, Kinoshita Y, *et al.* Association analysis of group II metabotropic glutamate receptor genes (GRM2 and GRM3) with mood disorders and fluvoxamine response in a Japanese population. Progress in neuro-psychopharmacology & biological psychiatry 2009, 33:875-9.

[242] Laje G, Paddock S, Manji H, Rush AJ, Wilson AF, Charney D, *et al.* Genetic markers of suicidal ideation emerging during citalopram treatment of major depression. The American journal of psychiatry 2007, 164:1530-8.

[243] Menke A, Lucae S, Kloiber S, Horstmann S, Bettecken T, Uhr M, *et al.* Genetic markers within glutamate receptors associated with antidepressant treatment-emergent suicidal ideation. The American journal of psychiatry 2008, 165:917-8.

[244] Laje G, Allen AS, Akula N, Manji H, John Rush A, McMahon FJ. Genome-wide association study of suicidal ideation emerging during citalopram treatment of depressed outpatients. Pharmacogenetics and genomics 2009, 19:666-74.

[245] Spina E, Santoro V, D'Arrigo C. Clinically relevant pharmacokinetic drug interactions with second-generation antidepressants: an update. Clinical therapeutics 2008, 30:1206-27.

[246] Jin Y, Pollock BG, Frank E, Cassano GB, Rucci P, Muller DJ, *et al.* Effect of age, weight, and CYP2C19 genotype on escitalopram exposure. Journal of clinical pharmacology 2010, 50:62-72.

[247] Ververs FF, Voorbij HA, Zwarts P, Belitser SV, Egberts TC, Visser GH, *et al.* Effect of cytochrome P450 2D6 genotype on maternal paroxetine plasma concentrations during pregnancy. Clinical pharmacokinetics 2009, 48:677-83.

[248] Cordon-Cardo C, O'Brien JP, Casals D, Rittman-Grauer L, Biedler JL, Melamed MR, *et al.* Multidrug-resistance gene (P-glycoprotein) is expressed by endothelial cells at blood-brain barrier sites. Proceedings of the National Academy of Sciences of the United States of America 1989, 86:695-8.

[249] Eichelbaum M, Fromm MF, Schwab M. Clinical aspects of the MDR1 (ABCB1) gene polymorphism. Therapeutic drug monitoring 2004, 26:180-5.

[250] Kato M, Fukuda T, Serretti A, Wakeno M, Okugawa G, Ikenaga Y, *et al.* ABCB1 (MDR1) gene polymorphisms are associated with the clinical response to paroxetine in patients with major depressive disorder. Progress in neuro-psychopharmacology & biological psychiatry 2008, 32:398-404.

[251] Nikisch G, Eap CB, Baumann P. Citalopram enantiomers in plasma and cerebrospinal fluid of ABCB1 genotyped depressive patients and clinical response: a pilot study. Pharmacol Res 2008, 58:344-7.

[252] Sarginson JE, Lazzeroni LC, Ryan HS, Ershoff BD, Schatzberg AF, Murphy GM, Jr. ABCB1 (MDR1) polymorphisms and antidepressant response in geriatric depression. Pharmacogenetics and genomics 2010, 20:467-75.

[253] Uhr M, Tontsch A, Namendorf C, Ripke S, Lucae S, Ising M, *et al.* Polymorphisms in the drug transporter gene ABCB1 predict antidepressant treatment response in depression. Neuron 2008, 57:203-9.

[254] Gex-Fabry M, Eap CB, Oneda B, Gervasoni N, Aubry JM, Bondolfi G, *et al.* CYP2D6 and ABCB1 genetic variability: influence on paroxetine plasma level and therapeutic response. Therapeutic drug monitoring 2008, 30:474-82.

[255] Mihaljevic Peles A, Bozina N, Sagud M, Rojnic Kuzman M, Lovric M. MDR1 gene polymorphism: therapeutic response to paroxetine among patients with major depression. Progress in neuro-psychopharmacology & biological psychiatry 2008, 32:1439-44.

[256] Peters EJ, Slager SL, Kraft JB, Jenkins GD, Reinalda MS, McGrath PJ, *et al.* Pharmacokinetic genes do not influence response or tolerance to citalopram in the STAR*D sample. PloS one 2008, 3:e1872.

[257] Laika B, Leucht S, Steimer W. ABCB1 (P-glycoprotein/MDR1) gene G2677T/a sequence variation (polymorphism): lack of association with side effects and therapeutic response in depressed inpatients treated with amitriptyline. Clinical chemistry 2006, 52:893-5.

[258] Roberts RL, Joyce PR, Mulder RT, Begg EJ, Kennedy MA. A common P-glycoprotein polymorphism is associated with nortriptyline-induced postural hypotension in patients treated for major depression. The pharmacogenomics journal 2002, 2:191-6.

[259] Menu P, Gressier F, Verstuyft C, Hardy P, Becquemont L, Corruble E. Antidepressants and ABCB1 gene C3435T functional polymorphism: a naturalistic study. Neuropsychobiology 2010, 62:193-7.

[260] Black JL, 3rd, O'Kane DJ, Mrazek DA. The impact of CYP allelic variation on antidepressant metabolism: a review. Expert Opin Drug Metab Toxicol 2007, 3:21-31.

[261] Lin JH, Lu AY. Inhibition and induction of cytochrome P450 and the clinical implications. Clinical pharmacokinetics 1998, 35:361-90.

[262] Desta Z, Zhao X, Shin JG, Flockhart DA. Clinical significance of the cytochrome P450 2C19 genetic polymorphism. Clinical pharmacokinetics 2002, 41:913-58.

[263] Porcelli S, Fabbri C, Spina E, Serretti A, De Ronchi D. Genetic polymorphisms of cytochrome P450 enzymes and antidepressant metabolism. Expert Opin Drug Metab Toxicol 2011, 7:1101-15.

[264] Steimer W, Zopf K, von Amelunxen S, Pfeiffer H, Bachofer J, Popp J, *et al.* Allele-specific change of concentration and functional gene dose for the prediction of steady-state serum concentrations of amitriptyline and nortriptyline in CYP2C19 and CYP2D6 extensive and intermediate metabolizers. Clinical chemistry 2004, 50:1623-33.

[265] Grasmader K, Verwohlt PL, Rietschel M, Dragicevic A, Muller M, Hiemke C, *et al.* Impact of polymorphisms of cytochrome-P450 isoenzymes 2C9, 2C19 and 2D6 on plasma concentrations and clinical effects of antidepressants in a naturalistic clinical setting. European journal of clinical pharmacology 2004, 60:329-36.

[266] Schenk PW, van Fessem MA, Verploegh-Van Rij S, Mathot RA, van Gelder T, Vulto AG, *et al.* Association of graded allele-specific changes in CYP2D6 function with imipramine dose requirement in a large group of depressed patients. Molecular psychiatry 2008, 13:597-605.

[267] Charlier C, Broly F, Lhermitte M, Pinto E, Ansseau M, Plomteux G. Polymorphisms in the CYP 2D6 gene: association with plasma concentrations of fluoxetine and paroxetine. Therapeutic drug monitoring 2003, 25:738-42.

[268] Sawamura K, Suzuki Y, Someya T. Effects of dosage and CYP2D6-mutated allele on plasma concentration of paroxetine. European journal of clinical pharmacology 2004, 60:553-7.

[269] Ueda M, Hirokane G, Morita S, Okawa M, Watanabe T, Akiyama K, *et al.* The impact of CYP2D6 genotypes on the plasma concentration of paroxetine in Japanese psychiatric patients. Progress in neuro-psychopharmacology & biological psychiatry 2006, 30:486-91.

[270] Fukuda T, Nishida Y, Zhou Q, Yamamoto I, Kondo S, Azuma J. The impact of the CYP2D6 and CYP2C19 genotypes on venlafaxine pharmacokinetics in a Japanese population. European journal of clinical pharmacology 2000, 56:175-80.

[271] Fukuda T, Yamamoto I, Nishida Y, Zhou Q, Ohno M, Takada K, *et al.* Effect of the CYP2D6*10 genotype on venlafaxine pharmacokinetics in healthy adult volunteers. British journal of clinical pharmacology 1999, 47:450-3.

[272] Ozdemir V, Tyndale RF, Reed K, Herrmann N, Sellers EM, Kalow W, *et al.* Paroxetine steady-state plasma concentration in relation to CYP2D6 genotype in extensive metabolizers. Journal of clinical psychopharmacology 1999, 19:472-5.

[273] Ohara K, Tanabu S, Ishibashi K, Ikemoto K, Yoshida K, Shibuya H. CYP2D6*10 alleles do not determine plasma fluvoxamine concentration/dose ratio in Japanese subjects. European journal of clinical pharmacology 2003, 58:659-61.

[274] Shimoda K, Someya T, Yokono A, Morita S, Hirokane G, Takahashi S, *et al.* The impact of CYP2C19 and CYP2D6 genotypes on metabolism of amitriptyline in Japanese psychiatric patients. Journal of clinical psychopharmacology 2002, 22:371-8.

[275] Rau T, Wohlleben G, Wuttke H, Thuerauf N, Lunkenheimer J, Lanczik M, *et al.* CYP2D6 genotype: impact on adverse effects and nonresponse during treatment with antidepressants-a pilot study. Clinical pharmacology and therapeutics 2004, 75:386-93.

[276] Tsai MH, Lin KM, Hsiao MC, Shen WW, Lu ML, Tang HS, *et al*. Genetic polymorphisms of cytochrome P450 enzymes influence metabolism of the antidepressant escitalopram and treatment response. Pharmacogenomics 2010, 11:537-46.

[277] Shams ME, Arneth B, Hiemke C, Dragicevic A, Muller MJ, Kaiser R, *et al*. CYP2D6 polymorphism and clinical effect of the antidepressant venlafaxine. J Clin Pharm Ther 2006, 31:493-502.

[278] Murphy GM, Jr., Kremer C, Rodrigues HE, Schatzberg AF. Pharmacogenetics of Antidepressant Medication Intolerance. The American journal of psychiatry 2003, 160:1830-5.

[279] Serretti A, Calati R, Massat I, Linotte S, Kasper S, Lecrubier Y, *et al*. Cytochrome P450 CYP1A2, CYP2C9, CYP2C19 and CYP2D6 genes are not associated with response and remission in a sample of depressive patients. International clinical psychopharmacology 2009, 24:250-6.

[280] Yin OQ, Wing YK, Cheung Y, Wang ZJ, Lam SL, Chiu HF, *et al*. Phenotype-genotype relationship and clinical effects of citalopram in Chinese patients. Journal of clinical psychopharmacology 2006, 26:367-72.

[281] Yu BN, Chen GL, He N, Ouyang DS, Chen XP, Liu ZQ, *et al*. Pharmacokinetics of citalopram in relation to genetic polymorphism of CYP2C19. Drug metabolism and disposition: the biological fate of chemicals 2003, 31:1255-9.

[282] Fudio S, Borobia AM, Pinana E, Ramirez E, Tabares B, Guerra P, *et al*. Evaluation of the influence of sex and CYP2C19 and CYP2D6 polymorphisms in the disposition of citalopram. European journal of pharmacology 2010, 626:200-4.

[283] de Vos A, van der Weide J, Loovers HM. Association between CYP2C19*17 and metabolism of amitriptyline, citalopram and clomipramine in Dutch hospitalized patients. The pharmacogenomics journal 2010.

[284] Rudberg I, Hendset M, Uthus LH, Molden E, Refsum H. Heterozygous mutation in CYP2C19 significantly increases the concentration/dose ratio of racemic citalopram and escitalopram (S-citalopram). Therapeutic drug monitoring 2006, 28:102-5.

[285] van der Weide J, van Baalen-Benedek EH, Kootstra-Ros JE. Metabolic ratios of psychotropics as indication of cytochrome P450 2D6/2C19 genotype. Therapeutic drug monitoring 2005, 27:478-83.

[286] de Leon J, Susce MT, Murray-Carmichael E. The AmpliChip CYP450 genotyping test: Integrating a new clinical tool. Molecular diagnosis & therapy 2006, 10:135-51.

[287] EGAPP. Recommendations from the EGAPP Working Group: testing for cytochrome P450 polymorphisms in adults with nonpsychotic depression treated with selective serotonin reuptake inhibitors. Genet Med 2007, 9:819-25.

[288] Kirchheiner J, Brosen K, Dahl ML, Gram LF, Kasper S, Roots I, *et al*. CYP2D6 and CYP2C19 genotype-based dose recommendations for antidepressants: a first step towards subpopulation-specific dosages. Acta Psychiatr Scand 2001, 104:173-92.

[289] Garriock HA, Kraft JB, Shyn SI, Peters EJ, Yokoyama JS, Jenkins GD, *et al*. A genomewide

association study of citalopram response in major depressive disorder. Biological psychiatry 2010, 67:133-8.

[290] Uher R, Perroud N, Ng MY, Hauser J, Henigsberg N, Maier W, *et al.* Genome-wide pharmacogenetics of antidepressant response in the GENDEP project. The American journal of psychiatry 2010, 167:555-64.

[291] Ising M, Lucae S, Binder EB, Bettecken T, Uhr M, Ripke S, *et al.* A genomewide association study points to multiple loci that predict antidepressant drug treatment outcome in depression. Archives of general psychiatry 2009, 66:966-75.

[292] Perroud N, Uher R, Ng MY, Guipponi M, Hauser J, Henigsberg N, *et al.* Genome-wide association study of increasing suicidal ideation during antidepressant treatment in the GENDEP project. The pharmacogenomics journal 2010.

[293] Slodkowska EA, Ross JS. MammaPrint 70-gene signature: another milestone in personalized medical care for breast cancer patients. Expert review of molecular diagnostics 2009, 9:417-22.

[294] Paik S, Tang G, Shak S, Kim C, Baker J, Kim W, *et al.* Gene expression and benefit of chemotherapy in women with node-negative, estrogen receptor-positive breast cancer. J Clin Oncol 2006, 24:3726-34.

[295] Sullivan PF. Spurious genetic associations. Biological psychiatry 2007, 61:1121-6.

[296] Lin PI, Vance JM, Pericak-Vance MA, Martin ER. No gene is an island: the flip-flop phenomenon. American journal of human genetics 2007, 80:531-8.

[297] Drago A, Crisafulli C, Serretti A. The genetics of antipsychotic induced tremors: a genome-wide pathway analysis on the STEP-BD SCP sample. Am J Med Genet B Neuropsychiatr Genet 2011, 156B:975-86.

[298] Tsuang M, S. F. The Genetics of Mood Disorders. Baltimore: MD: Johns Hopkins University Press, 1990.

[299] Cloninger C, Prybeck TR, *et al.* The Temperament and Character Inventory (TCI): A Guide to Its Development and Use: Center for Psychobiology of Personality, Washington University, St Louis, MO 1994.

[300] Smits KM, Smits LJ, Peeters FP, Schouten JS, Janssen RG, Smeets HJ, *et al.* The influence of 5-HTTLPR and STin2 polymorphisms in the serotonin transporter gene on treatment effect of selective serotonin reuptake inhibitors in depressive patients. Psychiatric genetics 2008, 18:184-90.

[301] Saeki Y, Watanabe T, Ueda M, Saito A, Akiyama K, Inoue Y, *et al.* Genetic and pharmacokinetic factors affecting the initial pharmacotherapeutic effect of paroxetine in Japanese patients with panic disorder. European journal of clinical pharmacology 2009, 65:685-91.

[302] Lotrich FE, Pollock BG, Kirshner M, Ferrell RF, Reynolds Iii CF. Serotonin transporter genotype interacts with paroxetine plasma levels to influence depression treatment response in geriatric patients. J Psychiatry Neurosci 2008, 33:123-30.

[303] Ruhe HG, Ooteman W, Booij J, Michel MC, Moeton M, Baas F, *et al.* Serotonin transporter gene

promoter polymorphisms modify the association between paroxetine serotonin transporter occupancy and clinical response in major depressive disorder. Pharmacogenetics and genomics 2009, 19:67-76.

[304] Yu YW, Tsai SJ, Chen TJ, Lin CH, Hong CJ. Association study of the serotonin transporter promoter polymorphism and symptomatology and antidepressant response in major depressive disorders. Molecular psychiatry 2002, 7:1115-9.

[305] Lee MS, Lee HY, Lee HJ, Ryu SH. Serotonin transporter promoter gene polymorphism and long-term outcome of antidepressant treatment. Psychiatric genetics 2004, 14:111-5.

[306] Kato M, Ikenaga Y, Wakeno M, Okugawa G, Nobuhara K, Fukuda T, *et al.* Controlled clinical comparison of paroxetine and fluvoxamine considering the serotonin transporter promoter polymorphism. Int Clin Psychopharmacol 2005, 20:151-6.

[307] Lewis G, Mulligan J, Wiles N, Cowen P, Craddock N, Ikeda M, *et al.* Polymorphism of the 5-HT transporter and response to antidepressants: randomised controlled trial. Br J Psychiatry 2011.

[308] Ng CH, Easteal S, Tan S, Schweitzer I, Ho BK, Aziz S. Serotonin transporter polymorphisms and clinical response to sertraline across ethnicities. Progress in neuro-psychopharmacology & biological psychiatry 2006, 30:953-7.

[309] Takahashi H, Yoshida K, Ito K, Sato K, Kamata M, Higuchi H, *et al.* No association between the serotonergic polymorphisms and incidence of nausea induced by fluvoxamine treatment. Eur Neuropsychopharmacol 2002, 12:477-81.

[310] Gressier F, Bouaziz E, Verstuyft C, Hardy P, Becquemont L, Corruble E. 5-HTTLPR modulates antidepressant efficacy in depressed women. Psychiatric genetics 2009, 19:195-200.

[311] Strohmaier J, Wust S, Uher R, Henigsberg N, Mors O, Hauser J, *et al.* Sexual dysfunction during treatment with serotonergic and noradrenergic antidepressants: Clinical description and the role of the 5-HTTLPR. World J Biol Psychiatry 2011.

[312] Stamm TJ, Adli M, Kirchheiner J, Smolka MN, Kaiser R, Tremblay PB, *et al.* Serotonin transporter gene and response to lithium augmentation in depression. Psychiatric genetics 2008, 18:92-7.

[313] Bishop JR, Moline J, Ellingrod VL, Schultz SK, Clayton AH. Serotonin 2A -1438 G/A and G-protein Beta3 subunit C825T polymorphisms in patients with depression and SSRI-associated sexual side-effects. Neuropsychopharmacology 2006, 31:2281-8.

[314] Yoshida K, Naito S, Takahashi H, Sato K, Ito K, Kamata M, *et al.* Monoamine oxidase A gene polymorphism, 5-HT_{2A} receptor gene polymorphism and incidence of nausea induced by fluvoxamine. Neuropsychobiology 2003, 48:10-3.

[315] Kang RH, Choi MJ, Paik JW, Hahn SW, Lee MS. Effect of serotonin receptor 2A gene polymorphism on mirtazapine response in major depression. Int J Psychiatry Med 2007, 37:315-29.

[316] Murphy G, Hollander S, Rodrigues H, Schatzberg A. Effects of the serotonin transporter promoter polymorphism on paroxetine and mirtazapine efficacy and side effects in geriatric major depression. In: Hospital TZH, editor. Pharmacogenetics in psychiatry meeting 2003 11-12, New York, 2003. p. green tab.

[317] Kishi T, Yoshimura R, Kitajima T, Okochi T, Okumura T, Tsunoka T, *et al.* HTR2A is Associated with SSRI Response in Major Depressive Disorder in a Japanese Cohort. Neuromolecular medicine 2009.

[318] Zhang X, Gainetdinov R, Beaulieu J-M, Sotnikova T, Burch L, Williams R, *et al.* Loss-of-Function Mutation in Tryptophan Hydroxylase-2 Identified in Unipolar Major Depression. Neuron 2005, 45(11-16).

[319] Garriock H, Allen J, Delgado P, Nahaz Z, Kling M, Carpenter L, *et al.* Lack of association of TPH2 exon XI polymorphisms with major depression and treatment resistance. Molecular psychiatry 2005, 10:976-7.

[320] Tsai SJ, Hong CJ, Yu YW, Chen TJ, Wang YC, Lin WK. Association study of serotonin 1B receptor (A-161T) genetic polymorphism and suicidal behaviors and response to fluoxetine in major depressive disorder. Neuropsychobiology 2004, 50:235-8.

[321] Gudayol-Ferre E, Herrera-Guzman I, Camarena B, Cortes-Penagos C, Herrera-Abarca JE, Martinez-Medina P, *et al.* The role of clinical variables, neuropsychological performance and SLC6A4 and COMT gene polymorphisms on the prediction of early response to fluoxetine in major depressive disorder. Journal of affective disorders 2010, 127:343-51.

[322] Yu YW, Tsai SJ, Hong CJ, Chen TJ, Chen MC, Yang CW. Association study of a monoamine oxidase a gene promoter polymorphism with major depressive disorder and antidepressant response. Neuropsychopharmacology 2005, 30:1719-23.

[323] Serretti A, Zanardi R, Franchini L, Artioli P, Dotoli D, Pirovano A, *et al.* Pharmacogenetics of selective serotonin reuptake inhibitor response: a 6-month follow-up. Pharmacogenetics 2004, 14:607-13.

[324] Domschke K, Hohoff C, Mortensen LS, Roehrs T, Deckert J, Arolt V, *et al.* Monoamine oxidase A variant influences antidepressant treatment response in female patients with Major Depression. Progress in neuro-psychopharmacology & biological psychiatry 2008, 32:224-8.

[325] Tsai SJ, Hong CJ, Chen TJ, Yu YW. Lack of supporting evidence for a genetic association of the FKBP5 polymorphism and response to antidepressant treatment. Am J Med Genet B Neuropsychiatr Genet 2007, 144B:1097-8.

[326] Zobel A, Schuhmacher A, Jessen F, Hofels S, von Widdern O, Metten M, *et al.* DNA sequence variants of the FKBP5 gene are associated with unipolar depression. The international journal of neuropsychopharmacology / official scientific journal of the Collegium Internationale Neuropsychopharmacologicum (CINP) 2010, 13:649-60.

[327] Sarginson JE, Lazzeroni LC, Ryan HS, Schatzberg AF, Murphy GM, Jr. FKBP5 polymorphisms and antidepressant response in geriatric depression. Am J Med Genet B Neuropsychiatr Genet 2010, 153B:554-60.

[328] Zou YF, Wang Y, Liu P, Feng XL, Wang BY, Zang TH, *et al.* Association of BDNF Val66Met polymorphism with both baseline HRQOL scores and improvement in HRQOL scores in Chinese major depressive patients treated with fluoxetine. Human psychopharmacology 2010, 25:145-52.

[329] Choi MJ, Kang RH, Lim SW, Oh KS, Lee MS. Brain-derived neurotrophic factor gene

polymorphism (Val66Met) and citalopram response in major depressive disorder. Brain Res 2006, 1118:176-82.

[330] Alexopoulos GS, Glatt CE, Hoptman MJ, Kanellopoulos D, Murphy CF, Kelly RE, Jr., *et al.* BDNF Val66met polymorphism, white matter abnormalities and remission of geriatric depression. Journal of affective disorders 2010.

[331] Taylor WD, McQuoid DR, Ashley-Koch A, Macfall JR, Bridgers J, Krishnan RR, *et al.* BDNF Val66Met genotype and 6-month remission rates in late-life depression. The pharmacogenomics journal 2010.

[332] Tsai SJ, Cheng CY, Yu YW, Chen TJ, Hong CJ. Association study of a brain-derived neurotrophic-factor genetic polymorphism and major depressive disorders, symptomatology, and antidepressant response. Am J Med Genet B Neuropsychiatr Genet 2003, 123B:19-22.

[333] Yoshida K, Higuchi H, Kamata M, Takahashi H, Inoue K, Suzuki T, *et al.* The G196A polymorphism of the brain-derived neurotrophic factor gene and the antidepressant effect of milnacipran and fluvoxamine. Journal of psychopharmacology (Oxford, England) 2007, 21:650-6.

[334] Kocabas NA, Antonijevic I, Faghel C, Forray C, Kasper S, Lecrubier Y, *et al.* Brain-derived neurotrophic factor gene polymorphisms: influence on treatment response phenotypes of major depressive disorder. International clinical psychopharmacology 2011, 26:1-10.

[335] Kang R, Chang H, Wong M, Choi M, Park J, Lee H, *et al.* Brain-derived neurotrophic factor gene polymorphisms and mirtazapine responses in Koreans with major depression. Journal of psychopharmacology (Oxford, England) 2009.

[336] Keers R, Bonvicini C, Scassellati C, Uher R, Placentino A, Giovannini C, *et al.* Variation in GNB3 predicts response and adverse reactions to antidepressants. Journal of psychopharmacology (Oxford, England) 2010.

[337] Baghai TC, Schule C, Zwanzger P, Minov C, Schwarz MJ, de Jonge S, *et al.* Possible influence of the insertion/deletion polymorphism in the angiotensin I-converting enzyme gene on therapeutic outcome in affective disorders. Molecular psychiatry 2001, 6:258-9.

[338] Baghai TC, Schule C, Zill P, Deiml T, Eser D, Zwanzger P, *et al.* The angiotensin I converting enzyme insertion/deletion polymorphism influences therapeutic outcome in major depressed women, but not in men. Neuroscience letters 2004, 363:38-42.

[339] Bondy B, Baghai T, Zill P, Schule C, Eser D, Deiml T, *et al.* Genetic variants in the angiotensin I-converting-enzyme (ACE) and angiotensin II receptor (AT1) gene and clinical outcome in depression. Progress in neuro-psychopharmacology & biological psychiatry 2005, 29:1094-99.

[340] Mendlewicz J, Oswald P, Claes S, Massat I, Souery D, Van Broeckhoven C, *et al.* Patient-control association study of substance P-related genes in unipolar and bipolar affective disorders. The international journal of neuropsychopharmacology / official scientific journal of the Collegium Internationale Neuropsychopharmacologicum (CINP). 2005, 8:505-13.

[341] Hong CJ, Wang YC, Tsai SJ. Association study of angiotensin I-converting enzyme polymorphism and symptomatology and antidepressant response in major depressive disorders. Journal of neural transmission 2002, 109:1209-14.

[342] Tsai SJ. Sipatrigine could have therapeutic potential for major depression and bipolar depression through antagonism of the two-pore-domain K+ channel TREK-1. Medical hypotheses 2008, 70:548-50.

[343] Adli M, Hollinde DL, Stamm T, Wiethoff K, Tsahuridu M, Kirchheiner J, *et al.* Response to lithium augmentation in depression is associated with the glycogen synthase kinase 3-beta -50T/C single nucleotide polymorphism. Biological psychiatry 2007, 62:1295-302.

[344] Cabanero M, Laje G, Detera-Wadleigh S, McMahon FJ. Association study of phosphodiesterase genes in the Sequenced Treatment Alternatives to Relieve Depression sample. Pharmacogenetics and genomics 2009, 19:235-8.

[345] Wong ML, Whelan F, Deloukas P, Whittaker P, Delgado M, Cantor RM, *et al.* Phosphodiesterase genes are associated with susceptibility to major depression and antidepressant treatment response. Proceedings of the National Academy of Sciences of the United States of America 2006, 103:15124-9.

[346] Teranishi KS, Slager SL, Garriock H, Kraft JB, Peters EJ, Reinalda MS, *et al.* Variants in PDE11A and PDE1A are not associated with citalopram response. Molecular psychiatry 2007, 12:1061-3.

[347] Serretti A, Cusin C, Benedetti F, Mandelli L, Pirovano A, Zanardi R, *et al.* Insomnia improvement during antidepressant treatment and CLOCK gene polymorphism. Am J Med Genet B Neuropsychiatr Genet 2005, 10:10.

[348] Kishi T, Kitajima T, Ikeda M, Yamanouchi Y, Kinoshita Y, Kawashima K, *et al.* CLOCK may predict the response to fluvoxamine treatment in Japanese major depressive disorder patients. Neuromolecular medicine 2009, 11:53-7.

[349] Yu YW, Chen TJ, Hong CJ, Chen HM, Tsai SJ. Association Study of the Interleukin-1beta (C-511T) Genetic Polymorphism with Major Depressive Disorder, Associated Symptomatology, and Antidepressant Response. Neuropsychopharmacology 2003, 28:1182-5.

[350] Tadic A, Rujescu D, Muller MJ, Kohnen R, Stassen HH, Szegedi A, *et al.* Association analysis between variants of the interleukin-1beta and the interleukin-1 receptor antagonist gene and antidepressant treatment response in major depression. Neuropsychiatric disease and treatment 2008, 4:269-76.

[351] Baune BT, Dannlowski U, Domschke K, Janssen DG, Jordan MA, Ohrmann P, *et al.* The interleukin 1 beta (IL1B) gene is associated with failure to achieve remission and impaired emotion processing in major depression. Biological psychiatry 2010, 67:543-9.

[352] Pae CU, Serretti A, Mandelli L, De Ronchi D, Patkar AA, Jun TY, *et al.* Dysbindin associated with selective serotonin reuptake inhibitor antidepressant efficacy. Pharmacogenetics and genomics 2007, 17:69-75.

[353] Arias B, Serretti A, Mandelli L, Gasto C, Catalan R, Ronchi DD, *et al.* Dysbindin gene (DTNBP1) in major depression: association with clinical response to selective serotonin reuptake inhibitors. Pharmacogenetics and genomics 2009, 19:121-8.

[354] Zill P, Baghai TC, Engel R, Zwanzger P, Schule C, Eser D, *et al*. The dysbindin gene in major depression: an association study. Am J Med Genet B Neuropsychiatr Genet 2004, 129:55-8.

[355] Perlis RH, Moorjani P, Fagerness J, Purcell S, Trivedi MH, Fava M, *et al*. Pharmacogenetic analysis of genes implicated in rodent models of antidepressant response: association of TREK1 and treatment resistance in the STAR(*)D study. Neuropsychopharmacology 2008, 33:2810-9.

[356] Liou YJ, Chen TJ, Tsai SJ, Yu YW, Cheng CY, Hong CJ. Support for the involvement of the KCNK2 gene in major depressive disorder and response to antidepressant treatment. Pharmacogenetics and genomics 2009, 19:735-41.

[357] Garriock HA, Tanowitz M, Kraft JB, Dang VC, Peters EJ, Jenkins GD, *et al*. Association of mu-opioid receptor variants and response to citalopram treatment in major depressive disorder. The American journal of psychiatry 2010, 167:565-73.

Send Orders for Reprints to reprints@benthamscience.net
Neurobiology of Mood Disorders, 2014, 107-126

CHAPTER 5

PATHOPHYSIOLOGY OF MOOD DISORDERS: NORADRENERGIC MECHANISMS

ELIYAHU DREMENCOV*

Institute of Molecular Physiology and Genetics, Slovak Academy of Sciences, Bratislava, Slovakia, and Neuroken Consulting, Healthy Ageing Campus Netherlands, Groningen, the Netherlands

Abstract: There are number of lines of evidence that the neurotransmitter norepinephrine (NE) might be very important in pathophysiology of anxiety and mood disorders. Firstly, NE projections innervate the limbic system, suggesting the involvement of NE in the regulation of emotions and cognition. Secondly, NE interacts with serotonin (5-HT) and dopamine (DA) systems, which also play very important roles in the regulation of mood. Thirdly, it has been shown that various agents for increasing NE availability, such as NE reuptake inhibitors, are also effective antidepressant drugs. And fourthly, the depletion of NE can result in the relapse of depression after successful treatment with antidepressant drugs. All these pieces of evidence suggest that the stimulation of NE transmission can be beneficial in the treatment of affective disorders. However, different psychiatric medications have distant effects on NE transmission. The current chapter analyses the effect of psychiatric medications on NE system and proposes how the treatment outcome might be improved.

Keywords: Norepinephrine (NE), serotonin (5-HT), locus coeruleus (LC), depression, anxiety, antidepressant drugs, mood stabilizers, selective serotonin reuptake inhibitors (SSRIs), electrophysiology, α2-adrenergic receptosr, serotonin-2A (5-HT2A) receptors.

1. INTRODUCTION

1.1. NEUROTRANSMITTER NOREPINEPHRINE

Norepinephrine, together with epinephrine and dopamine (DA), belongs to the catecholamine family of hormones and neurotransmitters. DA is synthesized in all catecholamine neurons by decarboxylation of levodopa. This process is catalyzed by aromatic amino acid decarboxylase and requires the presence of pyridoxal phosphate. Levodopa itself is synthesized by oxidation of the amino acid tyrosine. This oxidation is a rate-limited process and it is catalyzed by tyrosine hydroxylase. In the NE-releasing neurons (spinal neurons of the autonomic system, sympathetic ganglia neurons and brain NE neurons), the enzyme DA beta hydroxylase turns DA into NE. This process requires vitamin C as a cofactor. In the sympathetic ganglia neurons, and especially in the epinephrine-secreting cells of adrenal medulla, NE is partially transformed into epinephrine. This transformation is performed by the enzyme phenylethanolamine N-methyltransferase (PNMT) [1].

NE molecules are made inside into synaptic vesicles by the vesicular monoamine transporter (VMAT). This transport is an active, adenosine triphosphate (ATP)-requiring process. VMAT also transports DA, epinephrine and serotonin (5-HT). These hormones and transmitters are so-called monoamines (MO). Certain drugs, such as reserpine and tetrabenazine, inhibit the VMAT and suppress vesicular MO storage (Table **1**) [2,3].

***Address correspondence to Eliyahu Dremencov:** Neuroken Consulting, Healthy Ageing Campus Netherlands, Groningen, The Netherlands; E-mail: e.dremencov@neuroken.com

Disclosure: Part of information included in this chapter has been previously published in Current Drug Targets VOLUME: 10 ISSUE: 11 DOI:10.2175/138945009789735165

Bruno P Guiard and Eliyahu Dremencov (Eds)

Neuronal action potentials (APs), when they arrive to the nerve terminal, stimulate the fusion of the synaptic vesicles with the cellular membrane, and NE is released into the synaptic space. Certain compounds, such as methamphetamines or bupropion, increase NE release *via* an AP-independent release mechanism [4,5].

NE molecules released into the synaptic space are reabsorbed back into the presynaptic neuron by the membrane NE transporter (NET). This process requires ATP. The NET is a target for numerous drugs. Several tricyclic antidepressants (TCA), such as imipramine, non-specifically inhibit both NET and 5-HT (5-HTT) transporters [6]. Other TCAs, called norepinephrine reuptake inhibitors (NRIs), such as desipramine, specifically inhibit the NET [7,8]. There are also non-tricyclic selective inhibitors of the NET, called selective norepinephrine reuptake inhibitors (SNeRIs), and dual inhibitors of the NET and 5-HTT (SNRIs). The examples for SneRIs and SNRIs are reboxetine and venlafaxine, respectively [9-13].

After reuptake of it NE is stored again or it is degraded. The major metabolic pathway of NE is its oxidation into 3,4-dihydroxymandelic acid by the type A of the enzyme monoamine oxidize (MAO). Numerous drugs have MAO as their primary target. They can be divided into two groups: non-reversible MAO inhibitors (MAOIs) and reversible MAO inhibitors (RIMAs). Respective examples for these groups are phenelzine and moclobemide [14,15].

Process	Mediator	Drugs
Storage	Vesicular monoamine transporter	Reserpine (↓) Tetrabenazine (↓)
Release	Synaptic proteins	Methamphetamines (↑) Bupropion (↑)
Reuptake	Norepinephrine transporter	Tricyclic antidepressants (imipramine, ↓) Tricyclic norepinephrine reuptake inhibitors (desipramine, ↓) Selective norepinephrine reuptake inhibitors (reboxetine, ↓) Dual serotonin/ norepinephrine reuptake inhibitors (venlafaxine, ↓)
Negative autoregulation of norepinephrine neuronal firing activity	α_2-adrenergic autoreceptor	Idazoxan (↓) Noradrenergic and specific serotonergic antidepressants (Mirtazapine ,↓) Atipical antipsychotic drugs (Risperidone , ↓)
Metabolism	Monoamine oxidize A	(Reversible) monoamine oxidize inhibitors (phenelsine, moclobemide, ↓)

Table 1: Drugs affecting the storage, release, reuptake, autoregulation and metabolism of norepinephrine. (↓), inhibitory effect; (↑), excitatory effect.

2. NORADRENERGIC SYSTEM

There are several nuclei containing NE neurons in the pons and medulla oblongata (Figures **1**). The NE neurons of medulla oblongata are situated in the caudal raphe nuclei and project to the spinal cord (A1, A5 and A7 cell groups in rat) and hypothalamus (A2 group). These NE pathways regulate mostly sensory, motor and autonomic functions. The NE neurons of the pons are concentrated in the area called locus coeruleus (LC, A6 in rat). The NE system of the LC plays an important role in the regulation of sensory, motor, neuroendocrine, and cognitive functions of the brain [1,16,17]. In the current chapter only the NE system of LC will be discussed.

LC consists mostly of NE neurons. However, γ-aminobutyric acid (GABA)-secreting neurons are also found in the peripheries of the LC [18]. The NE neurons of LC have local and distant afferent and efferent connections. The local bilateral connections of LC arrive from and project to the GABA cells of periaqueductal gray (PAG) and acetylcholine (ACH) neurons of pontomesencephalic tegmentum (PMT) [19].

The major distant afferents to the LC arrive from the brainstem (nucleus paragigantocellularis, PGI) and telencephalon (central nucleus of amygdala, CEA, and prefrontal cortex, PFC). The efferents of the LC innervate literally all areas of the central neural system (CNS). The majority of the fibers, however, project to the hippocampus, dentate gyrus (DG), prefrontal cortex (PFC) and basolateral nucleus of amygdala (BLA) [1,16,17].

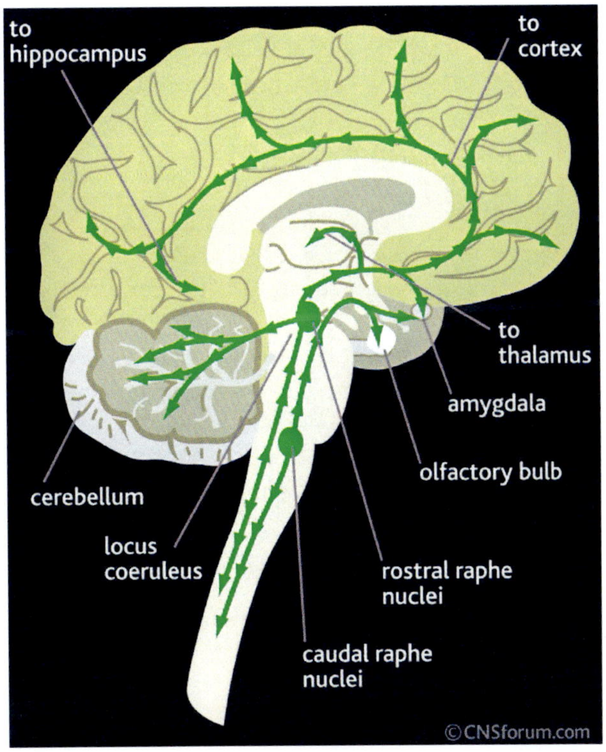

Figure 1. Norepinephrine pathways of human brain. Published with permission of Lundbeck Institute.

3. NORADRENERGIC RECEPTORS

All receptors for NE (adrenoceptors) are G-protein-coupled metabotropic receptors. However, they vary by their location (presynaptic autoreceptors and post-synaptic hetreroreceptors), pharmacology (three families α_1, α_2 and β with three subtypes in each family $\alpha_{1A/B/D}$, $\alpha_{2A/B/D}$ and $\beta_{1/2/3}$), signal transduction (G_{Q11}-α_1 family, G_I-α_2, and G_S-β), and physiology (excitatory of inhibitory effect on the postsynaptic neuron).

The only inhibitory adrenoceptors and only that are located on both pre- and post-synaptic neurons are a_2-adrenoceptors. These receptors are coupled to the G_I protein. Their activation results in $G_{I\alpha}$ dissociation into the $G_{I\alpha}$ and $G_{Ib\gamma}$. $G_{I\alpha}$ deactivates adenylyl cyclase (AC) and sodium (Ca^{2+}) channels, while $G_{Ib\gamma}$ opens potassium (K^+) channels. An increase in K^+- and decrease in Ca^{2+}-influx leads to hyperpolarisation. This decreases the rate of AP firing and inhibits NE release.

Both a_1 and β adrenoceptors are postsynaptic excitatory heteroreceptors. Their action is mediated *via* the activation of Ca^{2+} current. However, different mechanisms are involved: G_Q-mediated phospholipase C (PLC) activation and G_S-mediated AC stimulation, respectively [1]. When they present on glutamate pyramidal neurons, β-adrenoceptors receptors decrease the Ca^{2+}-activated after-hyperpolarization K^+ influx, making the neurons more responsive for excitatory inputs. The α_1 adrenoceptors, however, increase membrane conductance and make the pyramidal cells less excitable [20].

4. NOREPINEPHRINE NEURONS

NE neurons express mixed tonic/phasic firing activity. The firing rate is approximately 2 Hertz and it remains relatively constant. Short bursts containing two or three APs occur with a periodicity of one or two per minute (Figures **2**) [21-23]. The firing activity of NE neurons is auto-regulated as well as controlled by other transmitters. In the LC, NE the activation of a_2 adrenergic autoreceptors by NE suppresses the firing activity of NE neurons. In the nerve-terminal level, the activation α_2 adrenoceptors attenuates NE release without suppression of the firing activity [24].

The α_2 adrenoceptors are target for several drugs. Several of them, such as idozaxan, are selective antagonists of α_2-adrenoceptors. Others, such as mirtzapine, risperidone and paliperidone, antagonize α_2-adrenoceptors together with other receptors: α_1 adrenoceptors and 5-$HT_{2A/2C}$ serotonergic receptors [22,25-27].

NE neuronal firing activity is controlled by GABA and glutamate. GABA input to the NE neurons comes from both local (LC) and distant (such as PAG) neurons. GABA inhibits the firing activity of NE neurons *via* a $GABA_A$ receptor-mediated mechanism. The distant afferent inputs into the LC (PGI, CEA and PFC) are exclusively glutamatergic. Glutamate increases the firing activity of NE neurons [28].

The firing activity of NE neurons is negatively regulated by 5-HT and DA. The effect of 5-HT on NE neuronal firing activity is mediated *via* the 5-HT_{2A} and 5-HT_{1A} receptors. The 5-HT_{2A} receptors are situated on GABA neurons projecting to the LC. The 5-HT_{1A} receptors are located on the nerve terminals of glutamate afferents [29,30]. Their activation results in an increase of GABA and in a decrease of glutamate influx into the LC and in inhibition of firing activity of NE neurons [12,22,23,31,32,32]. It was reported that the specific lesion of DA neurons of the VTA results in an increase in firing activity of NE neurons in the LC [33]. However, local application of DA into the LC leads to the inhibition of firing activity of NE neurons [34]. It has been suggested that this inhibitory effect of DA on NE neurons is explained by direct activation of α2-adrenoceptors by DA [35].

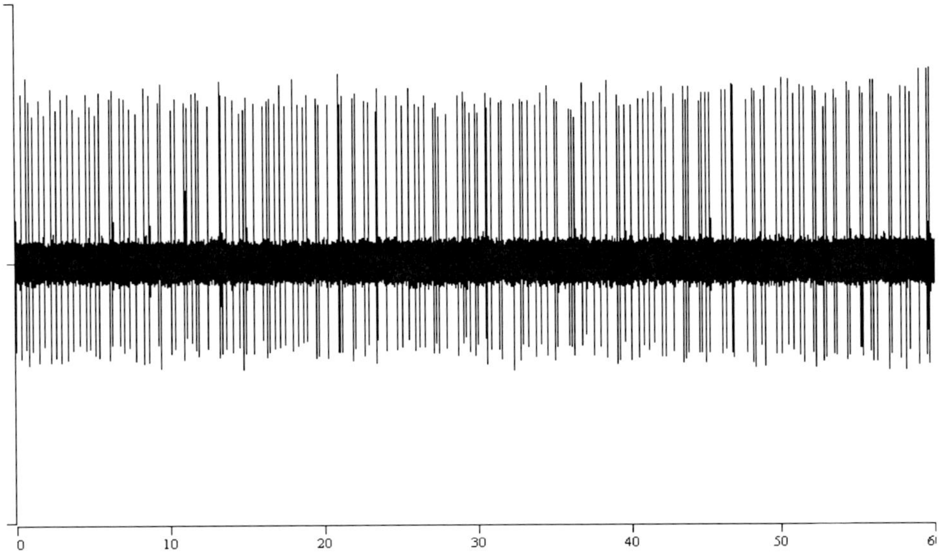

A. Normal firing of a norepinephrine neuron

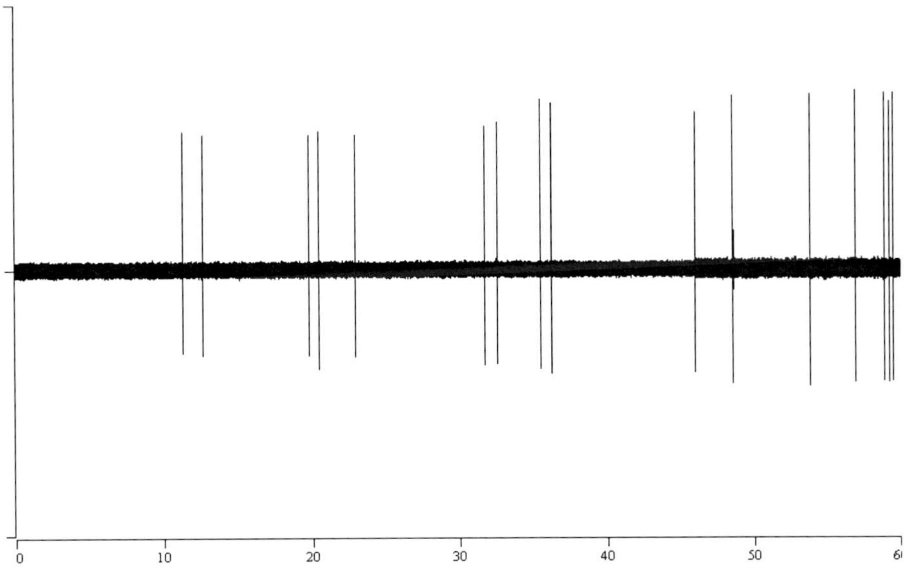

B. Firing of a norepinephrine neuron inhibited by serotonin

Figure 2. The effect of the selective serotonin reuptake inhibitor, escitalopram, on firing activity of norepinephrine neurons. Norepinephrine neurons exhibit tonic-phasic firing activity of 1.5-3.0 Hz, with small (2-3/min) number of short burst (*). Escitalopram inhibits the firing activity of norepinephrine neurons.

2. ROLE OF NOREPINEPHRINE IN MOOD AND COGNITION

2.1. PAIN AND NOCICEPTION

The NE system plays an important role in the perception, modulation, and response to the pain. Nociceptive stimuli arrive into the LC *via* the PGI pathway. NE neurons respond to the nociceptive stimuli by burst firing followed by silence [22,23,30,36-38]. The burst firing of NE results in an increase in NE releases [39].

The role of the NE system in pain response involves both the direct anti-nociception and the triggering on behavioral response to the pain as to an aversive event. The first is probably mediated *via* the NE efferents descending to the brain steam and spinal cord [40-44]. The second might be a function of the reciprocal LC-amygdala network.

The involvement of NE in pain modulation has been demonstrated in several studies. Thus, electrical stimulation of LC or its spinal cord-projecting efferents induces an anti-nociceptive effect in rats [45,46]. Paradoxically, lesioning of NE neurons is also increases the pain threshold [47]. Other studies demonstrated as well that NE can either enhance or suppress nociception in the spinal cord and brainstem levels. It has, therefore, been suggested that different receptors mediate nociceptive and anti-nociceptive effects of NE. Pain stimulation is probably mediated *via* the α_1-, and pain suppression *via* α_2-adrenoceptors [48]. Inflammation and sustained pain induce an increase in α_2-and a decrease in α_1-mediated NE transmission in the spinal cord. Thus, NE probably increases the sensitivity to acute pain and decreases it to chronic pain (Table **2**).

Target of pathway	Receptor	Physiological effect	Behavioral function
Brain steam and spinal cord	α_1 α_2	Excitation Inhibition	Nociception (acute pain) Anti-nociception (chronic pain)
Hypothalamus	α_2	Activation of HPA axis	Neuroendocrine response to the stress
Amygdala	β_1	Excitation	Fear feeling
Hippocampus	β_1, β_2 α_2	Excitation of pyramidal neurons. Induction of LTP. Inhibition of GABA basket cells	Emotional memory. Fear conditioning and extinction.
Prefrontal cortex	β_1 α_2	Excitation of pyramidal neurons. Inhibition of GABA basket cells	General activity, cognition, behavior flexibility, attention, concentration

Table 2. Norepinephrine pathways, their targets and functions.

2.2. EMOTIONS

NE transmission is fundamental in emotions, and in particular in fear and anxiety. Numerous animal and human studies support this paradigm. For example, exposure of rats to stressful stimuli increases NE release in various areas of brain, such as hypothalamus, stria terminalis, and supraoptic nucleus [49-57]. This response, however, desensitizes shortly when the stressful stimuli is repeated [58]. Neuroimaging studies in human subjects demonstrated that aversive emotional stimuli activate amygdala *via* a β-adrenoceptor-mediated mechanism [59]. Another study demonstrates that increase in brain NE reduces the taste threshold in humans, which indicates induction of anxiety [60].

Stress-related stimuli probably trigger NE neuronal activity, *via* the amygdala and PFC afferents. The activation of NE neurons results in an increase in NE transmission in the hypothalamus and limbic system. The increase in NE levels in hypothalamus results in activation of hypothalamus-hypophysis-adrenal (HPA) axis, *via* a β-adrenergic receptor-mediated mechanism. An increase in NE in the limbic system stimulates neuronal activity of glutamatergic pyramidal neurons and decreases the firing of GABA basket interneurons, *via* α_2- and β-adrenergic mechanisms, respectively.

NE-induced activation of the amygdala is probably involved in the emotional response to stress which includes behavior inhibition and freezing awareness. NE activation of hippocampus and PFC mediates the behavioral response to stress and danger. This response includes awareness, attention and activity.

Somewhat similar to the dual involvement of NE in the modulation of pain, this transmitter also paradoxically increases response to acute stress but decrease it to the chronic. This different effect on acute and chronic aversions increases the behavioral adaptation to the changing environmental conditions.

2.3. COGNITION

NE system plays an important role in various cognitive functions: attention, concentration, consolidation and retrieval of memory [61-63]. Studies in human and animal subjects demonstrated that proper NE function is critical for the spatial working memory [64]. In rodents, NE plays an important role in the olfactory memory [65]. NA reuptake inhibition improves the learning and behavior flexibility [66]. In humans, blocking of b_2-adrenoceptor-mediated cortical transmission suppress the numerical memory performance [67]. On the other hand, there is an increase in cortical NE during the spatial memory performance. There is also evidence for a critical role of cortical α_2-adrenoceptors in memory and cognition [68,69].

There are contradictory reports regarding the role of NE in probabilistic learning and decision making. Several suggest that the NE system involved in decision making [70,71]. However, other studies propose that 5-HT and DA mediate the estimation of probability and decision making rather than NE [72]. Its was also suggested that NE trigger on the formation and deformation of synchronized activity networks in the PFC. This effect of NE is probably mediated *via* the b_2-adrenergic receptor-mediated mechanism and mediates behavior adaptation and flexibility [17,73,74].

Several studies postulate that NE plays a central role in consolidation and retrieval of stress-related memory [75-78]. The role of this activity is fear conditioning and extinction. These behavioral effects of NE are probably mediated *via* hippocampal β_2 and α_2 receptors, respectively [79,80].

NE is fundamental in human attention and concentration. It has been demonstrated that idozaxan increase the attention in healthy volunteers [81]. To contrasy, the administration of α_2-adrenergic agonist clonidine results in attention lapses in humans. These clonidine-induced attention difficulties can be reversed by idozaxan [82].

3. NOREPINEPHRINE AND AFFECTIVE DISORDERS

3.1. STRESS AND ANXIETY DISORDERS

The important role of NE in stress response suggests that this transmitter might be involved in anxiety disorders [59]. An increased feeling of fear might be explained by hyper-functionality of the NE system, especially in the amygdala [83]. On the other hand, NE system of the hippocampus mediates fear extinction. Pathological inability to forget aversive events may be therefore explained by reduced NE transmission in the PFC [84]. Therefore, the NE system might play an important role in the pathology of generalized anxiety disorder (GAD), panic disorder (PD) and post-traumatic stress disorder (PTSD). However, different NE pathways may be involved.

Several studies demonstrated that anxiety disorders correlate with changes of NE activity. Fox example, GAD and melancholia are associated with increased plasma NE concentration. Clonidine challenge test studies demonstrated that anxiety associated with decreased activity of α_2-adrenergic autoreceptors, suggesting increased NE transmission. And indeed, increased plasma NE levels were observed in patients with anxiety and melancholia [85].

On the other side, PTSD does not correlate with an increase in basal NE transmission. However, robust increase in plasma concentrations of NE and its metabolites in PTSD patients are observed after their re-exposure to the traumatic contents. The administration of an a_2-adrenoceptor antagonist, yohimbine, resulted in a panic attack in PTSD patients. These observations suggest that an increased NE tone is involved in acute anxiety and panic attack, rather than in the cognitive aspect of PTSD. Further imaging studies are required to study the role of the hippocampal and/or cortical NE system in neuropathology of PTSD [86].

3.2. UNIPOLAR DEPRESSION AND BIPOLAR DISORDER

The NE system is involved in the feeling of energy, fear regulation, general activity, memory and cognition. It is therefore likely that NE is involved in depressive disorder, and in particular in anhedonia, reduced activity and cognition, and in increased anxiety observed in depressed patients. Increased nociception and chronic pain in depression may also be caused, at least in part, by impaired NE transmission [87-89].

Indeed, there is a correlation between impaired NE transmission and depressive behavior. Postmortem studies demonstrated increased NE levels in the brains of unipolar and bipolar suicide victims [90,91]. One positron emission tomography (PET) study suggested that depressive patients have an increased activity of MAO-A, which might result in reduced catecholamine levels [92]. Another imaging study showed correlation between the degree of loss of limbic NE innervation and severity of depressive symptoms in Parkinson patients [93,94].

Contrary to depression, the manic stage of bipolar disorder is characterized by increased energy and activity. Since the activity and energy feeling mediated by NE, an increase in NE transmission might contribute to manic behavior. Indeed, it has been reported that increased urine NE levels follow the manic episode of bipolar illness [87,91].

Based on the evidences, mentioned above, it can be concluded that NE is involved in both depression and mania. This involvement is based, at least in part, on the role of NE in the mediation of energy and activity. Decreased activity in depression might results from attenuation in NE transmission, and manic hyperactivity from an increase in NE tone.

4. EFFECT OF ANTIDEPRESSANT AND MOOD STABILIZING TREATMENTS ON NORADRENERGIC SYSTEM

4.1. ANTIDEPRESSANT DRUGS

Selective serotonin (5-HT) reuptake inhibitors (SSRIs) are used as a first-line treatment for depression and affective disorders. The primary mechanism of action of SSRIs is based on their ability to increase the extracellular levels of 5-HT in the brain. Because of the interactions between 5-HT and NE systems, this increase in 5-HT revels may results in the inhibition of NE neuronal firing activity. It was reported that short (2 days)- and long (14 days)-term administration a highly selective SSRI escitalopram results in suppression of the firing activity of NE neurons in the rat LC [95]. This suppression of NE neuronal firing activity by SSRIs can be reserved by co-administration of blockers of 5-HT_{2A} receptors [96]. It was also reported that the SSRI citalopram decrease extracellular levels of NE in rat LC and BLA [97].

It was demonstrated the acute administration of mirtazapine and short- or long-term regimen with quetiapine increase the firing activity of NE neurons in the rat LC, *via* an α_2-adrenoceptor-mediated mechanism [25,98]. It was also shown that mirtazapine increases extracellular NE levels in the rat brain[99].

It was reported that short-term regimen with trazadone stimulated NE neuronal firing activity in the rat LC, *via* a 5-HT_{2A}-receptor-mediated mechanism [100].

The tricyclic antidepressant desipramine, selective NE reuptake inhibitor reboxetine, dual 5-HT/NE reuptake inhibitor reboxetine, and NE/DA releaser bupropion increase extracellular NE levels in the brain[4,101-104]. This increase leads to the suppression of firing activity of NE neurons in the LC, *via* an α_2-adrenoceptor-mediated mechanism [7,37].

Novel dual NE/DA and triple 5-HT/NE/DA reuptake inhibitors inhibit the firing activity of NE neurons in the rat LC, *via* an α_2-adrenoceptor-mediated mechanism[105,106].

4.2. MOOD STABILIZERS AND ATYPICAL ANTIPSYCHOTIC DRUGS

Lithium (Li) is a common mood stabilizer and it used in the treatment of bipolar disorder. There are numerous evidences that the therapeutic effect of Li is mediated *via* an inositol triphosphate (IP_3) and protein kynase C (PKC)-mediated mechanism [107]. Since the IP_3 and PKC are involved the signal transduction pathway of α_1-adrenoceptors, it is possible that there receptor are target of Li treatment. Indeed, it has been observed that chronic Li suppress the α_1-mediated IP_3 formation and PKC activation. It has been also observed that chronic Li deregulates α_1, α_2 and β-adrenoceptors in the brain [108].

It has been observed that Li potentiates the SSRI milnacipran-induced elevation of extracellular NE levels in the rat PFC [109]. However, several studies suggest that Li might decrease the NE transmission when it is given alone. Chronic Li decreases the cAMP response to NE administration

[110]. Another study demonstrated that iontophoretic administration of Li antagonizes the action of NE on rat PFC neurons [111]. Based on the hypothesis that increased NE transmission is involved in manic episodes, it can be suggested that anti-manic effect of Li ix explained by its suppressive effect on the NE system.

Atypical antipsychotic drugs (AADs), in addition to their application as a first-line treatment in schizophrenia, are also effective mood stabilizers. AADs are successfully used in unipolar and bipolar mood disorders, either as solo treatment or as adjuncts to SSRIs [112-118]. It has been suggested that the beneficial effect of AADs as adjuncts to SSRIs is explained, at least in part, by their ability to reverse the SSRI-induced inhibition of NE neuronal firing activity in the LC [23,119,120]. The SSRI-induced inhibition of NE neuronal firing activity is mediated *via* 5-HT_{2A} receptors [36,121-123]. Thus, antagonists of these receptors might reverse the inhibitory effect of SSRIs on the firing of NE neurons. Indeed, it has been observed with the AADs risperidone and olanzapine co-administered with the SSRIs escitalopram and fluoxetine, respectively [22,124]. One study demonstrated that the AAD olanzapine not only reverses fluoxetine-induced inhibition of NE neuronal firing activity, but also stimulates the firing of NE neurons on its own [125].

In 1989, it was reported for the fist time that idozaxan is beneficial as a mood stabilizer [126]. It has been therefore suggested that α_2-adrenergic autoreceptors could be an important target for antipsychotic and mood-stabilizing treatments [127]. Indeed, certain AADs, such as risperidone, are potent antagonists of a_2-adrenoceptors [27,128]. As a result, risperidone not only reserve the SSRI-induced inhibition of NE neuronal firing activity but also increases it above the value observed in control animals [22]. The electrophysiological findings, demonstrating that the AADs increase and/or prevent the SSRI-induced decrease in the firing activity of NE neurons are consistent with an AAD-induced elevation in extracellular levels of NE, observed in microdialysis studies. The ability of AADs to stimulate the NE transmission might explain, at least in part, their beneficial effect in mood disorders.

4.3. NON-PHARMACEUTICAL TREATMENT STRATEGIES.

Electroconvulsive therapy has been used as antidepressive, mood-stabilizing and antipsychotic treatments [129,130]. It is reported that electroconvulsive shocks (ECS), an animal model for the ECT, affect the NE system. Thus, both acute and chronic ECS increase cortical and hippocampal NE release. Chronic ECS also desensitize α_2-adrenergic autoreceptors in the PFC [131]. Paradoxically, electrophysiological studies report that chronic ECS suppress the firing activity of NE neurons in the ECS [132]. Based on the evidences of ECS-induced increase in brain NE levels, it can be concluded that the beneficial effect of the ECT is mediated, at least in part, *via* NE system.

The vagus nerve stimulation (VNS) is a recently development non-pharmacological antidepressant and mood stabilizing treatment. It has been observed that VNS stimulates brain NE transmission *via* an a_1-adrenoceptor mediated mechanism [133].

5. CONCLUSIONS

The NE system mediates various autonomic, neuroendocrine, emotional and cognitive functions. One of the central roles of NE is response to stress and aversion. This role can be summarized as an activation of response to the acute stress and aversion, followed by decreased reaction to repeated or chronic aversion. Since the response to stress and aversion is a basic part in pathology of mood disorder, NE should play an important role in anxiety, depression and mania. Indeed, this role has been demonstrated in numerous animal and human studies. Majority of antidepressant drugs and mood stabilizers affect NE system as their direct or indirect target. Various medications have different effects on NE neuronal activity. The majority of antidepressants, Li and benzodiazepines suppress NE transmission. Other medications, such as AADs, activate NE neuronal firing activity and NE release. Appropriate combination of different medications, based on the consideration of their effect on NE system, might be critical to obtain good treatment outcome. The combination of SSRIs and AADs in bipolar or treatment-resistant depression is an example for such treatment strategies.

REFERENCES

[1] Kandel ER, Schwartz JH, Jessell TM. Principles of neural science. 2000,1414.

[2] Russo SM, Daniels AJ, Viveros OH, Reinhard JF,Jr. Differences in the reserpine-sensitive storage *in vivo* of 1-methyl-4-phenylpyridinium in rats and mice may explain differences in catecholamine toxicity to 1-methyl-4-phenyl-1,2,3,6-tetrahydropyridine. Neurotoxicology and teratology 1994, 16:277-281.

[3] Reinhard JF,Jr, Daniels AJ, Viveros OH. Potentiation by reserpine and tetrabenazine of brain catecholamine depletions by MPTP (1-methyl-4-phenyl-1,2,3,6-tetrahydropyridine) in the mouse; evidence for subcellular sequestration as basis for cellular resistance to the toxicant. Neuroscience letters 1988, 90:349-353.

[4] Piacentini MF, Clinckers R, Meeusen R, Sarre S, Ebinger G, Michotte Y. Effect of bupropion on hippocampal neurotransmitters and on peripheral hormonal concentrations in the rat. Journal of applied physiology (Bethesda, Md.: 1985) 2003, 95:652-656.

[5] Dong J, Blier P. Modification of norepinephrine and serotonin, but not dopamine, neuron firing by sustained bupropion treatment. Psychopharmacology 2001, 155:52-57.

[6] Corrodi H, Fuxe K. The effect of imipramine on central monoamine neurons. The Journal of pharmacy and pharmacology 1968, 20:230-231.

[7] Curet O, De Montigny C, Blier P. Effect of desipramine and amphetamine on noradrenergic neurotransmission: electrophysiological studies in the rat brain. European journal of pharmacology 1992, 221:59-70.

[8] Lacroix D, Blier P, Curet O, de Montigny C. Effects of long-term desipramine administration on noradrenergic neurotransmission: electrophysiological studies in the rat brain. The Journal of pharmacology and experimental therapeutics 1991, 257:1081-1090.

[9] Beique JC, de Montigny C, Blier P, Debonnel G. Venlafaxine: discrepancy between *in vivo* 5-HT and NE reuptake blockade and affinity for reuptake sites. Synapse (New York, N.Y.) 1999, 32:198-211.

[10] Beique JC, de Montigny C, Blier P, Debonnel G. Blockade of 5-hydroxytryptamine and noradrenaline uptake by venlafaxine: a comparative study with paroxetine and desipramine. British journal of pharmacology 1998, 125:526-532.

[11] Beique JC, Debonnel G, de Montigny C, Blier P. Discrepancies between the *in vitro* and *in*

vivo 5-HT and norepinephrine re-uptake blocking properties of venlafaxine. Annals of the New York Academy of Sciences 1998, 861:290-291.

[12] Szabo ST, Blier P. Effects of the selective norepinephrine reuptake inhibitor reboxetine on norepinephrine and serotonin transmission in the rat hippocampus. Neuropsychopharmacology: official publication of the American College of Neuropsychopharmacology 2001, 25:845-857.

[13] Dawson LA, Nguyen HQ, Geiger A. Effects of venlafaxine on extracellular concentrations of 5-HT and noradrenaline in the rat frontal cortex: augmentation *via* 5-HT1A receptor antagonism. Neuropharmacology 1999, 38:1153-1163.

[14] Blier P, de Montigny C. Serotoninergic but not noradrenergic neurons in rat central nervous system adapt to long-term treatment with monoamine oxidase inhibitors. Neuroscience 1985, 16:949-955.

[15] Blier P, De Montigny C, Azzaro AJ. Modification of serotonergic and noradrenergic neurotransmissions by repeated administration of monoamine oxidase inhibitors: electrophysiological studies in the rat central nervous system. The Journal of pharmacology and experimental therapeutics 1986, 237:987-994.

[16] Kiernan JA, Barr ML. Barr's The human nervous system: an anatomical viewpoint. 1998,518.

[17] Bouret S, Sara SJ. Network reset: a simplified overarching theory of locus coeruleus noradrenaline function. Trends in neurosciences 2005, 28:574-582.

[18] Iijima K, Ohtomo K. Immunocytochemical study using a GABA antiserum for the demonstration of inhibitory neurons in the rat locus ceruleus. The American Journal of Anatomy 1988, 181:43-52.

[19] Jones BE. Noradrenergic locus coeruleus neurons: their distant connections and their relationship to neighboring (including cholinergic and GABAergic) neurons of the central gray and reticular formation. Progress in brain research 1991, 88:15-30.

[20] Devilbiss DM, Waterhouse BD. Norepinephrine exhibits two distinct profiles of action on sensory cortical neuron responses to excitatory synaptic stimuli. Synapse (New York, N.Y.) 2000, 37:273-282.

[21] Aghajanian GK, Vandermaelen CP. Intracellular identification of central noradrenergic and serotonergic neurons by a new double labeling procedure. The Journal of neuroscience: the official journal of the Society for Neuroscience 1982, 2: 1786-1792.

[22] Dremencov E, El Mansari M, Blier P. Noradrenergic Augmentation of Escitalopram Response by Risperidone: Electrophysiologic Studies in the Rat Brain. Biological psychiatry 2007, 61:671-678.

[23] Dremencov E, El Mansari M, Blier P. Distinct electrophysiological effect of paliperidone and risperidone on the firing activity of rat serotonin and norepinephrine neurons. Psychopharmacology 2007, 194:63-72.

[24] Mongeau R, Blier P, de Montigny C. *In vivo* electrophysiological evidence for tonic activation by endogenous noradrenaline of alpha 2-adrenoceptors on 5-hydroxytryptamine terminals in the rat hippocampus. Naunyn-Schmiedeberg's archives of pharmacology 1993, 347:266-272.

[25] Haddjeri N, Blier P, de Montigny C. Effect of the alpha-2 adrenoceptor antagonist mirtazapine on the 5-hydroxytryptamine system in the rat brain. The Journal of pharmacology and experimental therapeutics 1996, 277:861-871.

[26] Haddjeri N, Blier P, de Montigny C. Noradrenergic modulation of central serotonergic neurotransmission: acute and long-term actions of mirtazapine. International clinical psychopharmacology 1995, 10 Suppl 4:11-17.

[27] Richelson E, Souder T. Binding of antipsychotic drugs to human brain receptors focus on newer generation compounds. Life Sciences 2000, 68:29-39.

[28] Torrecilla M, Ruiz-Ortega JA, Ugedo L, Pineda J. Excitatory regulation of noradrenergic neurons by L-arginine/nitric oxide pathway in the rat locus coeruleus *in vivo*. Naunyn-Schmiedeberg's archives of pharmacology 2007, 375:337-347.

[29] Szabo ST, Blier P. Effects of serotonin (5-hydroxytryptamine, 5-HT) reuptake inhibition plus 5-HT(2A) receptor antagonism on the firing activity of norepinephrine neurons. The Journal of pharmacology and experimental therapeutics 2002, 302:983-991.

[30] Szabo ST, Blier P. Serotonin (1A) receptor ligands act on norepinephrine neuron firing through excitatory amino acid and GABA(A) receptors: a microiontophoretic study in the rat locus coeruleus. Synapse (New York, N.Y.) 2001, 42:203-212.

[31] Szabo ST, de Montigny C, Blier P. Modulation of noradrenergic neuronal firing by selective serotonin reuptake blockers. British journal of pharmacology 1999, 126:568-571.

[32] Szabo ST, Blier P. Response of the norepinephrine system to antidepressant drugs. 2001, 6:679-684.

[33] Guiard BP, El Mansari M, Merali Z, Blier P.
Functional interaction between monoaminergic neurons. Biological psychiatry 2007, 61:125S-125S.

[34] Guiard BP, El Mansari M, Blier P. Cross-talk between dopaminergic and noradrenergic systems in the rat ventral tegmental area, locus ceruleus, and dorsal hippocampus. Molecular pharmacology 2008, 74:1463-1475.

[35] El Mansari M, Guiard BP, Chernoloz O, Ghanbari R, Katz N, Blier P. Relevance of norepinephrine-dopamine interactions in the treatment of major depressive disorder. CNS neuroscience & therapeutics 2010, 16:e1-17.

[36] Szabo ST, Blier P. Effects of serotonin (5-hydroxytryptamine, 5-HT) reuptake inhibition plus 5-HT(2A) receptor antagonism on the firing activity of norepinephrine neurons. The Journal of pharmacology and experimental therapeutics 2002, 302:983-991.

[37] Szabo ST, Blier P. Effect of the selective noradrenergic reuptake inhibitor reboxetine on the firing activity of noradrenaline and serotonin neurons. The European journal of neuroscience 2001, 13:2077-2087.

[38] Szabo ST, Blier P. Serotonin (1A) receptor ligands act on norepinephrine neuron firing through excitatory amino acid and GABA(A) receptors: a microiontophoretic study in the rat locus coeruleus. Synapse (New York, N.Y.) 2001, 42:203-212.

[39] Sajedianfard J, Khatami S, Semnanian S, Naghdi N, Jorjani M. *In vivo* measurement of noradrenaline in the locus coeruleus of rats during the formalin test: a microdialysis study. European journal of pharmacology 2005, 512:153-156.

[40] Clark FM, Proudfit HK. The projection of noradrenergic neurons in the A7 catecholamine cell group to the spinal cord in the rat demonstrated by anterograde tracing combined with immunocytochemistry. Brain research 1991, 547:279-288.

[41] Clark FM, Proudfit HK. Projections of neurons in the ventromedial medulla to pontine catecholamine cell groups involved in the modulation of nociception. Brain research 1991, 540:105-115.

[42] Clark FM, Proudfit HK. The projection of locus coeruleus neurons to the spinal cord in the rat determined by anterograde tracing combined with immunocytochemistry. Brain research 1991, 538:231-245.

[43] Clark FM, Yeomans DC, Proudfit HK. The noradrenergic innervation of the spinal cord: differences between two substrains of Sprague-Dawley rats determined using retrograde tracers combined with immunocytochemistry. Neuroscience letters 1991, 125:155-158.

[44] Proudfit HK, Clark FM. The projections of locus coeruleus neurons to the spinal cord. Progress in brain research 1991, 88:123-141.

[45] West WL, Yeomans DC, Proudfit HK. The function of noradrenergic neurons in mediating antinociception induced by electrical stimulation of the locus coeruleus in two different sources of Sprague-Dawley rats. Brain research 1993, 626:127-135.

[46] Yeomans DC, Clark FM, Paice JA, Proudfit HK. Antinociception induced by electrical stimulation of spinally projecting noradrenergic neurons in the A7 catecholamine cell group of the rat. Pain 1992, 48:449-461.

[47] Hammond DL, Proudfit HK. Effects of locus coeruleus lesions on morphine-induced antinociception. Brain research 1980, 188:79-91.

[48] Wei H, Pertovaara A. Spinal and pontine alpha2-adrenoceptors have opposite effects on pain-related behavior in the neuropathic rat. European journal of pharmacology 2006, 551:41-49.

[49] Fendt M, Siegl S, Steiniger-Brach B. Noradrenaline transmission within the ventral bed nucleus of the stria terminalis is critical for fear behavior induced by trimethylthiazoline, a component of fox odor. The Journal of neuroscience: the official journal of the Society for Neuroscience 2005, 25:5998-6004.

[50] Onaka T, Ikeda K, Yamashita T, Honda K. Facilitative role of endogenous oxytocin in noradrenaline release in the rat supraoptic nucleus. The European journal of neuroscience 2003, 18:3018-3026.

[51] Otagiri A, Wakabayashi I, Shibasaki T. Selective corticotropin-releasing factor type 1 receptor antagonist blocks conditioned fear-induced release of noradrenaline in the hypothalamic paraventricular nucleus of rats. Journal of neuroendocrinology 2000, 12:1022-1026.

[52] Shekhar A, Katner JS, Sajdyk TJ, Kohl RR. Role of norepinephrine in the dorsomedial

hypothalamic panic response: an *in vivo* microdialysis study. Pharmacology, biochemistry, and behavior 2002, 71:493-500.

[53] Shekhar A, Katner JS, Rusche WP, Sajdyk TJ, Simon JR. Fear-potentiated startle elevates catecholamine levels in the dorsomedial hypothalamus of rats. Pharmacology, biochemistry, and behavior 1994, 48:525-529.

[54] Shimizu T, Tsuda A, Yokoo H, Mizoguchi K, Gondoh Y, Matsuguchi N, Tanaka M. Effects of stress, non-stress cyclicity on hypothalamic noradrenaline release in rats. The Kurume medical journal 1990, 37:49-53.

[55] Tanaka M. Emotional stress and characteristics of brain noradrenaline release in the rat. Industrial health 1999, 37:143-156.

[56] Yokoo H, Tanaka M, Tanaka T, Tsuda A. Stress-induced increase in noradrenaline release in the rat hypothalamus assessed by intracranial microdialysis. Experientia 1990, 46:290-292.

[57] Yokoo H, Tanaka M, Yoshida M, Tsuda A, Tanaka T, Mizoguchi K. Direct evidence of conditioned fear-elicited enhancement of noradrenaline release in the rat hypothalamus assessed by intracranial microdialysis. Brain research 1990, 536:305-308.

[58] Hajos-Korcsok E, Robinson DD, Yu JH, Fitch CS, Walker E, Merchant KM. Rapid habituation of hippocampal serotonin and norepinephrine release and anxiety-related behaviors, but not plasma corticosterone levels, to repeated footshock stress in rats. Pharmacology, biochemistry, and behavior 2003, 74:609-616.

[59] van Stegeren AH. The role of the noradrenergic system in emotional memory. Acta Psychologica 2008, 127:532-541.

[60] Heath TP, Melichar JK, Nutt DJ, Donaldson LF. Human taste thresholds are modulated by serotonin and noradrenaline. The Journal of neuroscience: the official journal of the Society for Neuroscience 2006, 26:12664-12671.

[61] Harley CW. Norepinephrine and dopamine as learning signals. Neural plasticity 2004, 11:191-204.

[62] Berridge CW, Waterhouse BD. The locus coeruleus-noradrenergic system: modulation of behavioral state and state-dependent cognitive processes. Brain research.Brain research reviews 2003, 42:33-84.

[63] van der Meulen JA, Joosten RN, de Bruin JP, Feenstra MG. Dopamine and noradrenaline efflux in the medial prefrontal cortex during serial reversals and extinction of instrumental goal-directed behavior. Cerebral cortex (New York, N.Y.: 1991) 2007, 17:1444-1453.

[64] Rossetti ZL, Carboni S. Noradrenaline and dopamine elevations in the rat prefrontal cortex in spatial working memory. The Journal of neuroscience: the official journal of the Society for Neuroscience 2005, 25:2322-2329.

[65] Veyrac A, Nguyen V, Marien M, Didier A, Jourdan F. Noradrenergic control of odor recognition in a nonassociative olfactory learning task in the mouse. Learning & memory (Cold Spring Harbor, N.Y.) 2007, 14:847-854.

[66] Seu E, Lang A, Rivera RJ, Jentsch JD. Inhibition of the norepinephrine transporter improves behavioral flexibility in rats and monkeys. Psychopharmacology 2008,

[67] Muller U, Mottweiler E, Bublak P. Noradrenergic blockade and numeric working memory in humans. Journal of psychopharmacology (Oxford, England) 2005, 19:21-28.

[68] Coull JT. Pharmacological manipulations of the alpha 2-noradrenergic system. Effects on cognition. Drugs & aging 1994, 5:116-126.

[69] Matthews KL, Chen CP, Esiri MM, Keene J, Minger SL, Francis PT. Noradrenergic changes, aggressive behavior, and cognition in patients with dementia. Biological psychiatry 2002, 51:407-416.

[70] Nieuwenhuis S, Aston-Jones G, Cohen JD. Decision making, the P3, and the locus coeruleus-norepinephrine system. Psychological bulletin 2005, 131:510-532.

[71] Cohen JD, Aston-Jones G. Cognitive neuroscience: decision amid uncertainty. Nature 2005, 436:471-472.

[72] Chamberlain SR, Muller U, Blackwell AD, Clark L, Robbins TW, Sahakian BJ. Neurochemical modulation of response inhibition and probabilistic learning in humans. Science (New York, N.Y.) 2006, 311:861-863.

[73] Aston-Jones G, Cohen JD. Adaptive gain and the role of the locus coeruleus-norepinephrine system in optimal performance. The Journal of comparative neurology 2005, 493:99-110.

[74] Aston-Jones G, Cohen JD. An integrative theory of locus coeruleus-norepinephrine function: adaptive gain and optimal performance. Annual Review of Neuroscience 2005, 28:403-450.

[75] Ouyang M, Thomas SA. A requirement for memory retrieval during and after long-term extinction learning. Proceedings of the National Academy of Sciences of the United States of America 2005, 102:9347-9352.

[76] Mueller D, Porter JT, Quirk GJ. Noradrenergic signaling in infralimbic cortex increases cell excitability and strengthens memory for fear extinction. The Journal of neuroscience: the official journal of the Society for Neuroscience 2008, 28:369-375.

[77] Hurlemann R, Hawellek B, Matusch A, Kolsch H, Wollersen H, Madea B, Vogeley K, Maier W, Dolan RJ. Noradrenergic modulation of emotion-induced forgetting and remembering. The Journal of neuroscience: the official journal of the Society for Neuroscience 2005, 25:6343-6349.

[78] van Stegeren AH. The role of the noradrenergic system in emotional memory. Acta Psychologica 2008, 127:532-541.

[79] Garelick MG, Storm DR. The relationship between memory retrieval and memory extinction. Proceedings of the National Academy of Sciences of the United States of America 2005, 102:9091-9092.

[80] Davies MF, Tsui J, Flannery JA, Li X, DeLorey TM, Hoffman BB. Activation of alpha2 adrenergic receptors suppresses fear conditioning: expression of c-Fos and phosphorylated CREB in mouse amygdala. Neuropsychopharmacology: official publication of the American College of Neuropsychopharmacology 2004, 29:229-239.

[81] Smith AP, Wilson SJ, Nutt DJ. The effects and after-effects of the alpha-2-adrenoceptor antagonist idazoxan on mood, memory and attention in normal volunteers. 1992, 6:376-381.

[82] Smith A, Nutt D. Noradrenaline and attention lapses. Nature 1996, 380:291.

[83] van Stegeren AH, Wolf OT, Everaerd W, Rombouts SA. Interaction of endogenous cortisol and noradrenaline in the human amygdala. Progress in brain research 2008, 167:263-268.

[84] Mueller D, Porter JT, Quirk GJ. Noradrenergic signaling in infralimbic cortex increases cell excitability and strengthens memory for fear extinction. The Journal of neuroscience: the official journal of the Society for Neuroscience 2008, 28:369-375.

[85] Nutt DJ. Neurobiological mechanisms in generalized anxiety disorder. The Journal of clinical psychiatry 2001, 62 Suppl 11:22-7; discussion 28.

[86] Newport DJ, Nemeroff CB. Neurobiology of posttraumatic stress disorder. Current opinion in neurobiology 2000, 10:211-218.

[87] Nutt DJ. The role of dopamine and norepinephrine in depression and antidepressant treatment. The Journal of clinical psychiatry 2006, 67 Suppl 6:3-8.

[88] Nutt DJ, Baldwin DS, Clayton AH, Elgie R, Lecrubier Y, Montejo AL, Papakostas GI, Souery D, Trivedi MH, Tylee A. Consensus statement and research needs: the role of dopamine and norepinephrine in depression and antidepressant treatment. The Journal of clinical psychiatry 2006, 67 Suppl 6:46-49.

[89] Strittmatter M, Ostertag D, Hoffmann KH, Paulus C, Fischer C, Meyer S. Monoaminergic transmitters in the cerebrospinal fluid of patients with acute, chronic, and intermittent pain Interface between pain and depression? Der Nervenarzt 2005, 76:443-452.

[90] Wiste AK, Arango V, Ellis SP, Mann JJ, Underwood MD. Norepinephrine and serotonin imbalance in the locus coeruleus in bipolar disorder. Bipolar disorders 2008, 10:349-359.

[91] Juckel G, Hegerl U, Mavrogiorgou P, Gallinat J, Mager T, Tigges P, Dresel S, Schroter A, Stotz G, Meller I, Greil W, Moller HJ. Clinical and biological findings in a case with 48-hour bipolar ultrarapid cycling before and during valproate treatment. The Journal of clinical psychiatry 2000, 61:585-593.

[92] Meyer JH, Ginovart N, Boovariwala A, Sagrati S, Hussey D, Garcia A, Young T, Praschak-Rieder N, Wilson AA, Houle S. Elevated monoamine oxidase a levels in the brain: an explanation for the monoamine imbalance of major depression. Archives of General Psychiatry 2006, 63:1209-1216.

[93] Brooks DJ, Piccini P. Imaging in Parkinson's disease: the role of monoamines in behavior. Biological psychiatry 2006, 59:908-918.

[94] Remy P, Doder M, Lees A, Turjanski N, Brooks D. Depression in Parkinson's disease: loss of dopamine and noradrenaline innervation in the limbic system. Brain: a journal of neurology 2005, 128:1314-1322.

[95] Dremencov E, El Mansari M, Blier P. Distinct electrophysiological effects of paliperidone and risperidone on the firing activity of rat serotonin and norepinephrine neurons. Psychopharmacology 2007,

[96] Dremencov E, El Mansari M, Blier P. Brain Norepinephrine System as a Target for Antidepressant and Mood Stabilizing Medications. Current Drug Targets 2009,

[97] Kawahara Y, Kawahara H, Kaneko F, Tanaka M. Long-term administration of citalopram reduces basal and stress-induced extracellular noradrenaline levels in rat brain. Psychopharmacology 2007, 194:73-81.

[98] Chernoloz O, El Mansari M, Blier P. Effects of sustained administration of quetiapine alone and in combination with a serotonin reuptake inhibitor on norepinephrine and serotonin transmission. Neuropsychopharmacology: official publication of the American College of Neuropsychopharmacology 2012, 37:1717-1728.

[99] Millan MJ, Gobert A, Rivet JM, Adhumeau-Auclair A, Cussac D, Newman-Tancredi A, Dekeyne A, Nicolas JP, Lejeune F. Mirtazapine enhances frontocortical dopaminergic and corticolimbic adrenergic, but not serotonergic, transmission by blockade of alpha2-adrenergic and serotonin2C receptors: a comparison with citalopram. The European journal of neuroscience 2000, 12:1079-1095.

[100] Ghanbari R, El Mansari M, Blier P. Electrophysiological impact of trazodone on the dopamine and norepinephrine systems in the rat brain. European neuropsychopharmacology: the journal of the European College of Neuropsychopharmacology 2012, 22:518-526.

[101] Fernandez-Pastor B, Mateo Y, Gomez-Urquijo S, Javier Meana J. Characterization of noradrenaline release in the locus coeruleus of freely moving awake rats by *in vivo* microdialysis. Psychopharmacology 2005, 180:570-579.

[102] Parini S, Renoldi G, Battaglia A, Invernizzi RW. Chronic reboxetine desensitizes terminal but not somatodendritic alpha2-adrenoceptors controlling noradrenaline release in the rat dorsal hippocampus. Neuropsychopharmacology: official publication of the American College of Neuropsychopharmacology 2005, 30:1048-1055.

[103] Sacchetti G, Bernini M, Bianchetti A, Parini S, Invernizzi RW, Samanin R. Studies on the acute and chronic effects of reboxetine on extracellular noradrenaline and other monoamines in the rat brain. British journal of pharmacology 1999, 128:1332-1338.

[104] Li SX, Perry KW, Wong DT. Influence of fluoxetine on the ability of bupropion to modulate extracellular dopamine and norepinephrine concentrations in three mesocorticolimbic areas of rats. Neuropharmacology 2002, 42:181-190.

[105] Katz NS, Guiard BP, El Mansari M, Blier P. Effects of acute and sustained administration of the catecholamine reuptake inhibitor nomifensine on the firing activity of monoaminergic neurons. Journal of psychopharmacology (Oxford, England) 2010, 24:1223-1235.

[106] Guiard BP, Chenu F, El Mansari M, Blier P. Characterization of the electrophysiological properties of triple reuptake inhibitors on monoaminergic neurons. The international journal of neuropsychopharmacology / official scientific journal of the Collegium Internationale Neuropsychopharmacologicum (CINP) 2011, 14:211-223.

[107] Arnsten AF. Ameliorating prefrontal cortical dysfunction in mental illness: inhibition of phosphotidyl inositol-protein kinase C signaling. Psychopharmacology 2008,

[108] Devaki R, Shankar Rao S, Nadgir SM. The effect of lithium on the adrenoceptor-mediated

second messenger system in the rat brain. Journal of psychiatry & neuroscience: JPN 2006, 31:246-252.

[109] Kitaichi Y, Inoue T, Nakagawa S, Izumi T, Koyama T. Effect of milnacipran on extracellular monoamine concentrations in the medial prefrontal cortex of rats pre-treated with lithium. European journal of pharmacology 2005, 516:219-226.

[110] Masana MI, Bitran JA, Hsiao JK, Mefford IN, Potter WZ. Lithium effects on noradrenergic-linked adenylate cyclase activity in intact rat brain: an *in vivo* microdialysis study. Brain research 1991, 538:333-336.

[111] Kovacs P, Hernadi I. Iontophoresis of lithium antagonizes noradrenergic action on prefrontal neurons of the rat. Brain research 2002, 947:150-156.

[112] Blier P, Dremencov E, El Mansari M. Pharmacological dissection of the effect of risperidone on SSRI-induced changes of norepinephrine neuronal firing. Neuropsychopharmacology 2005, 30:S99-S99.

[113] Kennedy SH, Lam RW, Cohen NL, Ravindran AV. Clinical guidelines for the treatment of depressive disorders. IV. Medications and other biological treatments. Canadian journal of psychiatry. Revue canadienne de psychiatrie 2001, 46 Suppl 1:38S-58S.

[114] Kennedy SH, Lam RW. Enhancing outcomes in the management of treatment resistant depression: a focus on atypical antipsychotics. Bipolar disorders 2003, 5 Suppl 2:36-47.

[115] Papakostas GI, Shelton RC, Smith J, Fava M. Augmentation of antidepressants with atypical antipsychotic medications for treatment-resistant major depressive disorder: a meta-analysis. The Journal of clinical psychiatry 2007, 68:826-831.

[116] Simon JS, Nemeroff CB. Aripiprazole augmentation of antidepressants for the treatment of partially responding and nonresponding patients with major depressive disorder. The Journal of clinical psychiatry 2005, 66:1216-1220.

[117] Tremblay P, Blier P. Catecholaminergic strategies for the treatment of major depression. Current Drug Targets 2006, 7:149-158.

[118] Uzun S, Kozumplik O, Mimica N, Folnegovic-Smalc V. Aripiprazole: an overview of a novel antipsychotic. 2005, 17:67-75.

[119] Blier P, Szabo ST. Potential mechanisms of action of atypical antipsychotic medications in treatment-resistant depression and anxiety. The Journal of clinical psychiatry 2005, 66 Suppl 8:30-40.

[120] Dremencov E, El Mansari M, Blier P. Distinct electrophysiological effect of paliperidone and risperidone on the firing activity of rat serotonin and norepinephrine neurons. 2007, in press: 0-0.

[121] Celada P, Puig M, Amargos-Bosch M, Adell A, Artigas F. The therapeutic role of 5-HT1A and 5-HT2A receptors in depression. Journal of psychiatry & neuroscience: JPN 2004, 29:252-265.

[122] El Mansari M, Blier P. Responsiveness of 5-HT(1A) and 5-HT2 receptors in the rat orbitofrontal cortex after long-term serotonin reuptake inhibition. Journal of psychiatry & neuroscience: JPN 2005, 30:268-274.

[123] Marek GJ, Martin-Ruiz R, Abo A, Artigas F. The selective 5-HT2A receptor antagonist M100907 enhances antidepressant-like behavioral effects of the SSRI fluoxetine. Neuropsychopharmacology: official publication of the American College of Neuropsychopharmacology 2005, 30:2205-2215.

[124] Seager MA, Barth VN, Phebus LA, Rasmussen K. Chronic coadministration of olanzapine and fluoxetine activates locus coeruleus neurons in rats: implications for bipolar disorder. Psychopharmacology 2005, 181:126-133.

[125] Dawe GS, Huff KD, Vandergriff JL, Sharp T, O'Neill MJ, Rasmussen K. Olanzapine activates the rat locus coeruleus: *in vivo* electrophysiology and c-Fos immunoreactivity. Biological psychiatry 2001, 50:510-520.

[126] Osman OT, Rudorfer MV, Potter WZ. Idazoxan: a selective alpha 2-antagonist and effective sustained antidepressant in two bipolar depressed patients. Archives of General Psychiatry 1989, 46:958-959.

[127] Nutt DJ. Putting the 'A' in atypical: does 2-adrenoceptor antagonism account for the therapeutic advantage of new antipsychotics. 1994, 8:193-195.

[128] Janssen PA, Niemegeers CJ, Awouters F, Schellekens KH, Megens AA, Meert TF. Pharmacology of risperidone (R 64 766), a new antipsychotic with serotonin-S2 and dopamine-D2 antagonistic properties. The Journal of pharmacology and experimental therapeutics 1988, 244:685-693.

[129] Eitan R, Lerer B. Nonpharmacological, somatic treatments of depression: electroconvulsive therapy and novel brain stimulation modalities. Dialogues in clinical neuroscience 2006, 8:241-258.

[130] Shapira B, Calev A, Lerer B. Optimal use of electroconvulsive therapy: choosing a treatment schedule. The Psychiatric clinics of North America 1991, 14:935-946.

[131] Thomas DN, Nutt DJ, Holman RB. Effects of acute and chronic electroconvulsive shock on noradrenaline release in the rat hippocampus and frontal cortex. British journal of pharmacology 1992, 106:430-434.

[132] Grant MM, Weiss JM. Effects of chronic antidepressant drug administration and electroconvulsive shock on locus coeruleus electrophysiologic activity. Biological psychiatry 2001, 49:117-129.

[133] Manta S, El Mansari M, Debonnel G, Blier P. Electrophysiological and neurochemical effects of long-term vagus nerve stimulation on the rat monoaminergic systems. The international journal of neuropsychopharmacology / official scientific journal of the Collegium Internationale Neuropsychopharmacologicum (CINP) 2012,1-12.

Send Orders for Reprints to reprints@benthamscience.net
Neurobiology of Mood Disorders, 2014, 127-138

CHAPTER 6

PATHOPHYSIOLOGY OF MOOD DISORDERS: DOPAMINERGIC MECHANISMS

OLGA CHERNOLOZ*

Toronto, ON, Canada

Abstract: The serendipitous discovery of the antidepressant potential of inhibitors of monoamine oxidase (MAO, protein facilitating catabolism of the monoamines) in 1950 led to the development of the monoamine theory of depression. This theory was based on the correlation between the buildup of monoamines serotonin (5-HT), norepinephrine (NE) and dopamine (DA) in CNS, achieved with blockade of their cellular degradation by the above pharmacological agents, and the observed antidepressant effect. While the role of norepinephrine and serotonin in the pathophysiology and/or treatment of depression received a significant attention and was studied in detail in years following that discovery, DA remained a 'forgotten child' for some time. In past two decades, however, the relationship between the function/state of the DA system and depression has been studied from various perspectives

This section will be devoted to the review of evidence suggesting the important role of the DA system in pathophysiology and/or treatment of depression. The main features of DA system neuroanatomy and neurotransmission, critical for the proper understanding of physiological basis of depression, its treatment and applicable research methods, will be outlined. The focus will be made on the principal findings elucidating the involvement of DA in etiology of mood disorders, particularly depression. The findings from both clinical and animal studies will be discussed.

Keywords: Dopamine (DA), serotonin (5-HT), norepinephrine (NE), depression, ventral tegmental area (VTA), tricyclic antidepressant drugs (TCA), selective serotonin reuptake inhibitors (SSRIs), electrophysiology, dopamine-1/2 (D1/D2) receptors, dopamine transporter (DAT), serotonin-2C (5-HT2C) receptors.

1. DOPAMINERGIC SYSTEM

After Carlsson and his group have shown that despite presence of both NE and DA in the CNS, their regional distribution varied significantly, the role of DA as a neurotransmitter was established [1]. Up until then DA was only viewed as a NE precursor. In rats the number of DA cells in the mesencephalic tegmentum has been estimated at about 15,000–20,000 on each side of the brain [2,3]: some 9,000 in the ventral tegmental area (VTA) and the remainder in the zona compacta of the substantia nigra and retrorubral field [3]. Unlike 5-HT and NE, the general neuronal organization of the DA system is rather compartmentalized with DA neurons distributed across several nuclei. In the rat CNS, four major DA projection subsystems have been described — mesocortical, mesolimbic, nigrostriatal and tuberoinfundibular. Additionally, several parts of the diencephalon (A11-A15) as well as both the olfactory bulb (A16) and retina (A17), contain DA neurons. The VTA (A8, A10) projections to the cingulate and medial prefrontal cortex constitute the mesocortical pathway, while VTA afferents to the limbic structures like nucleus accumbens, amygdala, hippocampus and olfactory tubercle form the mesolimbic pathway. Together these two pathways mediate regulation of the emotional control, motivation, reward and cognition. Therefore, their malfunction is believed to be involved in etiology of several psychiatric conditions including affective disorders, depression,

***Address correspondence to Olga Chernoloz:** Toronto, ON, Canada; E-mail: olga4e@yahoo.ca

schizophrenia and addiction. The substantia nigra pars compacta DA neurons innervate the dorsal striatal structures like caudate, putamen and globus pallidus forming the nigrostriatal DA pathway. The proper function of this system is crucial for the sensomotor coordination; degradation of DA cells within this pathway underlies pathophysiology of Parkinson's Disease (PD). The tuberoinfundibular DA system is comprised by DA projections from the hypothalamus arcuate and periventricular nuclei to the anterior of pituitary, and is involved in the hormonal regulation. Disruption of its function may produce (unfavorable) neuroendocrine effects. The descending DA projection to the spinal cord originates from DA neurons (A11) in hypothalamus.

Synthesis of DA predominates in the nerve terminals but also occurs everywhere in the cytosol of DA neurons. There are two enzymatic steps involved in the synthesis process [4]. In the brain cathecholamine precursor L-tyrosine is hydroxilated to L-DOPA by the enzyme tyrosine hydroxylase (TH). Dopamine synthesis is completed in the next step, when L-aromatic amino acid decarboxylase converts L-DOPA to DA [5]. Tyrosine hydroxylase is the rate-limiting step in synthesis of DA and thus controls the neuronal concentrations of DA. The physiological tyrosine concentrations saturate TH and its increase usually does not elevate the rate of DA synthesis. The activation of DA neurons leads to the increase of TH activity; its expression can be either upregulated or downregulated by different drugs such as nicotine, caffeine, morphine, or antidepressants *via* modulation of the transcriptional regulatory elements of TH gene promoter [6].

Accumulation of DA in the vesicles depends on the operation of the VMAT2 [7]. The driving force for uptake into the synaptic vesicles is an ATP-dependent proton electrochemical gradient generated in the synaptic vesicle membrane. Thus, VMAT2 decreases cytoplasmic concentration of DA and prevents its metabolism by MAO. Administration of reserpine that competes with 5-HT,NE and DA for the VMAT binding site, thus preventing their effective storage, produces drastic reduction in the release of monoamines [8]. Two vesicular compartments of DA believed to exist [9]. One vesicular pool is designated for rapid releasable of DA. This releasable compartment represents the vesicles located near the presynaptic membrane and contains 5– 20% of the total DA content. The larger pool is designed for the reserve transmitter storage and is inactive during most physiological processes.

The release of DA mainly occurs *via* exocytosis in a Ca^{2+}-dependent manner, when the action potential invades the terminal (Figure **1**). The extent of DA release is dependent on both rate and pattern of DA neuronal firing. Indeed, burst firing, characteristic for DA neurons, is believed to be a more efficient form of the signal propagation, as more transmitter is released per pulse fired in burst, than single-spike mode [10,11]. The reverse transport of DA across the membrane by DA transporter (DAT) represents another form of DA release [12]. It occurs in Ca^{2+}-independent manner, however its role in release under physiological conditions is not functionally significant.

The metabolism of DA occurs *via* enzymatic degradation by COMT (extracellularly) and by MAO (both extra- and intracellularly) [4]. The MAO oxidatively deaminates DA and its O-methylated derivative, 3-methoxytyramine, forming transient derivative 3,4-dihydroxyphenylacetaldehyde. This aldehyde is than rapidly catabolised by the aldehyde dehydrogenases to 3,4-dihydroxyphenylacetic acid (DOPAC). About 40% of DOPAC is eliminated from the brain, while other 60% get further metabolized by the COMT resulting in homovanilic acid (HVA) formation. Accumulation of DOPAC and HVA in the brain or cerebrospinal fluid (CSF) is often used as an index of functional activity of the DA system.

The termination of action of synaptically released DA is primarily mediated by the reuptake process carried out by the membrane carrier - DAT. Dopamine transporter is a 12-membrane spanning hydrophobic glycoprotein, member of the family of Na^+/Cl^--dependent plasma membrane transporters.

As follows from the receptor family name, DAT is dependent on the Na^+ co-transport and requires extracellular Cl^- [13]. As reuptake depends on the Na^+ gradient across the neuronal membrane, drugs that inhibit Na^+/K^--transporting adenosine triphosphase or open Na^+ channels subsequently decrease the DA reuptake. As Na^+ gradient across the plasma membrane varies by the neuron state, DAT may operate in a reverse-mode pumping out DA from the cell to the synaptic cleft [14]. The neuronal reuptake is saturable and energy-dependent.

The molecular characterization of the DAT showed that it exhibits 66% homology with NET and is highly conserved between species.

The DA carrier mRNA occurs in presynaptic brain areas in which DA is synthesized: it is highest in the substantia nigra and the VTA and also detected in arcuate nucleus, olfactory bulb, and the retina. The regional distribution of the carrier follows the expected localization of the distinct DA neurons; however, DAT expression varies greatly among DA cell groups and is not expressed in all DA neurons. For instance, the hypothalamic tuberoinfundibular DA cells that release DA into the pituitary portal blood stream, lack DAT mRNA and protein. The DAT expression is also low in primate prefrontal cortex where DA reuptake is predominantly carried out by NET [15]. Not only neurons, but glia also carries DAT [16]. However the functional significance of the glial DA reuptake is not clear.

As DAT maintains transmitter homeostasis its modulation plays an important role in neuropsychiatric disorders. Blockade of this protein by cocaine and other drugs of abuse leads to the drastic increase in synaptic DA concentration and thus underlies their reinforcing properties. However, the binding site of these molecules is distinct from the transmitter binding site. Thus, DAT blockers interacting with the neurotransmitter binding site are devote of addictive properties and were shown to possess the antidepressant potential.

The existence of two distinct groups of DA receptors was proposed based upon a combination of biochemical, pharmacological and anatomical criteria [17,18]. Thus, DA receptor family is comprised by D_1- like and D_2-like receptors. Subsequent molecular biological studies postulated that based on the sequence homology as well as similarity in function, D_1 group contained D_1 and D_5 receptors, and D_2 group was made of D_2, D_3 and D_4 receptors [17-19]. The D_1 receptors activate AC *via* coupling to a Gs protein and increase cAMP formation, whereas D_2 receptors inhibit AC *via* Gi coupling decreasing cAMP and/or increasing IP3 production [18]. Interestingly, despite opposite effects on the signal transduction, D_1 and D_2 receptors can form hetero-oligomeric complexes [19].

The distribution of D_1 receptors was determined by the autoradiography. The D_1 receptors are localized throughout the brain regions receiving DA afferents with highest densities in the nucleus accumbens, caudate-putamen, olfactory tubercule and substantia nigra, as well as thalamus, hypothalamus and cortex. The D_5 receptors are limited to thalamus, hypothalamus and hippocampus. Frontocortical localization of D_1 receptors implicates their importance in the cognitive function.

Similarly to D_1 receptors, binding sites for D_2 receptors were detected in numerous brain areas receiving DA innervation [20]. However, levels of D_2 expression were much greater in projecting loci - VTA and substinta nigra, and in pituitary gland. The somatodendritic localization of these receptors hints their involvement in autoregulation. Indeed, activation of D_2 autoreceptors located on the cell body of midbrain DA neurons decreases the firing activity of the latter, while stimulation of terminal D_2 autoreceptors inhibits synthesis and release of the neurotransmitter (Fig. **1**).

The D_2 receptors are believed to be important players in psychopathology and/or treatment of schizophrenia, depression, PD and attention deficit hyperactivity.

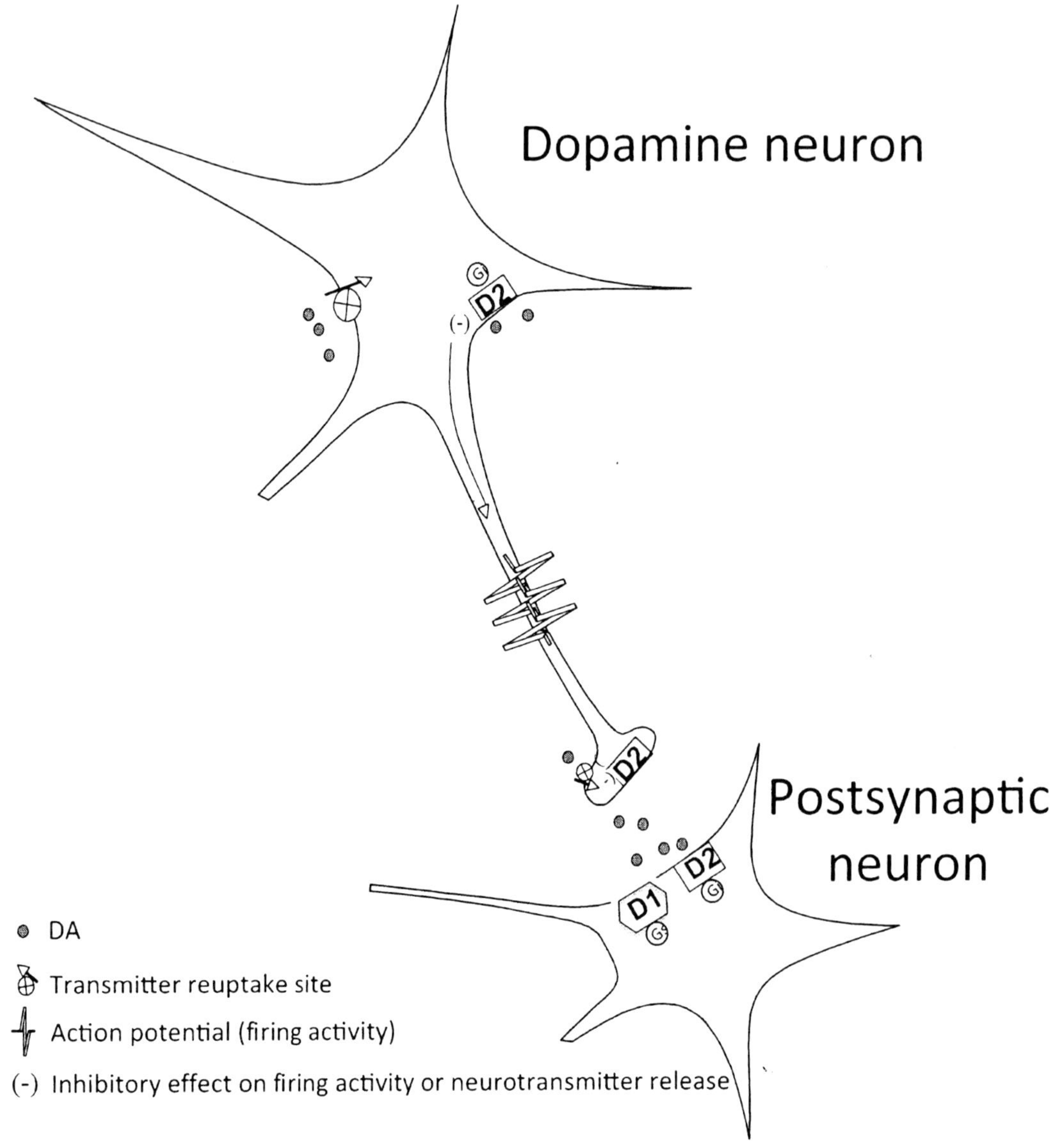
Dopamine neuron
D2
(-)
D2
Postsynaptic
neuron
D2
D1
DA
Transmitter reuptake site
Action potential (firing activity)
(-) Inhibitory effect on firing activity or neurotransmitter release

Figure 1.

2. DOPAMINERGIC DEREGULATION IN DEPRESSION

The validation of animal models of mood disorders is complicated by the emotional nature of their symptomatology in humans. However the greater degree of experimental control and flexibility of methodology, permitted by the animal studies, allow a unique tool for testing of the existing hypotheses of depression pathophysiology. In animals several approaches have been used for investigation of the role of DA system in depression. First, the changes in function of the DA system in modeled depressed sates were revealed in several studies. The levels of DA were found to be significantly decreased in caudate and nucleus accumbens of animals in the 'learned helplessness' depression model (where the state of behavioral despair is induced by the exposure to the inescapable stressor). The development of this state could be prevented by pretreatment with the DA agonists [21,22], whereas administration of DA blockers disallowed a beneficial action of antidepressants [23]. Similarly, in the 'forced swim test', used for prediction of the antidepressant activity of drugs, the antidepressant-like effect of TCAs, D_2-like receptor agonists and a NE/DA blocking drug nomifensine was reversed by the D_2-like receptor antagonists [24-27]. The 'chronic mild stress' depression model relies on induction of an anhedonic state in animals subjected to the low-level stressors over a prolonged period of time [28]. Rodents undergoing this testing paradigm present with a lower D_2/D_3 receptor binding within the nucleus accumbens. Interestingly, this decrease and the concomitant 'depressed' behavior can be reversed by the long-term administration of antidepressant drugs [29]. Analogously to the models described above, this antidepressant-like effect can, in turn, be prevented by co-administration of the agents blocking the D_2-like receptors [30,31].

Anhedonia – one of the core symptoms of depression is associated with the dysfunction of the DA reward system. In clinic the amphetamine challenge leading to the increased DA release was found to produce greater reward response and altered activation of brain regions mediating it, in depressed individuals, than controls [32,33]. Such effect suggests the diminished basal function of DA neurotransmission in depression. Furthermore, the increased sensitivity to the psychostimulant-induced DA release was found to be potentiated by the glucocorticoids [34]. As glucocorticoid levels are known to be increased in depressed patients, alternations in DA function may be in part influenced by this neuroendocrine pathology.

Further confirmation substantiating the involvement of the DA system in depression comes from the genetic studies. Metaanalysis combining the data from 12 studies totaling 2071 patients showed a consistent association between the D_4 receptor polymorphism and the vulnerability for depression [35]. Two more studies have documented the increased risk of affective disorders in individuals with D_3 receptor polymorphism [36,37].

Another line of evidence of DA malfunction in major depressive disorder (MDD) comes from the neuroimaging studies. The binding towards D_2 receptor was found to be enhanced in patients hospitalized with depression [38-40]. However, it is not clear whether this alternation in D_2 neuronal population is secondary to depression, or psychomotor retardation, often comorbid with it. This raise may indicate sensitization of the receptors and/or increase in their number and/or decrease of the synaptically available endogenous DA which competes with the testing agent for the binding site. In fact, the increase in sensitivity of D_2 receptors was linked to the treatment resistance [41]. In addition, PET studies revealed a decrease in the DAT density in patients suffering from depression, in comparison to controls [42,43]. Interestingly, the same changes were produced by the induced DA depletion [44,45]. The results of histopathological research closely follow the findings documented in the above neuroimaging studies: the levels of D_2 receptor binding were found to be significantly greater, whereas those of DAT - significantly lower in amygdala of depressed patients, compared to the non-depressed individuals postmortem [46]. The increase in binding for D_2 receptors, paralleled by the decrease in binding for DAT, observed in depression sufferers, likely reflects an adaptive change secondary to the drop in levels of available DA.

The biochemical studies represent another line of evidence confirming the DA deficiency in MDD. The turnover of DA can be estimated by measurement of the main metabolite levels in cerebrospinal fluid (CSF) and plasma. Several clinical studies have documented the decrease of HVA and other DA metabolites in patients diagnosed with MDD, compared to the age-matched controls [47-49]. Indeed, the level of HVA was found to be negatively correlated with the severity of depression [50,51]. In contrast, the levels of HVA in plasma and CSF of patients diagnosed with MDD with psychotic features was found to be significantly greater than in controls. Additionally, HVA levels were found to be elevated in suicide attempters and victims [52,53]. Indeed, the longitudinal study put into evidence an increase in risk of suicide attempts in MDD patients with low CSF HVA levels [54].

The high incidence of MDD comorbidity in Parkinson's disease, characterized by the progressive degeneration of nigrostriatal DA system and a consecutive denervation of the target brain regions, again emphasizes the importance of the DA system in depression. In fact, almost 50% of parkinsonian patients present with depressive symptoms, which improve after treatment with pro-dopaminergic agents [55]. While it has been suggested that the increased occurrence of depressive symptoms in patients suffering from PD is a mere result of the behavioral discomfort associated with a chronic illness diagnosis, several lines of evidence indicate otherwise. Most importantly, the depressive symptoms precede the deregulation of the motor system, thus clearly showing that the mood worsening is not a result of the reported serious clinical condition. Moreover, other debilitating chronic illnesses not associated with the DA system degradation, are not bearing such a great degree of comorbidity with depression [56,57].

The efficacy of drugs selectively targeting the DA system against the depressive symptoms, serves as yet another example of strong involvement of DA in depression neurobiology and/or treatment. Pramipexole is a selective D_2-like receptor agonist approved for the treatment of Parkinson's disease and restless legs syndrome [58-60]. Aside from its use in the above neurological conditions, this drug was also shown to be efficacious in the treatment of major depressive disorder, both as a monotherapy [61,62] and as an augmenting agent in treatment-resistant depressed patients [63-65]. Furthermore, not only pramipexole, but other D_2 receptor agonists with unrelated chemical structures, such as pergolide, piribedil and bromocriptine have also been shown to possess antidepressant-like properties in animal studies and a therapeutic action in depressed patients [66-69]. Imaging studies provided evidence that in depressed patients who achieve remission using pramipexole, the metabolic activity in brain areas affected by MDD was normalized [70]. Moreover, prolonged pramipexole treatment not only brought brain metabolism to the control level, it was also found to restore cortical plasticity in patients suffering from restless leg syndrome [71]. Furthermore, chronic administration of D_2 receptor agonists was found to promote neuronal proliferation in rat hippocampus [72,73]. This finding is of crucial importance as enhancement of neurogenesis appears to be one of the common changes occurring with drugs endowed with the antidepressant properties.

The changes in the state/function of the DA system induced by the antidepressant treatments (both pharmacological and non-pharmacological) represent another piece of data supporting the involvement of the discussed system in the pathophysiology and/or treatment of depression. Several animal studies suggest an increase in the functional sensitivity of postsynaptic D_2-like receptors located in the ventral striatum [74,75]. This hypothesis is evidenced by potentiation of the behavioral effects of DA agonists by antidepressants, administered in a chronic manner, as well as repeated electro-convulsive shocks and sleep deprivation (known to possess an antidepressant properties in animals and humans) [76]. Moreover, the concentrations of DA in rodent nucleus accumbens were found to increase following administration of TCAs and SSRIs [77]. Similarly, transcarnial magnetic stimulation of frontocortical areas elevated the levels of DA in both animals and humans [78-80]. In addition, the expression of D_3 receptor in rodent nucleus accumbens was found to rise following the long-term administration of antidepressants and repeated electro-convulsive shocks. [81].

Taking together these changes clearly indicate a decrease in the function of DA system in depression. Though it is not always clear if the alterations described above are causative of the neurobiological and behavioral changes observed in depression, or are consecutive of them, they reflect a strong link between the deficiency in function of DA system and the depression pathophysiology. Further development of the research techniques may enable more precise understanding of the processes underlying the development of depression and the role of DA in this process.

REFERENCES

[1] Carlsson A. The contribution of drug research to investigating the nature of endogenous depression. Pharmakopsychiatrie und Neuropsychopharmakologie 1976, 9:2-10.

[2] Hedreen JC, Chalmers JP. Neuronal degeneration in rat brain induced by 6-hydroxydopamine; a histological and biochemical study. Brain Res 1972, 47:1-36.

[3] Swanson LW. The projections of the ventral tegmental area and adjacent regions: A combined fluorescent retrograde tracer and immunofluorescence study in the rat. Brain Res Bull 1982, 9:321-353.

[4] Von Bohlen Und Halbach O, Krieglstein K, Schober A, Schulz JB. The dopaminergic nigrostriatal system: Development, physiology, disease. Cell Tissue Res 2004, 318:3.

[5] Deutch AY, Roth RH. Calcitonin gene-related peptide in the ventral tegmental area: Selective modulation of prefrontal cortical dopamine metabolism. Neurosci Lett 1987, 74:169-174.

[6] Kilbourne, E.J., Nankova, B.B., Lewis, E.J., McMahon, A., Osaka, H., Sabban, D.B., Sabban, E.L. Regulated expression of the tyrosine hydroxylase gene by membrane depolarization. Identification of the responsive element and possible second messengers. Journal of Biological Chemistry 1992, 267:7563-756

[7] Weihe E, Eiden LE. Chemical neuroanatomy of the vesicular amine transporters. FASEB Journal 2000, 14:2435-2449.

[8] Henry J-, Scherman D. Radioligands of the vesicular monoamine transporter and their use as markers of monoamine storage vesicles. Biochem Pharmacol 1989, 38:2395-2404.

[9] Pieribone, V.A., Shupliakov, O., Brodin, L., Hilfiker-Rothenfluh, S., Czernik, A.J., Greengard, P. Distinct pools of synaptic vesicles in neurotransmitter release. Nature 1995, 375:493-497

[10] Gonon FG. Nonlinear relationship between impulse flow and dopamine released by rat midbrain dopaminergic neurons as studied by *in vivo* electrochemistry. Neuroscience 1988, 24:19-28.

[11] Garris PA, Ciolkowski EL, Pastore P, Wightman RM. Efflux of dopamine from the synaptic cleft in the nucleus accumbens of the rat brain. Journal of Neuroscience 1994, 14:6084-6093.

[12] Raiteri M, Cerrito F, Cervoni AM, Levi G. Dopamine can be released by two mechanisms

differentially affected by the dopamine transport inhibitor nomifensine. J Pharmacol Exp Ther 1979, 208:195-202.

[13] Norregaard L, Gether U. The monoamine neurotransmitter transporters: Structure, conformational changes and molecular gating. Current Opinion in Drug Discovery and Development 2001, 4:591-601.

[14] Gainetdinov RR, Sotnikova TD, Caron MG. Monoamine transporter pharmacology and mutant mice. Trends Pharmacol Sci 2002, 23:367-373.

[15] Gresch PJ, Sved AF, Zigmond MJ, Finlay JM. Local influence of endogenous norepinephrine on extracellular dopamine in rat medial prefrontal cortex. J Neurochem 1995, 65:111-116.

[16] Meng, S.Z., Ozawa, Y., Itoh, M., Takashima, S. Developmental and age-related changes of dopamine transporter, and dopamine D_1 and D_2 receptors in human basal ganglia. Brain Research 1999, 843:136-144

[17] Garau L, Govoni S, Stefanini E. Dopamine receptors: Pharmacological and anatomical evidences indicate that two distinct dopamine receptor populations are present in rat striatum. Life Sci 1978, 23:1745-1750.

[18] Kebabian JW, Calne DB. Multiple receptors for dopamine. Nature 1979, 277:93-96.

[19] Rashid AJ, So CH, Kong MMC, Furtak T, El-Ghundi M, Cheng R, *et al.* D_1-D_2 dopamine receptor heterooligomers with unique pharmacology are coupled to rapid activation of Gq/11 in the striatum. Proc Natl Acad Sci U S A 2007, 104:654-659.

[20] Meador-Woodruff JH, Mansour A, Healy DJ, Kuehn R, Zhou Q-, Bunzow JR, *et al.* Comparison of the distributions of D1 and D2 dopamine receptor mRNAs in the rat brain. Neuropsychopharmacology 1991, 5:231-242.

[21] Anisman H, Irwin J, Sklar LS. Deficits of escape performance following catecholamine depletion: Implications for behavioral deficits induced by uncontrollable stress. Psychopharmacology (Berl) 1979, 64:163-170.

[22] Anisman H, Remington G, Sklar LS. Effect of inescapable shock on subsequent escape performance: Catecholaminergic and cholinergic mediation of response initiation and maintenance. Psychopharmacology (Berl) 1979, 61:107-124.

[23] Muscat R, Sampson D, Willner P. Dopaminergic mechanism of imipramine action in an animal model of depression. Biol Psychiatry 1990, 28:223-230.

[24] Basso AM, Gallagher KB, Bratcher NA, Brioni JD, Moreland RB, Hsieh GC, *et al.* Antidepressant-like effect of $D_{2/3}$ receptor-, but not D_4 receptor-activation in the rat forced swim test. Neuropsychopharmacology 2005, 30:1257-1268.

[25] Borsini F, Meli A. The forced swimming test: Its contribution to the understanding of the mechanisms of action of antidepressants. Dopamine and Mental Depression 1990:63-76.

[26] Renard CE, Dailly E, Nic Dhonnchadha BA, Hascoet M, Bourin M. Is dopamine a limiting factor of the antidepressant-like effect in the mouse forced swimming test? Prog Neuro-Psychopharmacol Biol Psychiatry 2004, 28:1255-1259.

[27] Cervo L, Grignaschi G, Samanin R. The role of the mesolimbic dopaminergic system in the desipramine effect in the forced swimming test. Eur J Pharmacol 1990, 178:129-133.

[28] D'Aquila PS, Collu M, Pani L, Gessa GL, Serra G. Antidepressant-like effect of selective dopamine D1 receptor agonists in the behavioural despair animal model of depression. Eur J Pharmacol 1994, 262:107-111.

[29] Papp M, Klimek V, Willner P. Parallel changes in dopamine D_2 receptor binding in limbic forebrain associated with chronic mild stress-induced anhedonia and its reversal by imipramine. Psychopharmacology (Berl) 1994, 115:441-446.

[30] Willner P, Muscat R, Papp M. Chronic mild stress-induced anhedonia: A realistic animal model of depression. Neurosci Biobehav Rev 1992, 16:525-534.

[31] Cheeta S, Broekkamp C, Willner P. Stereospecific reversal of stress-induced anhedonia by mianserin and its [+]-enantiomer. Psychopharmacology (Berl) 1994, 116:523-528.

[32] Tremblay LK, Naranjo CA, Cardenas L, Herrmann N, Busto UE. Probing brain reward system function in major depressive disorder: Altered response to dextroamphetamine. Arch Gen Psychiatry 2002, 59:409-416.

[33] Tremblay LK, Naranjo CA, Graham SJ, Herrmann N, Mayberg HS, Hevenor S, *et al.* Functional neuroanatomical substrates of altered reward processing in major depressive disorder revealed by a dopaminergic probe. Arch Gen Psychiatry 2005, 62:1228-1236.

[34] Oswald LM, Wong DF, McCaul M, Zhou Y, Kuwabara H, Choi L, *et al.* Relationships among ventral striatal dopamine release, cortisol secretion, and subjective responses to amphetamine. Neuropsychopharmacology 2005, 30:821-832.

[35] López León S, Croes EA, Sayed-Tabatabaei FA, Claes S, Van Broeckhoven C, Van Duijn CM. The dopamine D_4 receptor gene 48-base-pair-repeat polymorphism and mood disorders: A meta-analysis. Biol Psychiatry 2005, 57:999-1003.

[36] Chiaroni P, Azorin JM, Dassa D, Henry JM, Giudicelli S, Malthiéry Y, *et al.* Possible involvement of the dopamine D3 receptor locus in subtypes of bipolar affective disorder. Psychiatr Genet 2000, 10:43-49.

[37] Dikeos DG, Papadimitriou GN, Avramopoulos D, Karadima G, Daskalopoulou EG, Souery D, *et al.* Association between the dopamine D_3 receptor gene locus [DRD3] and unipolar affective disorder. Psychiatr Genet 1999, 9:189-195.

[38] D'haenen HA, Bossuyt A. Dopamine D_2 receptors in depression measured with single photon emission computed tomography. Biol Psychiatry 1994, 35:128-132.

[39] Ebert D, Feistel H, Loew T, Pirner A. Dopamine and depression - Striatal dopamine D_2 receptor SPECT before and after antidepressant therapy. Psychopharmacology (Berl) 1996, 126:91-94.

[40] Shah PJ, Ogilvie AD, Goodwin GM, Ebmeier KP. Clinical and psychometric correlates of dopamine D_2 binding in depression. Psychol Med 1997, 27:1247-1256.

[41] Healy E, McKeon P. Dopaminergic sensitivity and prediction of antidepressant response. Journal of Psychopharmacology 2000, 14:152-156.

[42] Martinot M-P, Bragulat V, Artiges E, Dollé F, Hinnen F, Jouvent R, *et al*. Decreased presynaptic dopamine function in the left caudate of depressed patients with affective flattening and psychomotor retardation. Am J Psychiatry 2001, 158:314-316.

[43] Meyer JH, Krüger S, Wilson AA, Christensen BK, Goulding VS, Schaffer A, *et al*. Lower dopamine transporter binding potential in striatum during depression. Neuroreport 2001, 12:4121-4125.

[44] Kilbourn MR, Sherman PS, Pisani T. Repeated reserpine administration reduces *in vivo* [18F] GBR 13119 binding to the dopamine uptake site. Eur J Pharmacol 1992, 216:109-112.

[45] Gordon I, Weizman R, Rehavi M. Modulatory effect of agents active in the presynaptic dopaminergic system on the striatal dopamine transporter. Eur J Pharmacol 1996, 298:27-30.

[46] Klimek V, Schenck JE, Han H, Stockmeier CA, Ordway GA. Dopaminergic abnormalities in amygdaloid nuclei in major depression: A postmortem study. Biol Psychiatry 2002, 52:740-748.

[47] Van Praag HM, Korf J, Lakke JPWF, Schut T. Dopamine metabolism in depressions, psychoses, and Parkinson's disease: the problem of the specificity of biological variables in behaviour disorders. Psychol Med 1975, 5:138-146.

[48] Mendels J, Frazer A, Fitzgerald RG, Ramsey TA, Stokes JW. Biogenic amine metabolites in cerebrospinal fluid of depressed and manic patients. Science 1972, 175:1380-1382.

[49] Roy A, De Jong J, Linnoila M. Cerebrospinal fluid monoamine metabolites and suicidal behavior in depressed patients. A 5-year follow-up study. Arch Gen Psychiatry 1989, 46:609-612.

[50] Roy A, Pickar D, Linnoila M, Potter WZ. Plasma norepinephrine level in affective disorders. Relationship to melancholia. Arch Gen Psychiatry 1985, 42:1181-1185.

[51] Hamner MB, Diamond BI. Plasma dopamine and norepinephrine correlations with psychomotor retardation, anxiety, and depression in non-psychotic depressed patients: A pilot study. Psychiatry Res 1996, 64:209-211.

[52] Engström G, Alling C, Blennow K, Regnéll GO, Träskman-Bendz L. Reduced cerebrospinal HVA concentrations and HVA/5-HIAA ratios in suicide attempters: Monoamine metabolites in 120 suicide attempters and 47 controls. European Neuropsychopharmacology 1999, 9:399-405.

[53] Roy A, Karoum F, Pollack S. Marked reduction in indexes of dopamine metabolism among patients with depression who attempt suicide. Arch Gen Psychiatry 1992, 49:447-450.

[54] Roy A, De Jong J, Linnoila M. Cerebrospinal fluid monoamine metabolites and suicidal behavior in depressed patients. A 5-year follow-up study. Arch Gen Psychiatry 1989, 46:609-612.

[55] Tandberg E, Larsen JP, Aarsland D, Cummings JL. The occurrence of depression in Parkinson's disease: A community-based study. Arch Neurol 1996, 53:175-179.

[56] Cummings JL. Psychosomatic aspects of movement disorders. Adv Psychosom Med 1985, 13:111-132.

[57] Sano M, Stern Y, Cote L, Williams JB, Mayeux R. Depression in Parkinson's disease: A biochemical model. J Neuropsychiatry Clin Neurosci 1990, 2:88-92.

[58] Guttman M, Jaskolka J. The use of pramipexole in Parkinson's disease: Are its actions D3 mediated? Parkinsonism and Related Disorders 2001, 7:231-234.

[59] Piercey MF. Pharmacology of pramipexole, a dopamine D3-preferring agonist useful in treating Parkinson's disease. Clin Neuropharmacol 1998, 21:141-151.

[60] Reichmann H, Odin P, Brecht HM, Köster J, Kraus PH. Changing dopamine agonist treatment in Parkinson's disease: Experiences with switching to pramipexole. Journal of Neural Transmission, Supplement 2006:17-25.

[61] Corrigan MH, Denahan AQ, Eugene Wright C, Ragual RJ, Evans DL. Comparison of praahpexole, fluoxetine, and placebo in patients with major depression. Depress Anxiety 2000, 11:58-65.

[62] Lattanzi L, Dell'Osso L, Cassano P, Pini S, Rucci P, Houck PR. Pramipexole in treatment-resistant depressive illness: Evidence in support of the cathecholamine hypothesis of mood disorders. Arch Gen Psychiatry 2002, 57:787-793.

[63] Sporn J, Ghaemi SN, Sambur MR, Rankin MA, Recht J, Sachs GS, *et al.* Pramipexole augmentation in the treatment of unipolar and bipolar depression: A retrospective chart review. Annals of Clinical Psychiatry 2000, 12:137-140.

[64] Cassano P, Lattanzi L, Soldani F, Navari S, Battistini G, Gemignani A, *et al.* Pramipexole in treatment-resistant depression: An extended follow-up. Depress Anxiety 2004, 20:131-138.

[65] Goldberg JF, Burdick KE, Endick CJ. Preliminary Randomized, Double-Blind, Placebo-Controlled Trial of Pramipexole Added to Mood Stabilizers for Treatment-Resistant Bipolar Depression. Am J Psychiatry 2004, 161:564-566.

[66] Brocco M, Dekeyne A, Papp M, Millan MJ. Antidepressant-like properties of the anti-Parkinson agent, piribedil, in rodents: Mediation by dopamine D2 receptors. Behav Pharmacol 2006, 17:559-572.

[67] Izumi T, Inoue T, Kitagawa N, Nishi N, Shimanaka S, Takahashi Y, *et al.* Open pergolide treatment of tricyclic and heterocyclic antidepressant-resistant depression. J Affect Disord 2000, 61:127-132.

[68] Muscat R, Papp M, Willner P. Antidepressant-like effects of dopamine agonists in an animal model of depression. Biol Psychiatry 1992, 31:937-946.

[69] Waehrens J, Gerlach J. Bromocriptine and imipramine in endogenous depression. A double-blind controlled trial in outpatients. J Affect Disord 1981, 3:193-202.

[70] Mah L, Zarate CA, Nugent AC, Singh JB, Manji HK, Drevets WC. Neural mechanisms of antidepressant efficacy of the dopamine receptor agonist pramipexole in treatment of bipolar depression. International Journal of Neuropsychopharmacology 2010:1-7.

[71] Rizzo V, Aricò I, Mastroeni C, Morgante F, Liotta G, Girlanda P, *et al.* Dopamine agonists restore cortical plasticity in patients with idiopathic restless legs syndrome. Movement Disorders 2009, 24:710-715.

[72] Hiramoto T, Kanda Y, Satoh Y, Takishima K, Watanabe Y. Dopamine D2 receptor stimulation

promotes the proliferation of neural progenitor cells in adult mouse hippocampus. Neuroreport 2007, 18:659-664.

[73] Höglinger GU, Rizk P, Muriel MP, Duyckaerts C, Oertel WH, Caille I, *et al.* Dopamine depletion impairs precursor cell proliferation in Parkinson disease. Nat Neurosci 2004, 7:726-735.

[74] Willner P. The mesolimbic dopamine system as a target for rapid antidepressant action. Int Clin Psychopharmacol 1997, 12[SUPPL.3]:S7-S14.

[75] Spyraki C, Fibiger HC. Behavioural evidence for supersensitivity of postsynaptic dopamine receptors in the mesolimbic system after chronic administration of desipramine. Eur J Pharmacol 1981, 74:195-206.

[76] D'Aquila PS, Collu M, Gessa GL, Serra G. The role of dopamine in the mechanism of action of antidepressant drugs. Eur J Pharmacol 2000, 405:365-373.

[77] Ichikawa J, Meltzer HY. Relationship between dopaminergic and serotonergic neuronal activity in the frontal cortex and the action of typical and atypical antipsychotic drugs. Eur Arch Psychiatry Clin Neurosci 1999, 249[SUPPL. 4]:IV90-IV98.

[78] Keck ME, Welt T, Müller MB, Erhardt A, Ohl F, Toschi N, *et al.* Repetitive transcranial magnetic stimulation increases the release of dopamine in the mesolimbic and mesostriatal system. Neuropharmacology 2002, 43:101-109.

[79] Strafella AP, Paus T, Barrett J, Dagher A. Repetitive transcranial magnetic stimulation of the human prefrontal cortex induces dopamine release in the caudate nucleus. The Journal of neuroscience : the official journal of the Society for Neuroscience 2001, 21[15].

[80] Strafella AP, Paus T, Fraraccio M, Dagher A. Striatal dopamine release induced by repetitive transcranial magnetic stimulation of the human motor cortex. Brain 2003, 126:2609-2615.

[81] Lammers C-, Diaz J, Schwartz J-, Sokoloff P. Selective increase of dopamine D3 receptor gene expression as a common effect of chronic antidepressant treatments. Mol Psychiatry 2000, 5:378-388.

Send Orders for Reprints to reprints@benthamscience.net
Neurobiology of Mood Disorders, 2014, 139-173

CHAPTER 7

ROLE OF PREFRONTAL CORTEX IN THE PATHOPHYSIOLOGY AND TREATMENT OF DEPRESSION AND SCHIZOPHRENIA

XAVIER LÓPEZ-GIL*, LAURA JIMÉNEZ-SÁNCHEZ, ALBERT ADELL

Centro de Investigación Biomédica en Red de Salud Mental (CIBERSAM), Barcelona, Spain

Abstract: The prefrontal cortex represents the brain region with the highest hierarchical level among the association cortices and stands as the most evolved cortex, responsible of the superior mental functions. The representation, planning and execution of actions, cognition, behavior and emotional control, adaptation to the environment and the working memory are dependent on the integrity of the prefrontal cortex and its interconnections with cortical and subcortical areas. Schizophrenia and depression generate profound changes in the patient's behavior, disabling them for a normal adaptation to society. In addition, treatments are far from being optimal for both illnesses; their effectiveness has a high degree of variation, and severe secondary effects usually emerge. Alterations of higher brain functions can be observed, thus indicating that depression and schizophrenia have in common a damage or dysfunction of the prefrontal cortex circuitry. Particularly, disruption of prefrontal neurotransmission of serotonin and dopamine is a shared feature. Furthermore, both psychiatric diseases present marked mood alterations. Hence, the characteristic negative symptoms of schizophrenia (apathy, lack of motivation) are key features of depression.In the present chapter we review the changes and alterations observed in the prefrontal cortex of patients of depression and schizophrenia in terms of cytoarchitecture, connections and functions, and how they are disrupted in both disorders. Some important preclinical findings are also reviewed. We also discuss how different treatments normalize the altered cortical neurotransmission and how this could be reflected by an improvement of the patient's symptomatology.

Keywords: Orbital (oPFC), medial (mPFC) and lateral (lPFC) prefrontal cortex, depression, schizophrenia, deep brain stimulation (DBS), NMDA receptor, antidepressant and antipsychotic drugs, glutamate, γ-aminobutyric acid (GABA).

1. THE PREFRONTAL CORTEX

The prefrontal cortex (PFC) is the most rostral area of the frontal lobe, which also includes the motor and premotor cortex. While those two areas are related with the movement generation, the prefrontal cortex is implicated in cognitive and motivational/emotional processes [1]. The functioning of the brain cortex has a hierarchical structure. At the lowest level, sensory information arrives to the sensory and motor areas. At the following level, other areas, more complex and evolved such as the association cortices, receive the information from the primary sensory and motor areas and carry out more integrative functions. The prefrontal cortex represents the highest level in this hierarchy, being responsible for the representation, planning and execution of actions. Consequently, the PFC does not make connections with sensory or motor areas, but only with associative cortices [1] (Figure **1**).

The prefrontal cortex can be divided in three major areas: orbital, medial and lateral. The orbital and medial regions are related to the emotional behavior while the lateral cortex, which in humans

***Address correspondence to Xavier López-Gil:** Centro de Investigación Biomédica en Red de Salud Mental (CIBERSAM), Barcelona, Spain; E-mail: xavier.lopez.gil@gmail.com

Bruno P Guiard and Eliyahu Dremencov (Eds)

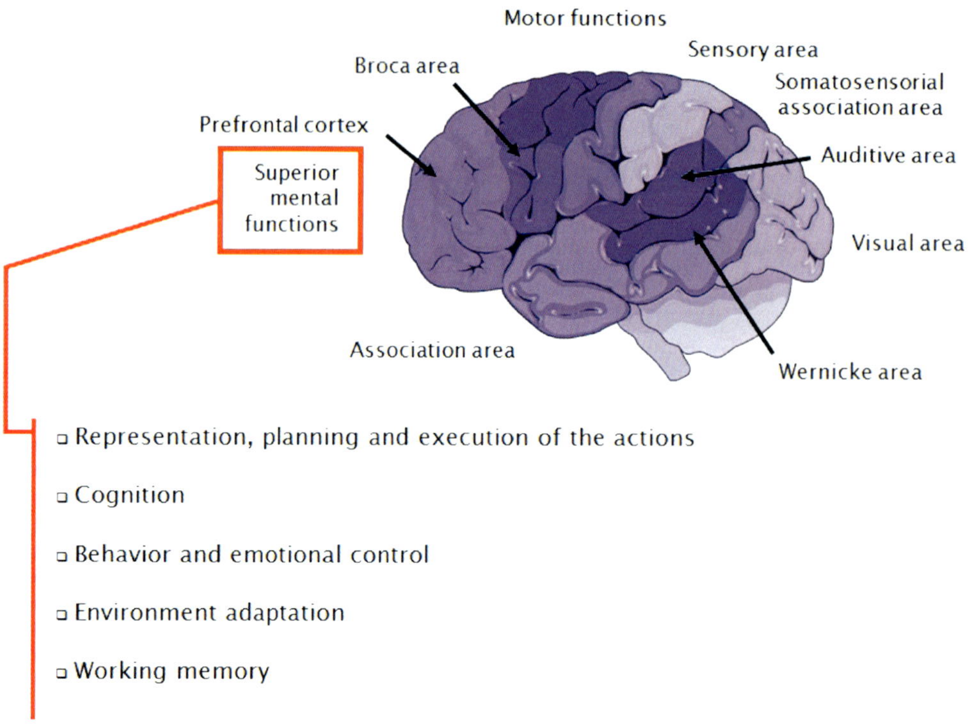

Figure 1: Scheme of some of the sensory and integration areas of the human brain and prefrontal cortex main functions.

reaches its greatest development, is implicated in cognitive functions like the timely organization of behavior, speech and reasoning [1]. Obviously, functions as complex as those described herein are not limited to only a specific area of the brain. Instead, connections of the prefrontal cortex with other cortical and subcortical structures shape the prefrontal cortex operation.

The prefrontal cortex is the most evolved cortex phylogenetically. In humans it constitutes the largest region of the cerebral hemispheres, up to approximately a 30% of the neocortex [1,2]. The prefrontal cortex develops late in life and reaches its maturity in the adolescence, when myelinization and creation of synapses is completed [1,2]. This lapse is coincident with the emergence of the superior cognitive functions, like reasoning and executive processes, which underscores the crucial role of the PFC in those complex behaviors.

In rodents, the prefrontal cortex can also be divided into three main regions: lateral, orbital and medial (the latter subdivided in three more areas, *i.e.,* anterior cingulate, prelimbic and infralimbic). There exists an obvious difficulty in comparing prefrontal regions between rodents and humans, but as a rule, the precise connectivity of the PFC with other structures is what defines its functions [1]. Thus, the prelimbic region would be more implicated in limbic and cognitive functions while the infralimbic cortex would regulate autonomous functions.

2. CYTOARCHITECTURE OF THE PREFRONTAL CORTEX

The prefrontal cortex consists of six cortical layers. Ontogenetically, the first layers formed are VI and V. Although the cytoarchitecture of the human prefrontal cortex is already established at birth, the process of maturation continues and is completed at the end of adolescence. The upper most layer (layer I) is devoid of pyramidal somas although it contains processes derived from apical dendrites. A few GABAergic neurons can also be found. Layer II contains small pyramidal cells that synapse with other neurons within the ipsilateral cortex, and double-bouquet GABAergic interneurons expressing calbindin (CB) and calretinin (CR). In layer III there is a larger number of pyramidal cells that project to the contralateral cortex. PV-containing GABAergic interneurons can also be found in this layer. Layer IV is devoid of pyramidal cells, but contains a notable amount of GABAergic interneurons. It is important to note that in the prefrontal cortex of rodents, layer IV is lacking [3]. Layer V also contains large pyramidal cells that project to striatum, brainstem and spinal cord. Finally, layer VI is also enriched in pyramidal cells that project to the thalamus, the input of which arrives to upper layers, mainly III and IV.

Cortical neurons can belong to a two different classes of cellular types, *i.e.,* pyramidal (glutamatergic) cells and GABAergic interneurons, which are excitatory and inhibitory, respectively. Pyramidal cells represent about the 75-80 % of the total number of neurons and establish synapses within the prefrontal cortex and/or project to other cortical and subcortical regions of the brain. These synapses are called asymmetric because, under the microscope, the postsynaptic component exhibits a prominent density in comparison with the presynaptic button. A single apical dendrite emerges from the apex of the pyramidal soma and extends to upper layers thereby integrating multiple synaptic inputs. In addition, several basal dendrites emerge from the base of the pyramidal soma. Each basal dendrite branches up to several times before terminating.

GABAergic interneurons represent 20-25 % of total number of cortical neurons. They are local inhibitory neurons, in that they do not project to other areas of the brain, and form symmetrical synapses that do not contain a prominent postsynaptic density. GABAergic interneurons can be classified according to their morphological, physiological and neurochemical features [4]. Despite this diversity, they have some characteristics in common. *First*, they receive both inhibitory and excitatory synapses. *Second*, they have aspiny dendrites. *Third*, their axons usually arborize within and between layers. It is of note that every segment of a pyramidal neuron, such as the soma, dendritic branches and spines, and the initial axonal segment, receives dense GABAergic synaptic innervation.

Morphological classification:

- Basket cells: They provide inhibitory input to the soma of pyramidal neurons.

- Chandelier cells: They target the axon initial segment of pyramidal cells forming numerous arrays of terminals called "cartridges", which are positioned to produce a short-circuiting of action potential propagation and thus play a major role in modulating the pyramidal neuron output activity.

- Martinotti cells: The soma is usually located in deep layers and their axons provide inhibitory inputs to the distal dendrites of pyramidal neurons across the layer I.

- Double bouquet cells: They target different segments of the apical dendritic arbor and other GABA neurons.

- Neurogliaform cells: They contact different parts of pyramidal neurons and are of particular interest because they are, together with basket neurons, the only interneuron subtype known to be contacted directly by thalamo-cortical afferents and are thus thought to play a major role in shaping the receptive fields properties of cortical neurons.

Physiological classification:

- Fast spiking (FS) cells: called so by their high rate of firing. - They show repetitive firing by synaptic activation of depolarized potentials. FS neurons have been shown to be connected to each other both through chemical synapses as well as through electrical synapses (gap junctions) so that they form networks that contribute to the synchronization of electrical activity in cortical neurons.

- Low-threshold-spiking (LTS) cells: - These neurons show typical burst-like discharges after a hyperpolarizing pre-pulse and are found in layer V (which also contains many bursting pyramidal cells).

- Regular-spiking (RS) cells: - These cells discharge in a manner that resembles regular-spiking pyramidal cells and have been found in layers II/III and V.

Neurochemical classification: It refers to their content in calcium-binding proteins.

Calcium-binding proteins (CBPs): Three proteins form this family, *i.e.*, calbindin (CB), parvalbumin (PV) and calretinin (CR). They are mutually exclusive in that each interneuron expresses only one calcium-binding protein. CB neurons are LTS cells, PV neurons are FS cells, and CR neurons are irregular-spiking interneurons (Figure **2**).

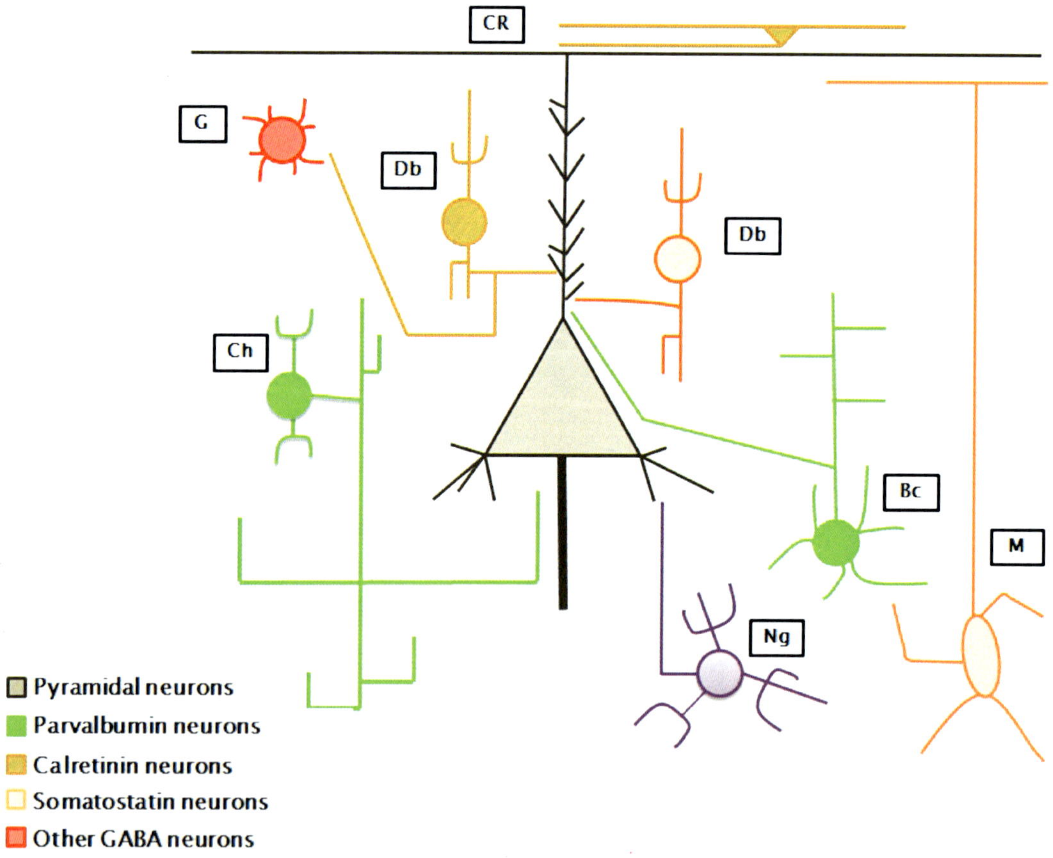

Figure 2: Schematic illustration of the different classes of GABAergic interneurons present in the prefrontal cortex. Adapted from Lewis *et al.* (2005).

3. FUNCTIONS OF THE PREFRONTAL CORTEX

The working memory is the one of the fundamental processes rooted in the prefrontal cortex. This concept refers to a type of memory that is active and relevant only during a short period of time, usually only a few seconds [5], in which the PFC "retrieves" previously acquired information and uses it to solve a task (Figure **3**). Experiments carried out in monkeys show that pyramidal neurons of the PFC remain active without external stimuli when the animal has to remember previous experience in order to resolve a task. However, in sensorymotor areas the neurons are only active when a determined stimulus is presented [6].

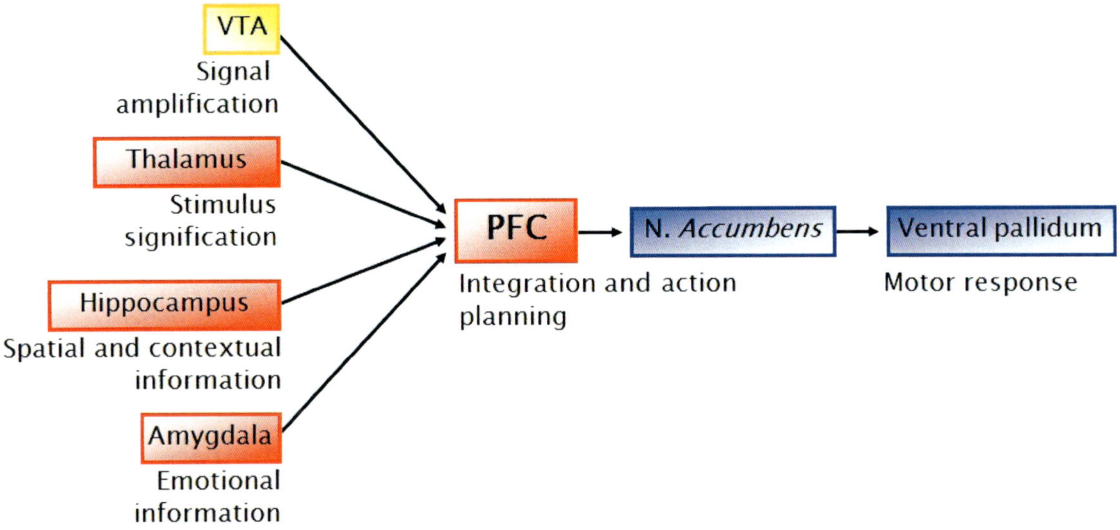

Figure 3: Scheme of the main circuits implicated in the working memory process and their respective function, according to [10].

The knowledge that we actually have about the functions of the different regions of the prefrontal cortex arise from psychological studies as well as from lesions that allow us to observe which processes are altered [1]. Thus, it has been shown that lesions of the orbital PFC induce large changes in personality (impulsivity, irritability, disinhibition, high-risk behavior, *etc.*). This indicates the role of this region in the emotional behavior and its regulation for a correct social interaction. Instead, lesions of the medial PFC have revealed its implication in attention and concentration processes. Damage to this area provokes problems in speech, the initiation of movements, as well as apathy, lack of interest and difficulties to concentrate [7]. With regard to the lateral PFC, lesions in this area induce an inability to formulate and execute plans, representation and construction of sentences and to carry out action sequences in a correct manner, which suggests the importance of this region in the temporal organization of behavior [1].

4. CONNECTIVITY OF THE PREFRONTAL CORTEX

Classically, the prefrontal cortex has been defined as the area that receives a prominent innervation from the mediodorsal nucleus of the thalamus [1], but it is also interconnected with a large number of cortical and subcortical structures. The prefrontal cortex project mainly to the thalamus, the monoaminergic nuclei of the brainstem (dorsal raphe nucleus, locus coeruleus, ventral tegmental area), lateral hypothalamus, limbic system (amygdala and, indirectly, the hippocampus), basal ganglia (caudate-putamen, nucleus accumbens) and lateral habenula [3,8]. A large part of these connections are reciprocal.

The main afferents to the PFC originate in the thalamus, hippocampus and monoaminergic nuclei of the brainstem. The connections from the brainstem, the diencephalon and the limbic system provide the PFC with the information from the internal condition of the body, motivation, and the most visceral part of the cognition. The amygdala and the hippocampus complete this information with the emotional significance of the different sensory stimuli [9]. Almost all the PFC regions receive projections (directly or indirectly) from the hippocampus, which supplies data related to the spatial context of actions [10]. Indeed, the hippocampus has been classically associated to learning and long-term memory processes and is also responsible for the processing of spatial and contextual information.

Due to the implication of serotonin (5-HT) in depression and in the treatment of schizophrenia, of all the subcortical connections of PFC, in this chapter a special attention will be paid to the connection between PFC and the dorsal raphe nucleus. All the brain serotonergic neurons have their cell bodies located in the raphe nuclei of the brainstem. The dorsal and the median raphe nucleus innervate virtually all areas of the brain, which includes a strong projection to the PFC. Therefore, it is logical to conclude that serotonin can play an important role in the modulation of the prefrontal cortex, mainly through inhibitory 5-HT_{1A} and excitatory 5-HT_{2A} serotonin receptors. Both receptors are present in the PFC, and are expressed in pyramidal and GABAergic neurons. Hence the release of 5-HT in the PFC as a consequence of the activation of the raphe nuclei can theoretically induce an activation or an inhibition of the prefrontal output [11-13]. However, the predominant effect on the PFC is inhibition, possibly because of the high density of 5-HT_{1A} receptors in the axonal hillock of pyramidal neurons, where they can strongly interfere with the propagation of action potentials [13,14].

On the other hand, the prefrontal cortex elicits a reciprocal, strong control of the activity of 5-HT cells within the dorsal raphe nucleus, which is carried out by a subpopulation (~5%) of layer V pyramidal neurons that projects directly to this nucleus [15]. Thus, due to the large number of brain areas innervated by the dorsal raphe nucleus, the prefrontal cortex can modulate an important number of brain functions [3]. Thus, the PFC excitation provokes an activation of the serotonergic neurons of the raphe nucleus and, consequently, an increase of the serotonin release in the prefrontal cortex [16,17]. According with that, the administration of drugs (like DOI) that stimulates the cortical pyramidal neurons produces a increase in the activity of serotonergic neurons and, consequently, an increase in the cortical extracellular levels of 5-HT. Overall, the cortical concentration of 5-HT can be taken as an indirect measure of the activity of the prefrontal cortex.

One of the most important issues for the integration of information and the correct functioning of the prefrontal cortex is the communication between the prefrontal cortices of both hemispheres. It is logical to think that the high-level of association and integration tasks carried out by the prefrontal cortex requires a distinct organization of the interhemispheric cortico-cortical communication.

The reciprocal connectivity between the two prefrontal cortices is furnished by layer III pyramidal neurons, the axons of which aggregate in a structure called corpus callosum. The corpus callosum is the larger white matter tract composed of more than 190 million axons in humans [18,19], and is one of the brain structures more developed during mammalian evolution [18]. It is the only fiber tract devoted to the connection of the two cortical hemispheres [18]. This strong interconnectivity underscores the importance of the coordination between both prefrontal cortices for to their correct efficiency. Indeed, the integrity of those axons is needed for the generation of the gamma oscillations between the two hemispheres [20]. The deep-layer callosal projection neurons make contacts with both the contralateral cortex as well as subcortical structures (contra or ipsilateral striatum, primary somatosensorial cortex and frontal premotor cortex) [18]. The later-born, evolutionary newer, superficial-layer callosal projection neurons, instead, participate in local circuitry within cortical columns. They send axons to the contralateral cortex through the corpus callosum to homotopic regions and ipsilaterally, they send collaterals to contact pyramidal neurons of layers II/III and, more strongly, to layer V. Thus, callosal projetion neurons are responsible not only of the communication between the cortical hemispheres, but also play a very important role in the association and integration of information, both ipsi- and contralaterally [18] (Figure **4**).

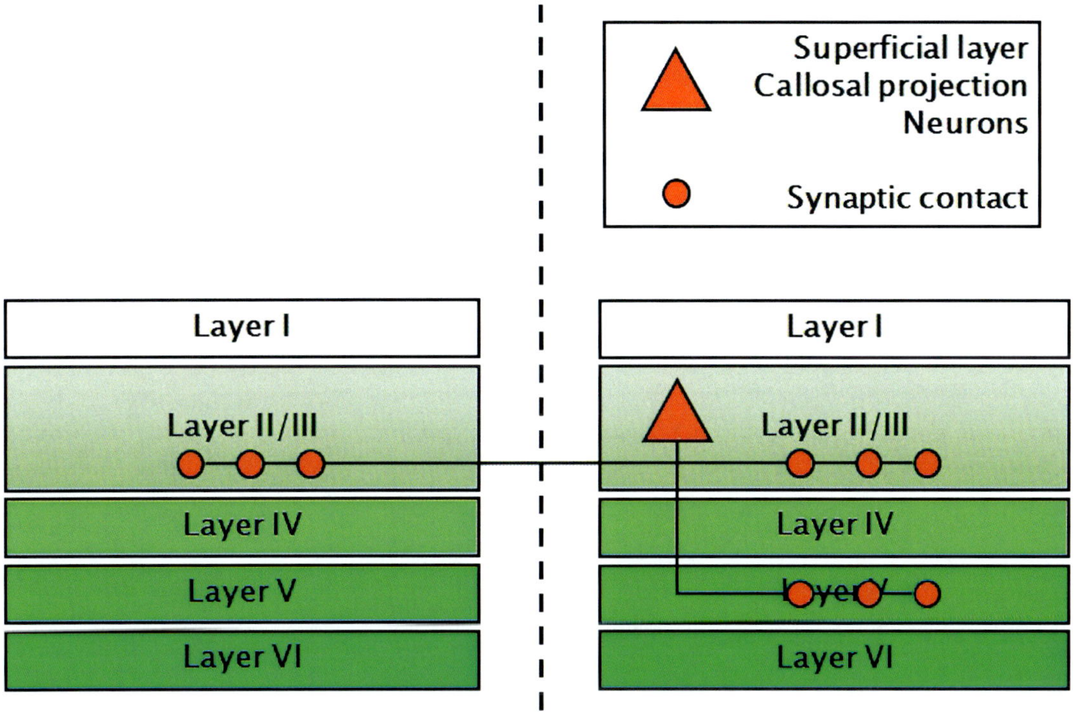

Figure 4: Scheme of the connections of the superficial-layer callosal projection neurons in the prefrontal cortex. These neurons not only are responsible of the interhemispheric coordination, they play a crucial role in the association and integration functions, both ipsi- and contralaterally.

5. DEPRESSION

Depression is a severe mental illness that affects ~120 million people and is among the leading causes of disability worldwide because only 25% of depressed people have access to effective treatments (WHO, 2011). Depressive individuals do not all experience the same symptoms. The severity, frequency, and duration of symptoms are highly variable. According to the American Psychiatric Association (2000), signs and symptoms include:

Persistent sad, anxious, or "empty" feelings

Feelings of hopelessness or pessimism

Feelings of guilt, worthlessness, or helplessness

Irritability, restlessness

Loss of interest in activities or hobbies once pleasurable, including sex

Fatigue and decreased energy

Difficulty concentrating, remembering details, and making decisions

Insomnia, early-morning wakefulness, or excessive sleeping

Overeating, or appetite loss

Thoughts of suicide, suicide attempts

Aches or pains, headaches, cramps, or digestive problems that do not ease even with treatment.

Actually, despite the prevalence of depression, the pathophysiology of the disease is not completely understood. It is likely that many brain regions mediate the diverse symptoms of depression, *i.e.,* anhedonia (nucleus accumbens), fear and anxiety (amygdaloid complex), depressed mood (limbic system) and somatic symptoms, such as changes in hormone secretion, appetite, sexual drive, sleep, etc (hypothalamus). In addition, as other psychiatric illnesses (schizophrenia, bipolar disorder), depression affects complex higher brain functions (cognitive performance), which suggests the implication of prefrontal cortex. In fact, abnormalities of prefrontal circuitry, revealed by structural and functional imaging studies, are associated with key symptoms of depression [21]. Thus, postmortem and neuroimaging studies of depressed patients have reported reductions in grey-matter volume and glial density in the prefrontal cortex and the hippocampus [22-24], regions thought to mediate the cognitive aspects of depression, such as feelings of guilt, worthlessness, or helplessness. This and the fact that the prefrontal cortex has extensive connections with the amygdala, nucleus accumbens, hypothalamus, and the noradrenaline, 5-HT and dopamine systems of the brainstem underscores the importance of prefrontal cortex in the pathophysiology of depression. More specifically, neuroimaging studies of resting state activity have associated depression with abnormally high levels of ventromedial prefrontal cortex activity [25,26], but abnormally low levels of dorsolateral prefrontal cortex activity [27,28]. In concordance with this neuroimaging findings, studies using patients with brain lesions have shown that bilateral ventromedial prefronto-cortical lesions are associated with low levels of depression, whereas bilateral dorsal prefronto-cortical lesions (involving dorsomedial and dorsolateral areas in both hemispheres) are associated with prominently higher levels of depression [29].

6. NEUROTRANSMITTERS AND DEPRESSION: HISTORY AND PHARMACOLOGY

Many of the current treatments for depression act by increasing serotonergic and noradrenergic neurotransmission, and such data form the basis for the monoamine hypothesis of the illness, i.e that depression is caused by too little monoaminergic activity. Consistent with this hypothesis, depression is related to changes in sleep and fatigue, eating alterations, *etc.*, behaviors that are regulated by noradrenaline and 5-HT. Prefrontal cortex is implicated in working memory, attention, impulse control and other aspects of executive function. Abnormalities in these cognitive domains are certainly seen in depression. Furthermore, serotonergic and noradrenergic pathways converge in the prefrontal cortex, thus suggesting that these prefrontal monoamines may probably play an important role in these functions. Although the exact contribution of each monoamine remains to be fully understood, some behaviors have been attributed to a particular transmission. For instance, serotonin has been involved in sleep and drive, and noradrenaline in alertness and energy mechanisms. In addition, impairment of motivation, psychomotor speed, attention, and the ability to experience pleasure are prominent features of depression which are thought to be regulated in part by dopaminergic circuitry [30]. In this regard, an increase in the dopamine release in prefrontal cortex may be responsible for the profound antidepressant effect observed in patients with treatment-resistant depression [31]. For this reason, it has been hypothesized that a triple reuptake inhibitor that activates dopamine neurotransmission in addition to serotonin and noradrenaline circuitries may result in enhanced antidepressant effects (Figure **5**). In fact, it has been shown that bupropion, a dopamine reuptake inhibitor, enhaces the antidepressant actions of SSRIs [32,33].

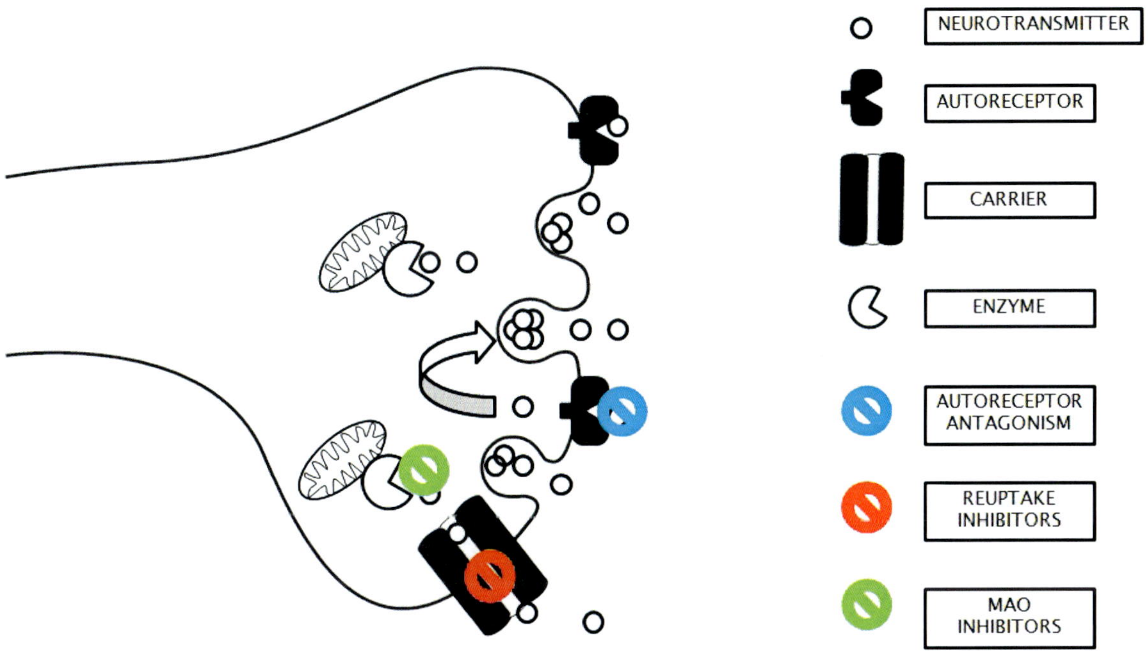

Figure 5: Diagram of a monoaminergic presynaptic terminal showing the different sites where antidepressant drugs can exert their effects.

In spite of the fact that >90% prescribed antidepressant drugs enhance monoaminergic transmission by inhibiting reuptake mechanisms, the monoamine hypothesis falls short in explaining all features of depression. For instance, blockade of reuptake occurs shortly after drug administration, but therapeutic effects are seen only after some weeks of sustained treatment. Several mechanisms have been postulated to explain this therapeutic delay. On the one hand, a prolonged administration of SSRis would lead to the desensitization of the negative feedback mechanisms driven by 5-HT_{1A} autoreceptors in the dorsal raphe [34,35], thus allowing a true enhancement of 5-HT availability at nerve endings. On the other hand, [36] has suggested that antidepressant actions are related to neuronal plasticity, neurotrophic factors, and neurogenesis. Depression is related to a reduction in brain-derived neurotrophic factor (BDNF), which may lead to hippocampal atrophy and inhibited neurogenesis. Serotonin enhances BDNF and neurogenesis in the hippocampus [37]. Thus, the delay in the effectiveness of antidepressants would be accounted for by the time it takes for new neurons to be produced and incorporated into hippocampal circuitry. Obviously these two hypotheses are not mutually exclusive.

7. NEW APPROACHES TO THE TREATMENT OF DEPRESSION

At present time, a major concern in depression therapy is that an important proportion of patients (20-30%) fail to respond to conventional medications [38], and it appears clear that market penetration will only be gained, at least initially, in the treatment of refractory patients. Given that the prefrontal cortex modulates the function of the temporolimbic cortical and subcortical regions involved in mood and affect, it has been hypothesized that the stimulation of this area may be useful for the treatment of depression. This beneficial effect could be due to an increase of the firing of descending projection neurons that target other limbic brain regions as well as subcortical monoaminergic nuclei.

In the last five years, deep brain stimulation (DBS) of the subgenual cingulate region (Brodmann area 25, Cg25) has emerged as a new strategy for treatment-resistant depression [39]. Although invasive, the procedure is well tolerated and thus it gives promise for patients with depression that proves refractory to standard pharmacological treatments. The main characteristics of this novel treatment are delineated in the following section.

8. DEEP BRAIN STIMULATION

Deep brain stimulation (DBS) is a surgical technique that involves the stereotaxical implantation of stimulating electrodes that are connected to an impulse generator implanted in the chest wall, and deliver a high frequency stimulation current (~130 Hz). In Parkinson's disease (PD), it has been demonstrated that chronic high-frequency DBS in pathologically overactive brain areas produces profound clinical benefits [40,41].

Functional neuroimaging studies have consistently shown a hyperactivity in the Cg25 of depressed patients [39]. Even when healthy humans are asked to recall sad episodes of their lives or are depleted of tryptophan, an augmentation of blood flow in this area is found [42,43]. For this reason the hypothesis was tested that the application of high frequency stimulation to this area would produce clinical benefits in patients with treatment-resistant depression (TRD). The first study carried out with only six patients revealed a clear amelioration of depressive symptomatology in these patients, which was accompanied by a reduction of the Cg25 blood flow [39]. These data were consistent with previous studies showing a decrease in Cg25 activity after clinical response to different antidepressant treatments including SSRIs, electroconvulsive therapy (ECT), repetitive transcranial magnetic stimulation (rTMS), and ablative surgery [44-46]. In addition, advantages of DBS over lesioning include potential reversibility, revisability, and adjustability [47]. On the other hand, these positive results have lead to the proposal that an unchanged Cg25 hyperactivity is a predictor of a lack of response to antidepressant treatment [48,49]. These initial clinical effects of DBS in TRD have been recently confirmed by another group of eight patients (Puigdemont *et al.* 2011). Furthermore, a recent follow-up study after 3 to 6 years has reported that DBS remains a safe and effective treatment for TRD [50].

Although nowadays DBS is used for TRD in a few hospitals, little is known about its mechanism(s) of action. However, several possible mechanisms have been proposed. For instance, one of them postulates a selective activation of specific axonal pathways. It is well known that axons are more excitable than soma or dendrites [51]. Thus, when DBS is applied selective pathways will be activated. The activation of the pathways lateral and medial to the ventral striatum or dorsal and lateral to the nucleus accumbens seems to be the best option to obtain a successful treatment [52]. But, the activation of pathways situated dorsal and lateral to the ventral striatum can deteriorate the clinical outcomes. Curiously, these inadequate pathways are activated in all non-responders [52].

Another possible mechanism is based in observations from neuroimaging studies and may explain the sudden mood improvement reported by some patients in the operating room shortly after initiation of DBS [53]. High frequency stimulation could silence neurons through inactivation of voltage-gated sodium and calcium channels or by means of a depolarization block [54,55]. The silencing of the neurons produced a decrease in the activity of Cg25, which eventually may improve mood. This mechanism is known as functional inactivation because the result is similar to a lesion-like effect [56,57].

However, more research is needed to decipher the precise mechanism of action of DBS. Of critical importance is the integrity of serotonergic system in the antidepressant effects of DBS. Indeed, [58] found that the antidepressant-like effects of prefrontal cortex DBS are absent in rats depleted of 5-HT. It is thus possible that in the clinical setting the high frequency stimulation of Cg25 produce an increase of monoamines in the PFC thereby improving mood. An increase in the serotonergic tone is related to a better affective response [59], and an increase in the dopaminergic tone may be responsible of a reduction in anhedonia [30], both being key features of depression (Figure **6**).

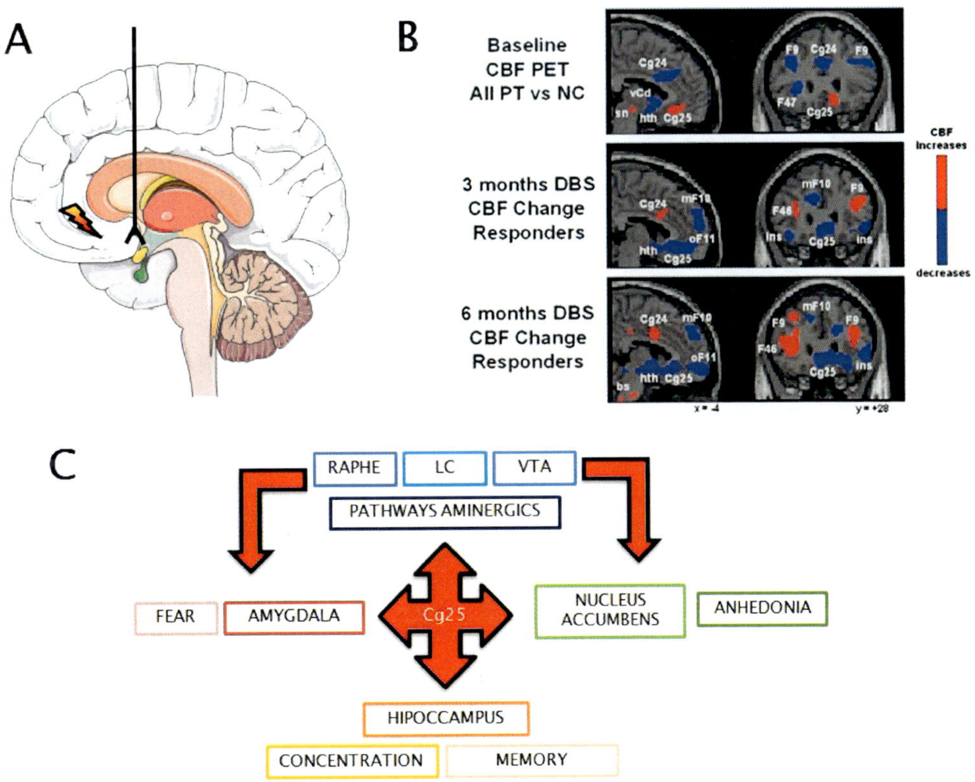

Figure 6: Deep brain stimulation (DBS). (A) Scheme of the electrode in the Cg25 of a human brain. (B) Regional cerebral blood flow in depressed patients, before DBS, 3 months and 6 months after the treatment. A decrease in the metabolic activity can be observed in the Cg25 after DBShe stimulation (reprinted from Neuron, vol. 45/5, Helen S.Mayberg, Andres M. Lozano, Valerie Voon, Heather E. McNeely, Jason M. Schwalb, Sidney H. Kennedy, "Deep Brain Stimulation for Treatment-Resistant Depression", 651-660, 2005, with permission from Elsevier). (C) Schematic illustration of Cg25 afferents and their relationship with different features of depression.

9. SCHIZOPHRENIA

The impairment of cortical connections with monoaminergic nuclei of the brainstem has been considered central in the pathophysiology of depression [60]. However, the very same circuitry has been also implicated in schizophrenia [61]. In fact, abnormal cortical serotonergic and dopaminergic transmission has been shown to occur in the brain of schizophrenia patients as well as in animal models of the illness [62,63].

Schizophrenia is a mental illness that causes profound alterations in the patients' behavior, disabling them for a normal life in society. Schizophrenia symptoms can be classified in positive symptoms (delusions, hallucinations, psychosis, *etc.*), negative symptoms (apathy, lack of motivation) and cognitive deficits (impairment of learning, executive functions and working memory). From a nosological viewpoint, negative symptoms of schizophrenia are also central features of depressive states, and so are cognitive deficits. Furthermore, an impaired functioning of the inhibitory GABAergic system has been reported in both pathologies [64,65].

Taken together, all these evidences suggest that both psychiatric diseases share a common anatomical substrate at both cellular and circuitry level.

10. INVOLVEMENT OF THE PREFRONTAL CORTEX IN SCHIZOPHRENIA

As mentioned above, the prefrontal cortex is the most important association area in the brain, responsible of high-level functions like working memory, planning ahead, conscious thought, emotions, *etc.* [1]. All these functions are dependent on the prefrontal cortex integrity and have been found to be impaired in schizophrenia [66]. For instance, deficits in the *Wisconsin Card Sorting Test*, a task used to examine cognitive functioning, are consistently found in schizophrenics. Other studies have also shown decreased cortical metabolism with a marked hypofrontality, *i.e.,* an insufficient activation of the prefrontal cortex when it is required for the execution of a working memory task [67-71]. Indeed, this hypofrontality correlated with the presence and severity of negative and cognitive symptoms [67,71,72], which underscores the role of PFC in this symptomatology. Interestingly, the atypical antipsychotic clozapine can normalize the changes in glucose metabolism observed in those patients [73]. Furthermore, it has been described a reduction of N-acetylaspartate (NAA, a marker of neuronal integrity) levels in the PFC, hippocampus and temporal lobe [74], which suggests the existence of damage to these areas in the schizophrenia brain.

Postmortem studies have also evidenced structural brain changes in schizophrenia consisting of a general reduction of the cortical, hippocampal and thalamic volume as well as an enlargement of the ventricles [75-78]. In addition, a reduction of serotonin transporter and an increase of 5-HT_{1A} receptors densities in the prefrontal cortex of schizophrenia patients [79] have been also found in postmortem tissue. One of the most robust alterations found in the PFC of the schizophrenia brain has been the reduction of the expression of GABAergic markers such as the mRNA coding for GAD_{67} and parvalbumin, which suggests an impairment of cortical inhibition, not generalized, but confined to parvalbumin-containing neurons [64,80,81].

An important tool to study schizophrenia is the use of animal models. Being a complex mental illness, it is obvious the difficulty in reproducing the great diversity of schizophrenia symptoms into an experimentation animal. However, some representative alterations in humans can be modeled in lab animals. Furthermore, an important characteristic of the so-called pharmacological models is that the administration of such drugs in humans provokes the emergence of schizophrenic symptoms, and the administration of antipsychotic drugs can reverse such changes both in humans and lab animals. Animal models also show notable alterations of neurotransmission and function in the PFC. Deficits in working memory can also be studied by means of behavioral tests such as T-maze, Morris water-maze and 5-CSRTT (5-choice serial reaction time task). Alterations in the release of neurotransmitters like serotonin (5-HT), dopamine and glutamate observed in these models can also provide valuable information on what might occur in the brain of human patients.

Two of such animal models take into account the neurodevelopmental origin of schizophrenia, which hypothesizes that environmental insults during gestation added to a genetic vulnerability would lead to the apparition of the illness [66]. In the first model the neurotoxin ibotenic acid is administered in the ventral hippocampus on postnatal day 7 [82,83]. This area projects heavily to the PFC and the ventral tegmental area (VTA), origin of the mesolimbic and mesocortical dopaminergic pathways [84]. In the adulthood, neonatally-lesioned rats exhibit cellular and functional disruptions of the PFC and related areas [85] as well as deficits in working memory [86]. The second model consists in the administration of methylazoxymethanol acetate (MAM) to pregnant rats. The adult offspring shows deficits in prefrontal neuronal synchronization [87,88], which has been associated with an hyperdopaminergic activity [89]. Indeed, an excess of dopaminergic activity has been a long-standing hypothesis of schizophrenia [90]. Several observations demonstrate the importance of dopamine in psychotic symptomatology. For example, psychostimulants like amphetamine can induce psychosis similar to that occurring in schizophrenia in healthy individuals and exacerbate the symptoms in patients [91]. A posterior revision of the dopaminergic theory proposed a hyperactivity of the mesolimbic pathway that would be responsible of positive symptoms and a hypofunction of the mesocortical pathway, which might be potentially associated with the negative symptoms and cognitive deficits [90,92-94]. More recently the animal models based in the administration of psychostimulants like amphetamine are less used because those models reproduce only the positive, but not the negative and cognitive symptoms of the illness. This suggests that a unique alteration in the dopaminergic neurotransmission is not sufficient to explain the diverse alterations observed in schizophrenia. In any case, however, there is an obvious relationship between cortical dopaminergic neurotransmission and schizophrenia inasmuch as almost all marketed antipsychotic drugs display antagonism at dopamine D2 receptor and their affinity for this receptor is correlated with their capacity to treat psychotic symptoms [95-98]. Indeed, conventional, first generation antipsychotics are characterized by their strong D2 antagonist action, whereas atypical, second generation antipsychotics possess a multi-target profile and show affinity for several dopaminergic and serotonergic receptors. According to the revised dopaminergic theory, blockade of the D2 receptors would be beneficial for the treatment of positive symptoms since they have been associated with an excess of dopamine [99]. However, these drugs would not be as efficacious to treat negative symptoms and cognitive deficits because these symptoms would be rather associated to a decrease in dopaminergic transmission. Interestingly, the prototypical atypical antipsychotic, clozapine, a drug with a relative weak D2 antagonism and a strong antagonism at serotonin 5-HT$_{2A}$ receptors is able to reduce the negative and cognitive deficits keeping its efficacy against the positive symptoms. This suggests the implication of other neurotransmitter systems in the pathophysiology of schizophrenia [100-103]. The antagonism at the 5-HT$_{2A}$ receptor depicted by atypical antipsychotics indicates the important implication of the serotonergic system in the schizophrenia and its treatment. The lesser blockade of dopamine D2 receptors exhibited by atypical antipsychotic drugs likely results in the reported diminution of the appearance of severe secondary effects of these drugs [104,105]. Accordingly with that, preclinical studies have shown that the 5-HT$_{2A}$ antagonism and the 5-HT$_{1A}$ agonism can diminish the cognitive deficits induced by the NMDA antagonism [106].

In fact, the 5-HT_{2A} receptor plays an important role in working memory process [107]. There is a higher number of those receptors in brain areas related with cognition and perception, especially in the PFC [11,108], where is expressed in pyramidal neurons as well as in GABAergic interneurons [109]. However, the higher proportion of these receptors in pyramidal neurons and the facilitatory action of DOI (5-$HT_{2A/2C}$ receptor antagonist) suggest a preferential effect on this compound on pyramidal cells [110].

11. THE NMDA RECEPTOR ANTAGONIST MODEL OF SCHIZOPHRENIA

Perhaps the most widely used animal model of schizophrenia, which is also in the basis of the glutamatergic theory, is the NMDA receptor antagonist pharmacological model of schizophrenia [111]. This model is based on the effects produced by the administration of non-competitive antagonists of the glutamate NMDA receptor: ketamine, phencyclidine (PCP) and MK-801 (dizocilpine). The administration of these drugs recreates schizophrenic symptoms in healthy individuals and exacerbate them in schizophrenia patients [112-116]. The most important feature of this model, that clearly deviate from other models, is that these compounds are able to reproduce the three types of symptoms present in schizophrenia, *i.e.,* positive, negative and cognitive deficits [113,117,118]. While other models such as the administration of psychostimulants (v.g. amphetamine) only produces psychotic symptoms, a single dose of PCP or ketamine can induce a psychotic state and cognitive deficits in healthy individuals that last for hours or even days [113,117,118]. This fact makes this model one of the best approaches for the study of schizophrenia [111] by reproducing more precisely the negative and cognitive deficits like the working memory disruption [112,119]. In fact, the administration of NMDA antagonists induces severe alterations of working memory and other cognitive functions -like the pre-pulse inhibition (PPI) of the startle response- that can be reversed by atypical antipsychotic drugs more efficiently than by classical antipsychotics [120-124]. Interestingly, children are resistant to the effects of the NMDA antagonists, which may reflect the fact that schizophrenia emerges later in life such as the beginning of adulthood [125].

In rats, the administration of ketamine, PCP and MK-801 produces hyperlocomotion and stereotypies like flat body posture, hindlimb abduction, head weaving, ataxia [62,126,127], behavioral alterations that are regarded as a surrogate for the positive symptoms of schizophrenia [111,128-130]. Furthermore, the systemic administration of NMDA antagonists induces marked increases of the extracellular concentration of glutamate [62,63,131-134], dopamine [62,135-137] and serotonin [62,63,131,138-140] in the prefrontal cortex. Moreover, electrophysiological experiments also evidence an increase in the activity of pyramidal neurons of the PFC after the systemic administration of NMDA antagonists [119,141-143] concurrently with the apparition of the behavioral alterations. This increase in the neuronal activity can also be measured with the formation of c-fos (an early gene considered to be a reliable marker of neuronal activation) in the cortex and the thalamus [141,142].

Altogether, these data appear paradoxical in that the blockade of an excitatory receptor results in an overt increment of prefrontal activity. The most accepted hypothesis to explain this is the disinhibition theory [118,134,144], which postulates that NMDA antagonists would block NMDA receptors located to tonically active GABAergic neurons that would control glutamatergic output. This would diminish GABAergic inhibition, thus disinhibiting glutamatergic neurotransmission (Figure **7**).

One of the most compelling postmortem findings in schizophrenia is the reduction of the expression of parvalbumin (PV) in several cortical areas. In the animal setting, this reduction has also been found

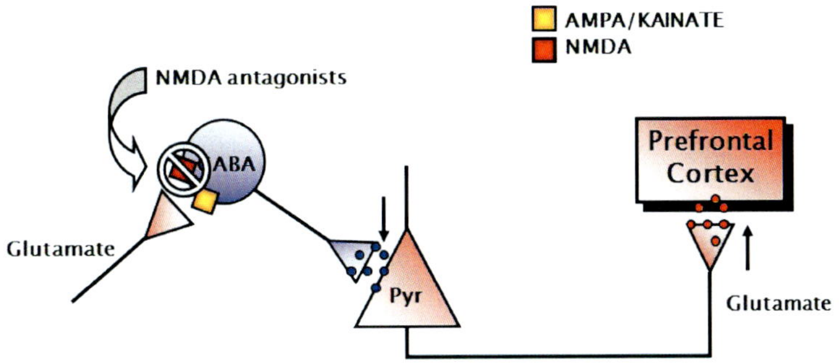

Figure 7: Scheme of the mechanism of action of NMDA antagonists. These drugs would block NMDA receptors in a population of tonically active GABAergic neurons. This would decrease the activity of these neurons, and the consequent decrease in GABA release would cause the disinhibition of glutamatergic neurotransmission that would lead to the described state of hyperactivity.

after acute [127] and chronic [64] administration of NMDA receptor antagonists. Furthermore, it has been described that the NMDA receptor of the PV positive GABAergic neurons are particularly sensitive to NMDA antagonism [125,145,146], which supports the view that NMDA antagonists would block the activity of PV-containing, GABAergic neurons, thus causing an overexcitation of pyramidal neurons.

12. ROLE OF PREFRONTAL CORTEX IN THE NMDA RECEPTOR ANTAGONISM MODEL

Although it is widely accepted that, in this model, NMDA receptor antagonists act preferentially on GABAergic cells, it remains to be determined the precise localization of these neurons in the brain. The systemic administration of NMDA receptor antagonists affects different transmitter systems in the prefrontal cortex and induces a marked behavioral activation. In contrast, the local perfusion of these compounds fails to alter the activity of pyramidal neurons or the behavior of the animals [143,147]. This would suggest that NMDA receptor antagonists produce their effects in areas outside the prefrontal cortex. In fact, it has been described that the local administration of PCP in the ventral hippocampus increases the firing of prefrontal pyramidal neurons [143]. On the other hand, an electrophysiological study has reported inhibition of cortical GABAergic neurons followed by an activation of pyramidal neurons in the PFC after the systemic administration of MK-801 [144]. This would rather suggest a preferential action of NMDA receptor antagonists in the prefrontal cortex. In this regard, as aforementioned, PV neurons are exceptionally responsive to NMDA receptor antagonists. In the PFC, the GABAergic neurons that express parvalbumin are the basket and chandelier cells. These two classes of neurons are responsible of the general activity of the prefrontal cortex circuits due to the large number of synaptic contacts they establish. In particular, these neurons play a primordial role in the generation of cortical oscillations, needed for the correct function of the PFC, and disrupted in schizophrenia patients [148,149].

The question remains as to why NMDA receptor antagonists act preferentially on cortical GABAergic neurons, given that both pyramidal cells and interneurons possess NMDA receptors. There are various possible explanations. On the one hand, the subunit composition of the NMDA receptors would need further consideration inasmuch as certain subunits can confer different sensitivity to NMDA receptor antagonists or different threshold for excitotoxicity. On the other hand, it is possible that a NMDA receptor antagonist would bind equally to both types of neurons, but the final effect would be rather associated to the activity state of the cell. Thus, a cell with a higher firing rate –such as fast-spiking GABAergic neurons- would be more responsive to NMDA receptor inhibition. It has been proposed that in the prefrontal cortex, the NMDA receptors would serve as "sensors" of the level of activity of the neural circuits, thus being the main responsible of the excitability of the GABA neuron [123,150]. In line with this hypothesis, electrophysiological studies have reported that NMDA receptors regulate tonically and preferentially the activity of interneurons whereas the basal condition of pyramidal cells would not be not controlled directly by such receptors, but would be sensitive to disinhibition [144-146,150]. Furthermore, with its "sensor" blocked by a NMDA receptor antagonist, the GABA neuron would not be able to cope with the hyperactivity of the cortical network and to restore a normal operation needed for a correct cognitive function [150].

Therefore, the administration of ketamine, PCP or MK-801 would block the NMDA receptor of the GABAergic neurons of the PFC, reducing their activity level. This would disinhibit the cortical pyramidal neurons and consequently, there would be an increase in the activity of the cortical circuitry, generating thus the neurotransmission alterations previously described (Figure **8**).

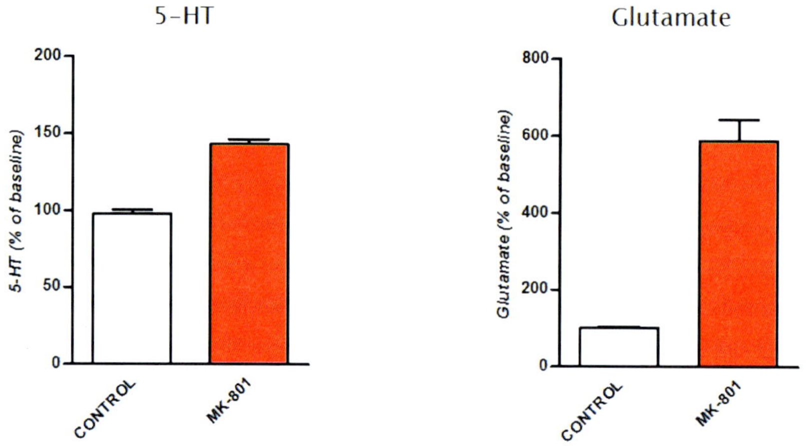

Figure 8: The systemic administration of the NMDA antagonist MK-801 (1mg/kg) induced a marked increase in the extracellular concentration of serotonin (5-HT) and glutamate in the prefrontal cortex.

13. THE IMPORTANCE OF THE CORPUS CALLOSUM IN SCHIZOPHRENIA

In our laboratory, we have shown that the systemic administration of noncompetitive NMDA receptor antagonists increased the extracellular concentration of 5-HT and glutamate in the PFC [63,140] whereas the local, unilateral perfusion of these compounds in the PFC did not provoke any change. This is in contrast with the data of [144] that suggests a direct effect of NMDA receptor antagonists on the GABAergic neurons of the prefrontal cortex. To reconcile such contradictory data, we hypothesized that NMDA receptor antagonists would need to block NMDA receptors located on GABAergic neurons of both prefrontal cortices (left and right hemispheres) to produce the neurochemical and behavioral alterations observed after their systemic administration. To test this possibility, two microdialysis probes were implanted (one in each prefrontal cortex), through which MK-801 or ketamine were given. The results confirmed that the bilateral administration of the NMDA receptor antagonists produced a marked increase in the extracellular concentration of serotonin in the PFC that was comparable to that seen after the systemic administration [151] (Figure **9**). However, the question remains as to whether this effect is accounted for by a larger application of the drugs or, indeed, the connection between both prefrontal cortices is needed. To test the mechanism underlying our results, we perfused tetrodotoxin (TTX) -a toxin that prevents the propagation of nerve impulses- in only one prefrontal cortex, while MK-801 and ketamine were administered systemically, so that these drugs reached the entire brain. The unilateral perfusion of TTX was able to block the increase of 5-HT both in the ipsilateral and in the contralateral prefrontal cortices, thus suggesting that a bilateral effect is needed to increase cortical serotonergic transmission [151] (Figure **10**). Furthermore, the unilateral administration of TTX also prevented the MK-801-induced formation of c-fos in the contralateral PFC without changing that in the dorsal raphe nucleus, which suggests a reduced activity of pyramidal cells. Overall, these results indicate that the effects of bilateral administration of NMDA receptor antagonists are not mediated by a greater activation of 5-HT neurons but by a bilateral disruption of the PFC [151].

In summary, these findings not only remark the importance of the prefrontal cortex in the NMDA hypofunction model of schizophrenia; but also the role played by callosal fibers connecting both prefrontal cortices. It is thus possible that at least some of the alterations induced by the NMDA receptor antagonists (like the cortical hyperactivity status) are mediated by the disruption of interhemispheric prefrontal connections [151] (Figure **11**).

The implication of the corpus callosum in schizophrenia agrees with the disconnectivity theory of the illness, which advocates that schizophrenia is caused by the abnormal communication between brain regions [152], thus leading to a wrong processing of the information [152]. As a matter of fact, in schizophrenia patients it has been found reductions of the volume of callosal fibers [152,153]

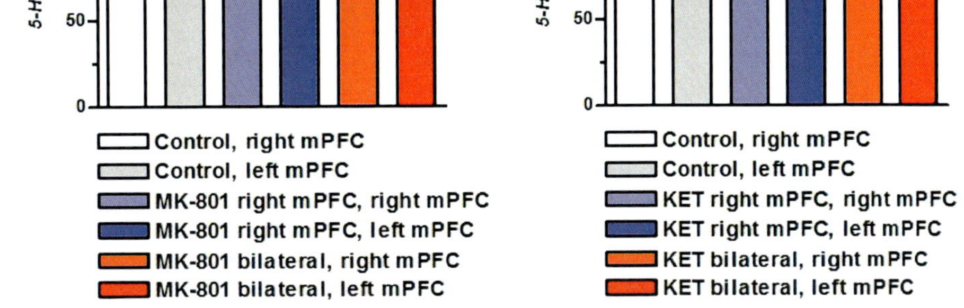

Figure 9: The bilateral (but not unilateral) perfusion of MK-801 (300μM; A) or ketamine (3mM; B) increased the extracellular level of 5-HT significantly both in the left and right medial prefrontal cortex.

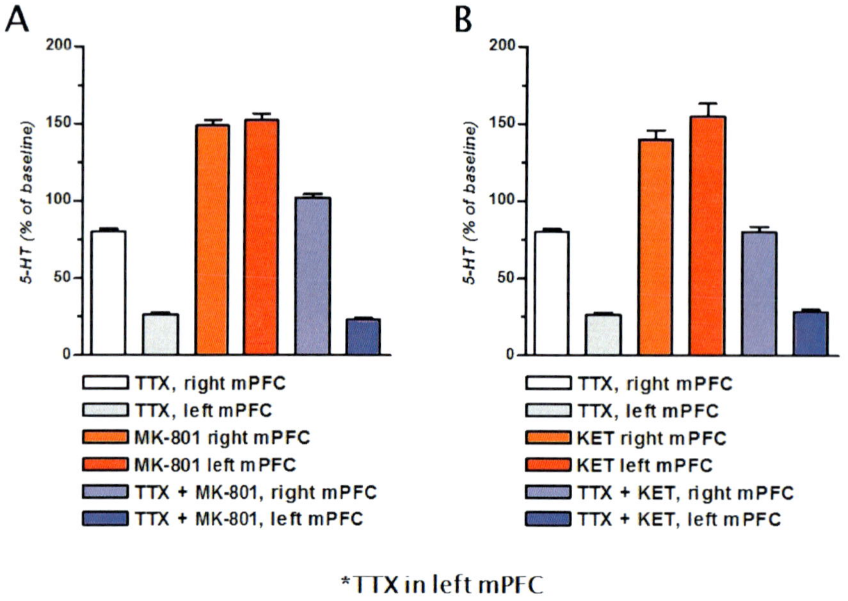

Figure 10: The local perfusion of TTX (1μM) in the left mPFC was able to block the increase of 5-HT concentration induced by the systemic administration of MK-801 in both the left and right mPFC.

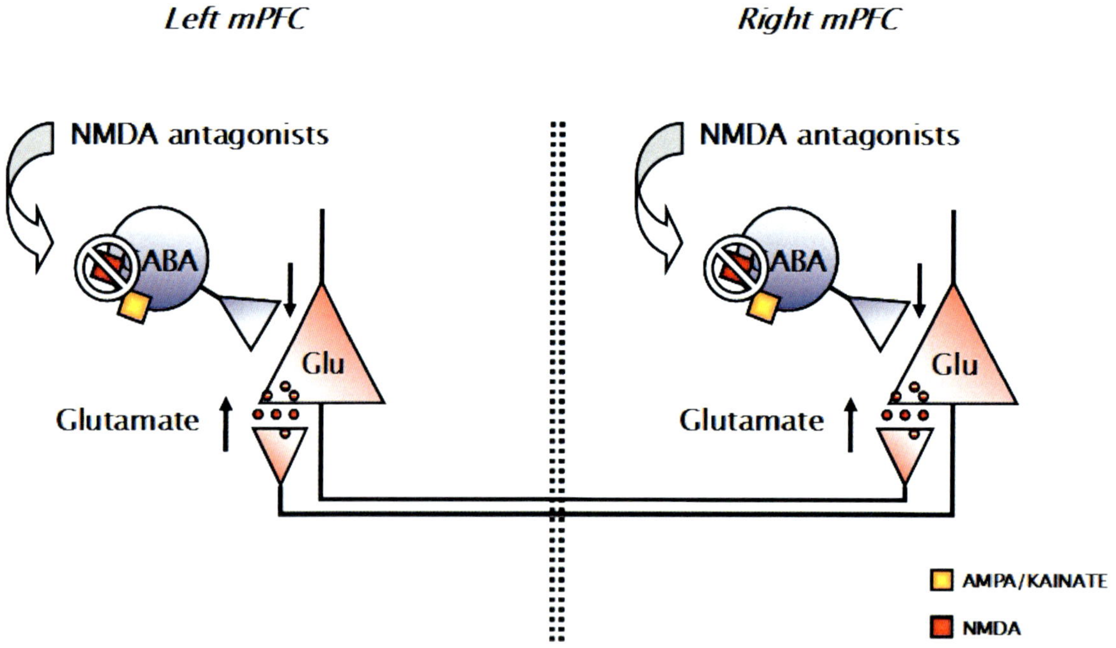

Figure 11: The bilateral perfusion of NMDA antagonists would reduce the activity of GABAergic neurons, which would result in an overstimulation of the cortico-cortical connection and, consequently, in the hyperactivity of pyramidal neurons (as reflected by the increase in extracellular 5-HT).

that correlated with the severity of psychotic symptoms [20,154]. Moreover, these reductions are prominent in the genu and anterior part of the corpus callosum, precisely the site where the prefrontal cortex fibers cross to the contralateral hemisphere [20,153]. Diffusion tensor imaging studies have also described a reduction of fractional anisotropy (FA) in the frontal fibers of the corpus callosum in schizophrenia patients [152]. FA is used as a measure of myelin integrity because FA reductions result from myelin or axon damage. Therefore, the observed decrease of the FA is suggestive of a demyelination process of these fibers, and evidences an impaired white matter integrity [152,155]. It is interesting to note that the myelination of callosal fibers in humans occurs postnatally and is completed in the adolescence/early adulthood [153,155-158], the same period of life when the first symptoms of schizophrenia usually appear.

The cells responsible for the formation of the myelin sheath of neurons are the oligodendrocytes. A down-regulation of genes related with oligodendrocytes and myelin has been consistently found in the dorsolateral prefrontal cortex of schizophrenia patients. Furthermore, post-mortem studies have revealed a reduction in the density and in the absolute numbers of oligodendrocytes in cortical areas 9 and 24, and anterior thalamic nuclei [155,159-161]. In line with this observations, electron microscopy studies have also reported the presence of apoptotic oligodendrocytes and a damaged myelin sheath in schizophrenia [162]. The oligodendrocytes play also an important role in synaptic plasticity (young rats raised in an enriched environment show a 27-33% increase of the number of oligodendrocytes in the occipital cortex), and in the modulation of conduction velocity [155], necessary for learning processes. Rats treated with cuprizone (a demyelinating toxin) exhibit deficits in working memory, disruptions of PPI, decreased social interaction and loss of oligodendrocytes [155]. It has been proposed that the demyelination of callosal axons could result in a reduction of excitatory inputs onto GABA interneurons, which would eventually lead to an excess of glutamatergic transmission, similar to that observed after treatment with NMDA antagonists [155]. It has also been described that the prenatal administration of PCP to rodents results in a reduced immunolabeling for myelin basic protein and NG2, which is suggestive of a decreased number of oligodendrocyte progenitors [156].

In humans, NMDA receptor antagonists induce alterations of the corpus callosum similar to those observed in schizophrenia. In this regard, chronic consumption of ketamine produced a reduction of the FA values in bilateral frontal and left temporoparietal white matter [163], thus indicating damaged integrity of the myelin sheath. Furthermore, this reduction correlates with total lifetime ketamine consumption. [163]. Altogether, these observations in the human and animal setting underscore 1) the ability of NMDA receptor antagonists to model of schizophrenia, and 2) the importance of integrity of the corpus callosum in the pathophysiology of schizophrenia. It is possible that some of the alterations observed in rodents (cortical overexcitability, stereotypies, *etc.*) and in schizophrenia patients (reality distortion, hallucinations, psychosis, *etc.*) are caused by a disrupted cortico-cortical communication and the subsequent impairment in the processing of the information between hemispheres.

14. ROLE OF THE PREFRONTAL CORTEX IN THE ACTION OF ANTIPSYCHOTIC DRUGS.

At present, no treatment is yet able to cure schizophrenia. Instead, all marketed drugs only relieve some symptoms of the illness, sometimes at risk of serious side effects. Chlorpromazine was the first drug of the so-called first generation (also called typical or classical) antipsychotics. This class of drugs is characterized by a strong antagonism of the dopamine D_2 receptor, which correlates with their clinical effectiveness [95-98]. The administration of these drugs is able to revert the psychotic symptoms of the illness (related to a hyperactivity of the mesolimbic dopaminergic pathway), but not the negative and cognitive symptoms (potentially associated to a decreased activity of the mesocortical dopaminergic pathway). Furthermore, blockade of the cortical dopaminergic neurotransmission carried out by the antipsychotics may worsen the cognitive functions of schizophrenia patients, and blockade of dopamine D_2 receptors in the striatum may produce extrapyramidal side effects such as parkinsonism, ataxia, etc [100-104,164,165].

Clozapine was discovered at mid 70s, and was the first of the so-called second generation (also called atypical) antipsychotics. The "atypicality" of such drugs consisted of an antagonism at the serotonin 5-HT_{2A} receptors coupled to a lower antagonism at dopamine D_2 receptor, compared to typical antipsychotic drugs. The lower occupation of D_2 receptors together with their ability to produce part of their actions through 5-HT_{2A} receptor allow these drugs to exert their therapeutic action without the motor adverse effects elicited by classical antipsychotics [102]. In addition, these drugs appear to improve the negative symptoms and cognitive deficits, probably through their distinct pharmacological profile. Besides their higher affinity for 5-HT_{2A} receptors relative to dopamine D_2 receptors [79], atypical antipsychotics form a heterogeneous group of drugs that exhibit affinity for other monoamine receptors, such as the serotonin 5-HT_{1A} dopamine D_1, α_1- and α_2- adrenergic receptors. Indeed, the better therapeutic profile of clozapine (and possibly of other atypical drugs) could be accounted for by its affinity for a large number of receptors, thus being able to regulate different neurotransmitter systems [101,166] (Figure **12**).

It has been described that drugs, like clozapine and olanzapine, that show antagonism at 5-HT_{2A} receptors increased the release of dopamine in the PFC of rodents, an effect dependent on the presence of operative 5-HT_{1A} receptors [167,168]. Furthermore, it has been observed that clozapine exerts a

	Classical		Atypical				
Receptor	Clorpromazine	Haloperidol	Clozapine	Olanzapine	Risperidone	Quetiapine	Ziprasidone
D_1	19.95	210	85	31	430	455	525
D_2	1.25	0.7	126	11	4	160	5
D_3		2	473	49	10		7
D_4		3	35	27	9		32
5-HT_{1A}		1100	875	>10 000	210	2800	3
5-HT_{2A}	7.94	45	16	4	0.5	295	0.4
5-HT_{2C}	12.59	>10 000	16	23	25		1
α_1	1	6	7	19	0.7	7	11
H_1		440	6	7	20	11	50
M_1		>1500	1.9	1.9	>10 000	120	>1000

Figure 12: Table resume of the *in vitro* affinity of some of the main classical and atypical antipsychotics (affinities in nanomolar, data from human cloned receptors [173-176].

differential effect on the firing of prefrontal pyramidal neurons that is dependent on the basal state of these cells. Thus, clozapine inhibits pyramidal cells firing at higher rates, and excites those with lower firing rates [169]. In contrast, haloperidol only produces inhibitions on this neuronal activity, independently of the basal firing rate. This dual action of clozapine suggests that the drug is able to modulate both hiperactivity and hipoactivity of cortical circuits. This fine-tuning regulation can represent the precise type of control needed for a therapeutic effect, able to improve the cortical processing in schizophrenia patients [169].

As we just have seen, the administration of antipsychotics induces changes in the activity of prefrontal cortex neurons, indeed in the case of clozapine we can talk about a complex modulation of cortical circuitry activity. Previously, we have shown the importance of prefrontal cortex in the NMDA antagonists model of schizophrenia: the neurochemical changes and the direct effect in this brain area. So the question now is which is the role of prefrontal cortex in the mechanism of action of antipsychotic drugs and its therapeutic effect?

It has been reported that some of the alterations induced by NMDA receptor antagonists can only be reversed by atypical –but not classical- antipsychotics [120-124]. In schizophrenia patients there are also differences between both class of antipsychotics: while both classes of drug are effective in the treatment of the positive (psychotic) symptoms, the atypical ones also improve the negative and cognitive deficits.

In the setting of the NMDA hypofunction, studies from our lab have shown that the atypical drugs, clozapine and olanzapine were able to prevent the excessive release of 5-HT induced by PCP and ketamine, an effect not shared with haloperidol [140]. Furthermore, as depicted in (Figure **13**), we

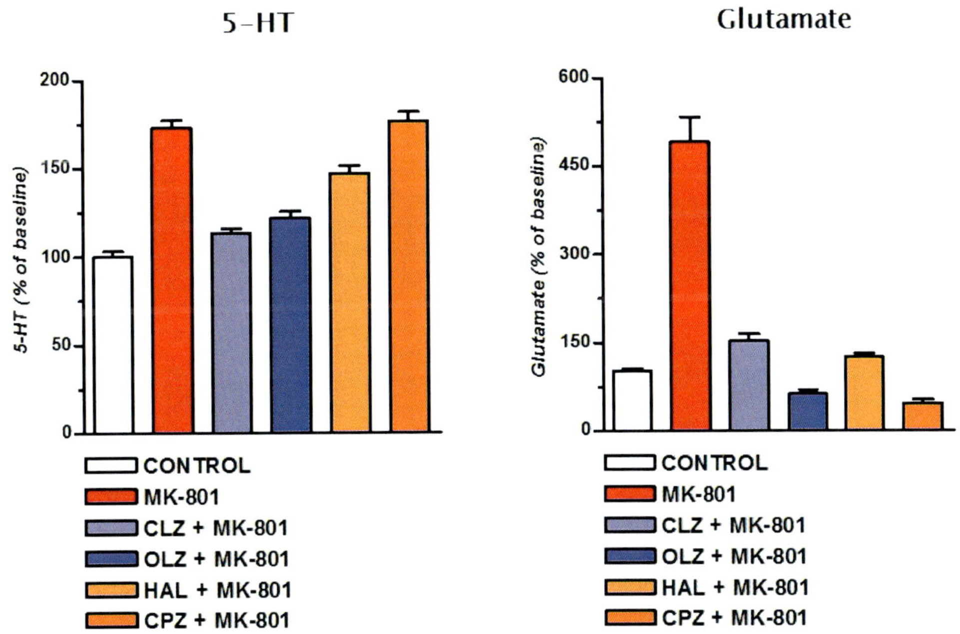

Figure 13: The cortical perfusion of the atypical antipsychotics clozapine (300μM) and olanzapine (300μM) were able to block the increase of both 5-HT and glutamate induced by the systemic administration of MK-801 (1mg/kg). In contrast, the local administration of the classical drugs haloperidol (30μM) and clorpromazine (300μM) only reversed the increase in the extracellular concentration of glutamate.

found that the local perfusion in the prefrontal cortex of clozapine and olanzapine were able to block the increases of both serotonin and glutamate in the prefrontal cortex elicited by MK-801 [63]. Instead, haloperidol and chlorpromazine were only able to block the increased cortical glutamate levels, but not those of 5-HT [63]. This is a very interesting difference in the effect of the two classes of antipsychotics: while the increased serotonin levels only respond to the atypical drugs, both classical and atypical antipsychotics are able to reverse the excessive cortical glutamate neurotransmission (Figure **14**). The ability to suppress the prefrontal glutamate increase shared by typical and atypical drugs could result from their inhibition of hyperactive pyramidal neurons of the PFC [169], perhaps through the blockade of dopamine D_2 receptors. Indeed, it is well known that the blockade of those receptors in the mesolimbic dopaminergic pathway reduced psychotic symptoms [170]. In contrast, the interaction of clozapine and olanzapine with 5-HT_{2A}, 5-HT_{2C}, 5-HT_{1A}, D_1, α-adrenergic, H_1, and M_1 receptors [173, 174] located in a subpopulation of layer V pyramidal neurons that project to the dorsal raphe nucleus would account for the capacity of atypical antipsychotics to modulate these particular neurons, thus diminishing their activity, thereby inhibiting the excessive serotonin neurotransmission.

A very important observation was that these effects were reproduced when these drugs were administered systemically (Figure **14**). The fact that the local perfusion in the prefrontal cortex and the systemic administration of the antipsychotics yielded comparable results suggests that the prefrontal cortex is a crucial area for the action of those drugs. This data also suggests that an important part of the therapeutic action of antipsychotic drugs is related to their local action on the prefrontal cortex.

As aforementioned, the prefrontal cortex is the most important association area of the brain, and is ultimately responsible of higher-level functions such as working memory, functions that are impaired in schizophrenia and following NMDA receptor blockade. In this regard, the administration of NMDA antagonists induces severe alterations of prefrontal neurotransmission that would probably occur in

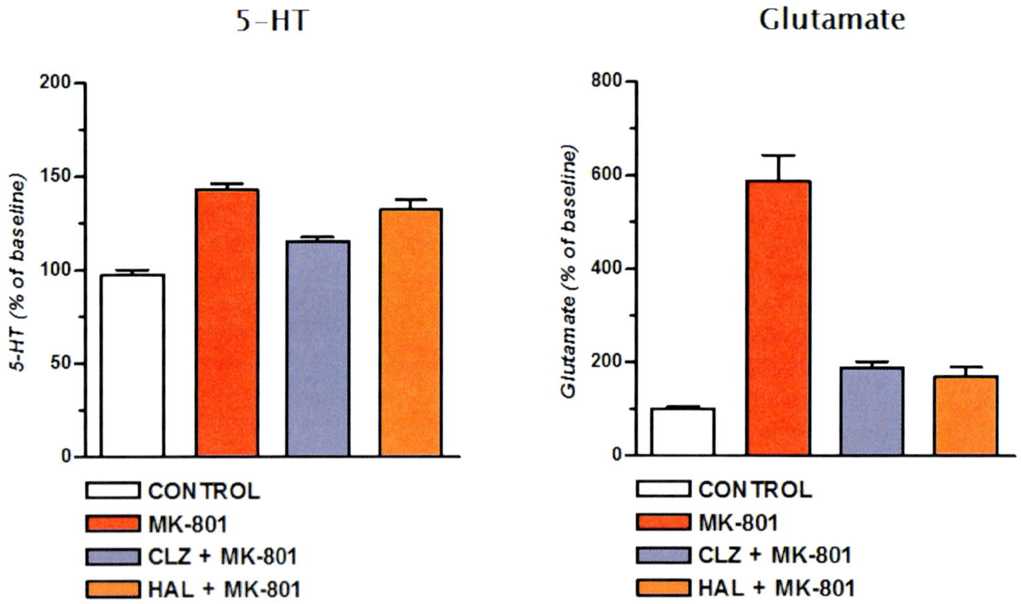

Figure 14: The systemic administration of clozapine (5 mg/kg) was able to reverse the cortical increase of both 5-HT and glutamate induced by the systemic administration of MK-801 (1mg/kg). Instead, the systemic administration of haloperidol (1 mg/kg) only blocked the increase in glutamate levels.

schizophrenia patients. Through a local action within the prefrontal cortex, antipsychotic drugs are able to block the NMDA antagonist-induced hyperactivity and restore the levels of serotonin and glutamate to normal values. This restoration of cortical neurotransmission and function is possibly a crucial part of their therapeutic effects. Furthermore, our results suggest that the increase of the glutamate neurotransmission in the prefrontal cortex would be reflective of positive, psychotic symptoms of the schizophrenia, effectively treated by all the antipsychotics [171], probably through the common blockade of the dopamine D2 receptor. Instead, an excessive prefrontal serotonin neurotransmission would be rather associated with the negative symptoms and cognitive deficits of the illness, which are better treated by the atypical drugs [102,103,172], probably due to their simultaneous interaction with multiple neurotransmitter receptors.

In summary, these data suggests that cortical serotonergic neurotransmission is regulated by different neurotransmitter systems (for which clozapine and olanzapine displays higher affinity) while glutamatergic transmission would be highly dependent on the activity of dopamine D_2 receptors. The modulation elicited by atypical antipsychotics of both cortical 5-HT and glutamate could be the key feature whereby those drugs have the ability to improve the negative and cognitive symptoms.

REFERENCES

[1] Fuster JM. The prefrontal cortex--an update: time is of the essence. Neuron 2001, 30:319-333.

[2] Uylings HB, van Eden CG. Qualitative and quantitative comparison of the prefrontal cortex in rat and in primates, including humans. Prog Brain Res 1990, 85:31-62.

[3] Groenewegen HJ, Uylings HB. The prefrontal cortex and the integration of sensory, limbic and autonomic information. Prog Brain Res 2000, 126:3-28.

[4] Markram H, Toledo-Rodriguez M, Wang Y, Gupta A, Silberberg G, Wu C. Interneurons of the neocortical inhibitory system. Nat Rev Neurosci 2004, 5:793-807.

[5] Goldman-Rakic PS. Cellular basis of working memory. Neuron 1995, 14:477-485.

[6] Goldman-Rakic PS. Regional and cellular fractionation of working memory. Proc Natl Acad Sci U S A 1996, 93:13473-13480.

[7] Cummings JL. Frontal-subcortical circuits and human behavior. Arch Neurol 1993, 50:873-880.

[8] Groenewegen HJ, Wright CI, Uylings HB. The anatomical relationships of the prefrontal cortex with limbic structures and the basal ganglia. J Psychopharmacol 1997, 11:99-106.

[9] LeDoux JE. Emotional memory systems in the brain. Behav Brain Res 1993, 58:69-79.

[10] Floresco SB, Braaksma DN, Phillips AG. Thalamic-cortical-striatal circuitry subserves working memory during delayed responding on a radial arm maze. J Neurosci 1999, 19:11061-11071.

[11] Amargos-Bosch M, Bortolozzi A, Puig MV, Serrats J, Adell A, Celada P *et al.* Co-expression and *in vivo* interaction of serotonin1A and serotonin2A receptors in pyramidal neurons of prefrontal cortex. Cereb Cortex 2004, 14:281-299.

[12] Hajos M, Gartside SE, Varga V, Sharp T. *In vivo* inhibition of neuronal activity in the rat ventromedial prefrontal cortex by midbrain-raphe nuclei: role of 5-HT1A receptors. Neuropharmacology 2003, 45:72-81.

[13] Puig MV, Artigas F, Celada P. Modulation of the activity of pyramidal neurons in rat prefrontal cortex by raphe stimulation *in vivo*: involvement of serotonin and GABA. Cereb Cortex 2005, 15:1-14.

[14] Puig MV, Celada P, Artigas F. [Serotonergic control of prefrontal cortex]. Rev Neurol 2004, 39:539-547.

[15] Gabbott PL, Warner TA, Jays PR, Salway P, Busby SJ. Prefrontal cortex in the rat: projections to subcortical autonomic, motor, and limbic centers. J Comp Neurol 2005, 492:145-177.

[16] Celada P, Puig MV, Casanovas JM, Guillazo G, Artigas F. Control of dorsal raphe serotonergic neurons by the medial prefrontal cortex: Involvement of serotonin-1A, GABA(A), and glutamate receptors. J Neurosci 2001, 21:9917-9929.

[17] Sesack SR, Deutch AY, Roth RH, Bunney BS. Topographical organization of the efferent projections of the medial prefrontal cortex in the rat: an anterograde tract-tracing study with Phaseolus vulgaris leucoagglutinin. J Comp Neurol 1989, 290:213-242.

[18] Fame RM, MacDonald JL, Macklis JD. Development, specification, and diversity of callosal projection neurons. Trends Neurosci 2011, 34:41-50.

[19] TOMASCH J. Size, distribution, and number of fibres in the human corpus callosum. Anat Rec 1954, 119:119-135.

[20] Innocenti GM, Ansermet F, Parnas J. Schizophrenia, neurodevelopment and corpus callosum. Mol Psychiatry 2003, 8:261-274.

[21] Krishnan V, Nestler EJ. The molecular neurobiology of depression. Nature 2008, 455:894-902.

[22] Drevets WC. Neuroimaging and neuropathological studies of depression: implications for the cognitive-emotional features of mood disorders. Curr Opin Neurobiol 2001, 11:240-249.

[23] Harrison NA, Brydon L, Walker C, Gray MA, Steptoe A, Critchley HD. Inflammation causes mood changes through alterations in subgenual cingulate activity and mesolimbic connectivity. Biol Psychiatry 2009, 66:407-414.

[24] Sheline YI, Gado MH, Kraemer HC. Untreated depression and hippocampal volume loss. Am J Psychiatry 2003, 160:1516-1518.

[25] Mayberg HS, Liotti M, Brannan SK, McGinnis S, Mahurin RK, Jerabek PA *et al.* Reciprocal limbic-cortical function and negative mood: converging PET findings in depression and normal sadness. Am J Psychiatry 1999, 156:675-682.

[26] Nofzinger EA, Buysse DJ, Germain A, Price JC, Meltzer CC, Miewald JM *et al.* Alterations in regional cerebral glucose metabolism across waking and non-rapid eye movement sleep in depression. Arch Gen Psychiatry 2005, 62:387-396.

[27] Galynker II, Cai J, Ongseng F, Finestone H, Dutta E, Serseni D. Hypofrontality and negative symptoms in major depressive disorder. J Nucl Med 1998, 39:608-612.

[28] Mayberg HS, Liotti M, Brannan SK, McGinnis S, Mahurin RK, Jerabek PA *et al.* Reciprocal limbic-cortical function and negative mood: converging PET findings in depression and normal sadness. Am J Psychiatry 1999, 156:675-682.

[29] Koenigs M, Huey ED, Calamia M, Raymont V, Tranel D, Grafman J. Distinct regions of prefrontal cortex mediate resistance and vulnerability to depression. J Neurosci 2008, 28:12341-12348.

[30] Dunlop BW, Nemeroff CB. The role of dopamine in the pathophysiology of depression. Arch Gen Psychiatry 2007, 64:327-337.

[31] Morita M, Nakayama K. Mirtazapine in combination with perospirone synergistically enhances dopamine release in the rat prefrontal cortex *via* 5-HT1A receptor activation. Psychiatry Clin Neurosci 2011, 65:246-253.

[32] Prica C, Hascoet M, Bourin M. Is co-administration of bupropion with SSRIs and SNRIs in forced swimming test in mice, predictive of efficacy in resistant depression? Behav Brain Res 2008, 194:92-99.

[33] Trivedi MH, Fava M, Wisniewski SR, Thase ME, Quitkin F, Warden D *et al.* Medication augmentation after the failure of SSRIs for depression. N Engl J Med 2006, 354:1243-1252.

[34] Artigas F, Romero L, de Montigny C, Blier P. Acceleration of the effect of selected antidepressant drugs in major depression by 5-HT1A antagonists. Trends Neurosci 1996, 19:378-383.

[35] Artigas F, Bel N, Casanovas JM, Romero L. Adaptative changes of the serotonergic system after antidepressant treatments. Adv Exp Med Biol 1996, 398:51-59.

[36] Duman RS, Malberg J, Thome J. Neural plasticity to stress and antidepressant treatment. Biol Psychiatry 1999, 46:1181-1191.

[37] Jacobs BL, van Praag H, Gage FH. Adult brain neurogenesis and psychiatry: a novel theory of depression. Mol Psychiatry 2000, 5:262-269.

[38] Fava M, McGrath PJ, Sheu WP. Switching to reboxetine: an efficacy and safety study in patients with major depressive disorder unresponsive to fluoxetine. J Clin Psychopharmacol 2003, 23(4):365-369.

[39] Mayberg HS, Lozano AM, Voon V, McNeely HE, Seminowicz D, Hamani C *et al.* Deep brain stimulation for treatment-resistant depression. Neuron 2005, 45:651-660.

[40] Lang AE, Lozano AM. Parkinson's disease. Second of two parts. N Engl J Med 1998, 339:1130-1143.

[41] Benabid AL. Deep brain stimulation for Parkinson's disease. Curr Opin Neurobiol 2003, 13:696-706.

[42] Damasio AR. Neuropsychology. Towards a neuropathology of emotion and mood. Nature 1997, 386:769-770.

[43] Liotti M, Mayberg HS, Brannan SK, McGinnis S, Jerabek P, Fox PT. Differential limbic--cortical correlates of sadness and anxiety in healthy subjects: implications for affective disorders. Biol Psychiatry 2000, 48:30-42.

[44] Dougherty DD, Weiss AP, Cosgrove GR, Alpert NM, Cassem EH, Nierenberg AA *et al.* Cerebral metabolic correlates as potential predictors of response to anterior cingulotomy for treatment of major depression. J Neurosurg 2003, 99:1010-1017.

[45] Mayberg HS, Brannan SK, Tekell JL, Silva JA, Mahurin RK, McGinnis S *et al.* Regional metabolic effects of fluoxetine in major depression: serial changes and relationship to clinical response. Biol Psychiatry 2000, 48:830-843.

[46] Malizia AL. The frontal lobes and neurosurgery for psychiatric disorders. J Psychopharmacol 1997, 11:179-187.

[47] Hirschfeld RM. Deep brain stimulation for treatment-resistant depression. Am J Psychiatry 2011, 168:455-456.

[48] Konarski JZ, Kennedy SH, Segal ZV, Lau MA, Bieling PJ, McIntyre RS *et al.* Predictors of nonresponse to cognitive behavioural therapy or venlafaxine using glucose metabolism in major depressive disorder. J Psychiatry Neurosci 2009, 34:175-180.

[49] Konarski JZ, Kennedy SH, McIntyre RS, Rafi-Tari S, Soczynska JK, Mayberg HS. Relationship between regional brain metabolism, illness severity and age in depressed subjects. Psychiatry Res 2007, 155:203-210.

[50] Kennedy SH, Giacobbe P, Rizvi SJ, Placenza FM, Nishikawa Y, Mayberg HS *et al.* Deep brain stimulation for treatment-resistant depression: follow-up after 3 to 6 years. Am J Psychiatry 2011, 168:502-510.

[51] Ranck JB, Jr. Which elements are excited in electrical stimulation of mammalian central nervous system: a review. Brain Res 1975, 98:417-440.

[52] Lujan JL, Chaturvedi A, Malone DA, Rezai AR, Machado AG, McIntyre CC. Axonal pathways linked to therapeutic and nontherapeutic outcomes during psychiatric deep brain stimulation. Hum Brain Mapp 2011.

[53] Ressler KJ, Mayberg HS. Targeting abnormal neural circuits in mood and anxiety disorders: from the laboratory to the clinic. Nat Neurosci 2007, 10:1116-1124.

[54] Bikson M, Lian J, Hahn PJ, Stacey WC, Sciortino C, Durand DM. Suppression of epileptiform activity by high frequency sinusoidal fields in rat hippocampal slices. J Physiol 2001, 531:181-191.

[55] Beurrier C, Bioulac B, Audin J, Hammond C. High-frequency stimulation produces a transient blockade of voltage-gated currents in subthalamic neurons. J Neurophysiol 2001, 85:1351-1356.

[56] Benazzouz A, Gross C, Feger J, Boraud T, Bioulac B. Reversal of rigidity and improvement in motor performance by subthalamic high-frequency stimulation in MPTP-treated monkeys. Eur J Neurosci 1993, 5:382-389.

[57] Deniau JM, Degos B, Bosch C, Maurice N. Deep brain stimulation mechanisms: beyond the concept of local functional inhibition. Eur J Neurosci 2010, 32:1080-1091.

[58] Hamani C, Diwan M, Macedo CE, Brandao ML, Shumake J, Gonzalez-Lima F *et al.* Antidepressant-like effects of medial prefrontal cortex deep brain stimulation in rats. Biol Psychiatry 2010, 67:117-124.

[59] Gingrich JA, Hen R. Dissecting the role of the serotonin system in neuropsychiatric disorders using knockout mice. Psychopharmacology (Berl) 2001, 155:1-10.

[60] Covington HE, III, Lobo MK, Maze I, Vialou V, Hyman JM, Zaman S *et al.* Antidepressant effect of optogenetic stimulation of the medial prefrontal cortex. J Neurosci 2010, 30:16082-16090.

[61] Tekin S, Cummings JL. Frontal-subcortical neuronal circuits and clinical neuropsychiatry: an update. J Psychosom Res 2002, 53(2):647-654.

[62] Adams BW, Moghaddam B. Effect of clozapine, haloperidol, or M100907 on phencyclidine-activated glutamate efflux in the prefrontal cortex. Biol Psychiatry 2001, 50:750-757.

[63] Lopez-Gil X, Babot Z, Amargos-Bosch M, Sunol C, Artigas F, Adell A. Clozapine and haloperidol differently suppress the MK-801-increased glutamatergic and serotonergic transmission in the medial prefrontal cortex of the rat. Neuropsychopharmacology 2007, 32:2087-2097.

[64] Cochran SM, Kennedy M, McKerchar CE, Steward LJ, Pratt JA, Morris BJ. Induction of metabolic hypofunction and neurochemical deficits after chronic intermittent exposure to phencyclidine: differential modulation by antipsychotic drugs. Neuropsychopharmacology 2003, 28:265-275.

[65] Hasler G, van der Veen JW, Tumonis T, Meyers N, Shen J, Drevets WC. Reduced prefrontal glutamate/glutamine and gamma-aminobutyric acid levels in major depression determined using proton magnetic resonance spectroscopy. Arch Gen Psychiatry 2007, 64:193-200.

[66] Lewis DA, Lieberman JA. Catching up on schizophrenia: natural history and neurobiology. Neuron 2000, 28:325-334.

[67] Andreasen NC, Rezai K, Alliger R, Swayze VW, Flaum M, Kirchner P *et al.* Hypofrontality in neuroleptic-naive patients and in patients with chronic schizophrenia. Assessment with xenon 133 single-photon emission computed tomography and the Tower of London. Arch Gen Psychiatry 1992, 49:943-958.

[68] Andreasen NC, O'Leary DS, Flaum M, Nopoulos P, Watkins GL, Boles Ponto LL *et al.* Hypofrontality in schizophrenia: distributed dysfunctional circuits in neuroleptic-naive patients. Lancet 1997, 349:1730-1734.

[69] Gao XM, Tamminga CA. An increase in NMDA-sensitive [3H]glutamate and [3H]kainate binding in hippocampus 24 hours after PCP. Neurosci Lett 1994, 174:149-153.

[70] Potkin SG, Alva G, Fleming K, Anand R, Keator D, Carreon D *et al.* A PET study of the pathophysiology of negative symptoms in schizophrenia. Positron emission tomography. Am J Psychiatry 2002, 159:227-237.

[71] Tamminga CA, Thaker GK, Buchanan R, Kirkpatrick B, Alphs LD, Chase TN *et al.* Limbic system abnormalities identified in schizophrenia using positron emission tomography with fluorodeoxyglucose and neocortical alterations with deficit syndrome. Arch Gen Psychiatry 1992, 49:522-530.

[72] Weinberger DR, Gallhofer B. Cognitive function in schizophrenia. Int Clin Psychopharmacol 1997, 12 Suppl 4:S29-S36.

[73] Potkin SG, Buchsbaum MS, Jin Y, Tang C, Telford J, Friedman G *et al.* Clozapine effects on glucose metabolic rate in striatum and frontal cortex. J Clin Psychiatry 1994, 55 Suppl B:63-66.

[74] Tsai G, Coyle JT. N-acetylaspartate in neuropsychiatric disorders. Prog Neurobiol 1995, 46:531-540.

[75] Benes FM. Emerging principles of altered neural circuitry in schizophrenia. Brain Res Brain Res Rev 2000, 31:251-269.

[76] Brown R, Colter N, Corsellis JA, Crow TJ, Frith CD, Jagoe R *et al.* Postmortem evidence of structural brain changes in schizophrenia. Differences in brain weight, temporal horn area, and parahippocampal gyrus compared with affective disorder. Arch Gen Psychiatry 1986, 43:36-42.

[77] Harrison PJ. The hippocampus in schizophrenia: a review of the neuropathological evidence and its pathophysiological implications. Psychopharmacology (Berl) 2004, 174:151-162.

[78] Selemon LD, Rajkowska G, Goldman-Rakic PS. Abnormally high neuronal density in the schizophrenic cortex. A morphometric analysis of prefrontal area 9 and occipital area 17. Arch Gen Psychiatry 1995, 52:805-818.

[79] Abi-Dargham A. Alterations of serotonin transmission in schizophrenia. Int Rev Neurobiol 2007, 78:133-164.

[80] Coyle JT. The GABA-glutamate connection in schizophrenia: which is the proximate cause? Biochem Pharmacol 2004, 68:1507-1514.

[81] Hashimoto T, Volk DW, Eggan SM, Mirnics K, Pierri JN, Sun Z *et al.* Gene expression deficits in a subclass of GABA neurons in the prefrontal cortex of subjects with schizophrenia. J Neurosci 2003, 23:6315-6326.

[82] Lipska BK, Weinberger DR. Delayed effects of neonatal hippocampal damage on haloperidol-induced catalepsy and apomorphine-induced stereotypic behaviors in the rat. Brain Res Dev Brain Res 1993, 75:213-222.

[83] Lipska BK, Weinberger DR. To model a psychiatric disorder in animals: schizophrenia as a reality test. Neuropsychopharmacology 2000, 23:223-239.

[84] Carr DB, Sesack SR. Hippocampal afferents to the rat prefrontal cortex: synaptic targets and relation to dopamine terminals. J Comp Neurol 1996, 369:1-15.

[85] Lipska BK, Halim ND, Segal PN, Weinberger DR. Effects of reversible inactivation of the neonatal ventral hippocampus on behavior in the adult rat. J Neurosci 2002, 22:2835-2842.

[86] Lipska BK. Using animal models to test a neurodevelopmental hypothesis of schizophrenia. J Psychiatry Neurosci 2004, 29:282-286.

[87] Goto Y, Grace AA. Alterations in medial prefrontal cortical activity and plasticity in rats with disruption of cortical development. Biol Psychiatry 2006, 60:1259-1267.

[88] Moore H, Jentsch JD, Ghajarnia M, Geyer MA, Grace AA. A neurobehavioral systems analysis of adult rats exposed to methylazoxymethanol acetate on E17: implications for the neuropathology of schizophrenia. Biol Psychiatry 2006, 60:253-264.

[89] Lodge DJ, Grace AA. Aberrant hippocampal activity underlies the dopamine dysregulation in an animal model of schizophrenia. J Neurosci 2007, 27:11424-11430.

[90] Carlsson A. The current status of the dopamine hypothesis of schizophrenia. Neuropsychopharmacology 1988, 1:179-186.

[91] Ellenbroek BA, Cools AR. Animal models with construct validity for schizophrenia. Behav Pharmacol 1990, 1:469-490.

[92] Abi-Dargham A, Rodenhiser J, Printz D, Zea-Ponce Y, Gil R, Kegeles LS *et al*. Increased baseline occupancy of D2 receptors by dopamine in schizophrenia. Proc Natl Acad Sci U S A 2000, 97:8104-8109.

[93] Davis KL, Kahn RS, Ko G, Davidson M. Dopamine in schizophrenia: a review and reconceptualization. Am J Psychiatry 1991, 148:1474-1486.

[94] Weinberger DR, Berman KF, Daniel DG. Mesoprefrontal cortical dopaminergic activity and prefrontal hypofunction in schizophrenia. Clin Neuropharmacol 1992, 15 Suppl 1 Pt A:568A-569A.

[95] Creese I, Burt DR, Snyder SH. Dopamine receptor binding predicts clinical and pharmacological potencies of antischizophrenic drugs. J Neuropsychiatry Clin Neurosci 1996, 8:223-226.

[96] Kapur S, Mamo D. Half a century of antipsychotics and still a central role for dopamine D2 receptors. Prog Neuropsychopharmacol Biol Psychiatry 2003, 27:1081-1090.

[97] Seeman P, Lee T, Chau-Wong M, Wong K. Antipsychotic drug doses and neuroleptic/dopamine receptors. Nature 1976, 261:717-719.

[98] Seeman P, Lee T. Antipsychotic drugs: direct correlation between clinical potency and presynaptic action on dopamine neurons. Science 1975, 188:1217-1219.

[99] Kapur S. How antipsychotics become anti-"psychotic"--from dopamine to salience to psychosis. Trends Pharmacol Sci 2004, 25:402-406.

[100] Meltzer HY, Matsubara S, Lee JC. Classification of typical and atypical antipsychotic drugs on the basis of dopamine D-1, D-2 and serotonin2 pKi values. J Pharmacol Exp Ther 1989, 251:238-246.

[101] Meltzer HY, Bastani B, Ramirez L, Matsubara S. Clozapine: new research on efficacy and mechanism of action. Eur Arch Psychiatry Neurol Sci 1989, 238:332-339.

[102] Meltzer HY. The role of serotonin in antipsychotic drug action. Neuropsychopharmacology 1999, 21:106S-115S.

[103] Meltzer HY. What's atypical about atypical antipsychotic drugs? Curr Opin Pharmacol 2004, 4:53-57.

[104] Kapur S, Zipursky RB, Remington G. Clinical and theoretical implications of 5-HT2 and D2 receptor occupancy of clozapine, risperidone, and olanzapine in schizophrenia. Am J Psychiatry 1999, 156:286-293.

[105] Meltzer HY, Park S, Kessler R. Cognition, schizophrenia, and the atypical antipsychotic drugs. Proc Natl Acad Sci U S A 1999, 96:13591-13593.

[106] Carli M, Baviera M, Invernizzi RW, Balducci C. Dissociable contribution of 5-HT1A and 5-HT2A receptors in the medial prefrontal cortex to different aspects of executive control such as impulsivity and compulsive perseveration in rats. Neuropsychopharmacology 2006, 31:757-767.

[107] Williams GV, Rao SG, Goldman-Rakic PS. The physiological role of 5-HT2A receptors in working memory. J Neurosci 2002, 22:2843-2854.

[108] Pompeiano M, Palacios JM, Mengod G. Distribution of the serotonin 5-HT2 receptor family mRNAs: comparison between 5-HT2A and 5-HT2C receptors. Brain Res Mol Brain Res 1994, 23:163-178.

[109] Santana N, Bortolozzi A, Serrats J, Mengod G, Artigas F. Expression of serotonin1A and serotonin2A receptors in pyramidal and GABAergic neurons of the rat prefrontal cortex. Cereb Cortex 2004, 14:1100-1109.

[110] Bortolozzi A, Amargos-Bosch M, Adell A, Diaz-Mataix L, Serrats J, Pons S *et al. In vivo* modulation of 5-hydroxytryptamine release in mouse prefrontal cortex by local 5-HT(2A) receptors: effect of antipsychotic drugs. Eur J Neurosci 2003, 18:1235-1246.

[111] Adell A, Jimenez-Sanchez L, Lopez-Gil X, Romon T. Is the Acute NMDA Receptor Hypofunction a Valid Model of Schizophrenia? Schizophr Bull 2011.

[112] Javitt DC, Zukin SR. Recent advances in the phencyclidine model of schizophrenia. Am J Psychiatry 1991, 148:1301-1308.

[113] Krystal JH, Karper LP, Seibyl JP, Freeman GK, Delaney R, Bremner JD *et al.* Subanesthetic effects of the noncompetitive NMDA antagonist, ketamine, in humans. Psychotomimetic, perceptual, cognitive, and neuroendocrine responses. Arch Gen Psychiatry 1994, 51:199-214.

[114] Malhotra AK, Pinals DA, Weingartner H, Sirocco K, Missar CD, Pickar D *et al.* NMDA receptor function and human cognition: the effects of ketamine in healthy volunteers. Neuropsychopharmacology 1996, 14:301-307.

[115] Newcomer JW, Farber NB, Jevtovic-Todorovic V, Selke G, Melson AK, Hershey T *et al.* Ketamine-induced NMDA receptor hypofunction as a model of memory impairment and psychosis. Neuropsychopharmacology 1999, 20:106-118.

[116] Tamminga CA. Schizophrenia and glutamatergic transmission. Crit Rev Neurobiol 1998, 12:21-36.

[117] Jardemark KE, Liang X, Arvanov V, Wang RY. Subchronic treatment with either clozapine, olanzapine or haloperidol produces a hyposensitive response of the rat cortical cells to N-methyl-D-aspartate. Neuroscience 2000, 100:1-9.

[118] Krystal JH, D'Souza DC, Mathalon D, Perry E, Belger A, Hoffman R. NMDA receptor antagonist effects, cortical glutamatergic function, and schizophrenia: toward a paradigm shift in medication development. Psychopharmacology (Berl) 2003, 169:215-233.

[119] Jackson ME, Homayoun H, Moghaddam B. NMDA receptor hypofunction produces concomitant firing rate potentiation and burst activity reduction in the prefrontal cortex. Proc Natl Acad Sci U S A 2004, 101:8467-8472.

[120] Abi-Saab WM, D'Souza DC, Moghaddam B, Krystal JH. The NMDA antagonist model for schizophrenia: promise and pitfalls. Pharmacopsychiatry 1998, 31 Suppl 2:104-109.

[121] Aultman JM, Moghaddam B. Distinct contributions of glutamate and dopamine receptors to temporal aspects of rodent working memory using a clinically relevant task. Psychopharmacology (Berl) 2001, 153:353-364.

[122] Geyer MA, Krebs-Thomson K, Braff DL, Swerdlow NR. Pharmacological studies of prepulse inhibition models of sensorimotor gating deficits in schizophrenia: a decade in review. Psychopharmacology (Berl) 2001, 156:117-154.

[123] Olney JW, Newcomer JW, Farber NB. NMDA receptor hypofunction model of schizophrenia. J Psychiatr Res 1999, 33:523-533.

[124] Tsai G, Coyle JT. Glutamatergic mechanisms in schizophrenia. Annu Rev Pharmacol Toxicol 2002, 42:165-179.

[125] Coyle JT. Glutamate and schizophrenia: beyond the dopamine hypothesis. Cell Mol Neurobiol 2006, 26:365-384.

[126] Hertel P, Mathe JM, Nomikos GG, Iurlo M, Mathe AA, Svensson TH. Effects of D-amphetamine and phencyclidine on behavior and extracellular concentrations of neurotensin and dopamine in the ventral striatum and the medial prefrontal cortex of the rat. Behav Brain Res 1995, 72:103-114.

[127] Homayoun H, Stefani MR, Adams BW, Tamagan GD, Moghaddam B. Functional Interaction Between NMDA and mGlu5 Receptors: Effects on Working Memory, Instrumental Learning, Motor Behaviors, and Dopamine Release. Neuropsychopharmacology 2004, 29:1259-1269.

[128] Jentsch JD, Roth RH. The neuropsychopharmacology of phencyclidine: from NMDA receptor hypofunction to the dopamine hypothesis of schizophrenia. Neuropsychopharmacology 1999, 20:201-225.

[129] Moghaddam B, Adams BW. Reversal of phencyclidine effects by a group II metabotropic glutamate receptor agonist in rats. Science 1998, 281:1349-1352.

[130] Mohn AR, Gainetdinov RR, Caron MG, Koller BH. Mice with reduced NMDA receptor expression display behaviors related to schizophrenia. Cell 1999, 98:427-436.

[131] Calcagno E, Carli M, Invernizzi RW. The 5-HT(1A) receptor agonist 8-OH-DPAT prevents prefrontocortical glutamate and serotonin release in response to blockade of cortical NMDA receptors. J Neurochem 2006, 96:853-860.

[132] Ceglia I, Carli M, Baviera M, Renoldi G, Calcagno E, Invernizzi RW. The 5-HT receptor antagonist M100,907 prevents extracellular glutamate rising in response to NMDA receptor blockade in the mPFC. J Neurochem 2004, 91:189-199.

[133] Lorrain DS, Baccei CS, Bristow LJ, Anderson JJ, Varney MA. Effects of ketamine and N-methyl-D-aspartate on glutamate and dopamine release in the rat prefrontal cortex: modulation by a group II selective metabotropic glutamate receptor agonist LY379268. Neuroscience 2003, 117:697-706.

[134] Moghaddam B, Adams B, Verma A, Daly D. Activation of glutamatergic neurotransmission by ketamine: a novel step in the pathway from NMDA receptor blockade to dopaminergic and cognitive disruptions associated with the prefrontal cortex. J Neurosci 1997, 17:2921-2927.

[135] Adams B, Moghaddam B. Corticolimbic dopamine neurotransmission is temporally dissociated from the cognitive and locomotor effects of phencyclidine. J Neurosci 1998, 18:5545-5554.

[136] Mathe JM, Nomikos GG, Blakeman KH, Svensson TH. Differential actions of dizocilpine (MK-801) on the mesolimbic and mesocortical dopamine systems: role of neuronal activity. Neuropharmacology 1999, 38:121-128.

[137] Schmidt CJ, Fadayel GM. Regional effects of MK-801 on dopamine release: effects of competitive NMDA or 5-HT2A receptor blockade. J Pharmacol Exp Ther 1996, 277:1541-1549.

[138] Martin P, Carlsson ML, Hjorth S. Systemic PCP treatment elevates brain extracellular 5-HT: a microdialysis study in awake rats. Neuroreport 1998, 9:2985-2988.

[139] Millan MJ, Brocco M, Gobert A, Joly F, Bervoets K, Rivet J *et al.* Contrasting mechanisms of action and sensitivity to antipsychotics of phencyclidine versus amphetamine: importance of nucleus accumbens 5-HT2A sites for PCP-induced locomotion in the rat. Eur J Neurosci 1999, 11:4419-4432.

[140] Amargos-Bosch M, Lopez-Gil X, Artigas F, Adell A. Clozapine and olanzapine, but not haloperidol, suppress serotonin efflux in the medial prefrontal cortex elicited by phencyclidine and ketamine. Int J Neuropsychopharmacol 2006, 9:565-573.

[141] Kargieman L, Santana N, Mengod G, Celada P, Artigas F. Antipsychotic drugs reverse the disruption in prefrontal cortex function produced by NMDA receptor blockade with phencyclidine. Proc Natl Acad Sci U S A 2007, 104:14843-14848.

[142] Kargieman L, Santana N, Mengod G, Celada P, Artigas F. NMDA antagonist and antipsychotic actions in cortico-subcortical circuits. Neurotox Res 2008, 14:129-140.

[143] Suzuki Y, Jodo E, Takeuchi S, Niwa S, Kayama Y. Acute administration of phencyclidine induces tonic activation of medial prefrontal cortex neurons in freely moving rats. Neuroscience 2002, 114:769-779.

[144] Homayoun H, Moghaddam B. NMDA receptor hypofunction produces opposite effects on prefrontal cortex interneurons and pyramidal neurons. J Neurosci 2007, 27:11496-11500.

[145] Grunze HC, Rainnie DG, Hasselmo ME, Barkai E, Hearn EF, McCarley RW *et al.* NMDA-dependent modulation of CA1 local circuit inhibition. J Neurosci 1996, 16:2034-2043.

[146] Li Q, Clark S, Lewis DV, Wilson WA. NMDA receptor antagonists disinhibit rat posterior cingulate and retrosplenial cortices: a potential mechanism of neurotoxicity. J Neurosci 2002, 22:3070-3080.

[147] Jodo E, Suzuki Y, Katayama T, Hoshino KY, Takeuchi S, Niwa S *et al.* Activation of medial prefrontal cortex by phencyclidine is mediated *via* a hippocampo-prefrontal pathway. Cereb Cortex 2005, 15:663-669.

[148] Cho RY, Konecky RO, Carter CS. Impairments in frontal cortical gamma synchrony and cognitive control in schizophrenia. Proc Natl Acad Sci U S A 2006, 103:19878-19883.

[149] Gonzalez-Burgos G, Lewis DA. GABA neurons and the mechanisms of network oscillations: implications for understanding cortical dysfunction in schizophrenia. Schizophr Bull 2008, 34:944-961.

[150] Lisman JE, Coyle JT, Green RW, Javitt DC, Benes FM, Heckers S *et al.* Circuit-based framework for understanding neurotransmitter and risk gene interactions in schizophrenia. Trends Neurosci 2008, 31:234-242.

[151] Lopez-Gil X, Jimenez-Sanchez L, Romon T, Campa L, Artigas F, Adell A. Importance of inter-hemispheric prefrontal connection in the effects of non-competitive NMDA receptor antagonists. Int J Neuropsychopharmacol 2011;1-12.

[152] Whitford TJ, Kubicki M, Schneiderman JS, O'Donnell LJ, King R, Alvarado JL *et al.* Corpus callosum abnormalities and their association with psychotic symptoms in patients with schizophrenia. Biol Psychiatry 2010, 68:70-77.

[153] Bersani G, Quartini A, Iannitelli A, Paolemili M, Ratti F, Di Biasi C *et al.* Corpus callosum abnormalities and potential age effect in men with schizophrenia: an MRI comparative study. Psychiatry Res 2010, 183:119-125.

[154] Aydin K, Ucok A, Guler J. Altered metabolic integrity of corpus callosum among individuals at ultra high risk of schizophrenia and first-episode patients. Biol Psychiatry 2008, 64:750-757.

[155] Takahashi N, Sakurai T, Davis KL, Buxbaum JD. Linking oligodendrocyte and myelin dysfunction to neurocircuitry abnormalities in schizophrenia. Prog Neurobiol 2011, 93:13-24.

[156] Lindahl JS, Kjellsen BR, Tigert J, Miskimins R. In utero PCP exposure alters oligodendrocyte differentiation and myelination in developing rat frontal cortex. Brain Res 2008, 1234:137-147.

[157] Pujol J, Vendrell P, Junque C, Marti-Vilalta JL, Capdevila A. When does human brain development end? Evidence of corpus callosum growth up to adulthood. Ann Neurol 1993, 34:71-75.

[158] Wang F, Kalmar JH, Edmiston E, Chepenik LG, Bhagwagar Z, Spencer L *et al.* Abnormal corpus callosum integrity in bipolar disorder: a diffusion tensor imaging study. Biol Psychiatry 2008, 64:730-733.

[159] Hof PR, Haroutunian V, Friedrich VL, Jr., Byne W, Buitron C, Perl DP *et al*. Loss and altered spatial distribution of oligodendrocytes in the superior frontal gyrus in schizophrenia. Biol Psychiatry 2003, 53:1075-1085.

[160] Stark AK, Uylings HB, Sanz-Arigita E, Pakkenberg B. Glial cell loss in the anterior cingulate cortex, a subregion of the prefrontal cortex, in subjects with schizophrenia. Am J Psychiatry 2004, 161:882-888.

[161] Byne W, Tatusov A, Yiannoulos G, Vong GS, Marcus S. Effects of mental illness and aging in two thalamic nuclei. Schizophr Res 2008, 106:172-181.

[162] Uranova N, Orlovskaya D, Vikhreva O, Zimina I, Kolomeets N, Vostrikov V *et al*. Electron microscopy of oligodendroglia in severe mental illness. Brain Res Bull 2001, 55:597-610.

[163] Liao Y, Tang J, Ma M, Wu Z, Yang M, Wang X *et al*. Frontal white matter abnormalities following chronic ketamine use: a diffusion tensor imaging study. Brain 2010, 133:2115-2122.

[164] Meltzer HY, Sumiyoshi T. Does stimulation of 5-HT(1A) receptors improve cognition in schizophrenia? Behav Brain Res 2008, 195:98-102.

[165] Millan MJ. Improving the treatment of schizophrenia: focus on serotonin (5-HT)(1A) receptors. J Pharmacol Exp Ther 2000, 295:853-861.

[166] Roth BL, Hanizavareh SM, Blum AE. Serotonin receptors represent highly favorable molecular targets for cognitive enhancement in schizophrenia and other disorders. Psychopharmacology (Berl) 2004, 174:17-24.

[167] Bortolozzi A, Diaz-Mataix L, Toth M, Celada P, Artigas F. *In vivo* actions of aripiprazole on serotonergic and dopaminergic systems in rodent brain. Psychopharmacology (Berl) 2007, 191:745-758.

[168] Diaz-Mataix L, Scorza MC, Bortolozzi A, Toth M, Celada P, Artigas F. Involvement of 5-HT1A receptors in prefrontal cortex in the modulation of dopaminergic activity: role in atypical antipsychotic action. J Neurosci 2005, 25:10831-10843.

[169] Homayoun H, Moghaddam B. Fine-tuning of awake prefrontal cortex neurons by clozapine: comparison with haloperidol and N-desmethylclozapine. Biol Psychiatry 2007, 61:679-687.

[170] Kapur S, Zipursky R, Jones C, Remington G, Houle S. Relationship between dopamine D(2) occupancy, clinical response, and side effects: a double-blind PET study of first-episode schizophrenia. Am J Psychiatry 2000, 157:514-520.

[171] Coyle JT, Tsai G. The NMDA receptor glycine modulatory site: a therapeutic target for improving cognition and reducing negative symptoms in schizophrenia. Psychopharmacology (Berl) 2004, 174:32-38.

[172] Kapur S, Seeman P. Does fast dissociation from the dopamine d(2) receptor explain the action of atypical antipsychotics?: A new hypothesis. Am J Psychiatry 2001, 158:360-369.

[173] Arnt J, Skarsfeldt T. Do novel antipsychotics have similar pharmacological characteristics? A review of the evidence. Neuropsychopharmacology 1998, 18:63-101.

[174] Bymaster FP, Calligaro DO, Falcone JF, Marsh RD, Moore NA, Tye NC *et al.* Radioreceptor binding profile of the atypical antipsychotic olanzapine. Neuropsychopharmacology 1996, 14:87-96.

[175] Daniel DG, Zimbroff DL, Potkin SG, Reeves KR, Harrigan EP, Lakshminarayanan M. Ziprasidone 80 mg/day and 160 mg/day in the acute exacerbation of schizophrenia and schizoaffective disorder: a 6-week placebo-controlled trial. Ziprasidone Study Group. Neuropsychopharmacology 1999, 20:491-505.

[176] Seeger TF, Seymour PA, Schmidt AW, Zorn SH, Schulz DW, Lebel LA *et al.* Ziprasidone (CP-88,059): a new antipsychotic with combined dopamine and serotonin receptor antagonist activity. J Pharmacol Exp Ther 1995, 275:101-113.

[177] Romon T, Mengod G, Adell A. Expression of parvalbumin and glutamic acid decarboxylase-67 after acute administration of MK-801. Implications for the NMDA hypofunction model of schizophrenia. Psychopharmacology (Berl) 2011, 217:231-238.

CHAPTER 8

PATHOPHYSIOLOGY OF MOOD DISORDERS: NEUROENDOCRINE MECHANISMS

CHRISTOPHER L. LA RICHE*, **DAVIDE PRESTIA, SAMANTHA G. BLOCK, CHARLES B. NEMEROFF**

University of Miami Miller School of Medicine, Miami, Florida, USA

Abstract: We review the major findings of the Hypothalamic-Pituatary-Adrenal (HPA) axis and depression. We give an overview of the HPA axis organization and its component parts, including cortisol, CRF and CRFBP, and interpret findings from the dexamethasone suppression test, dex/CRF and CRF-provocation tests in relation to depression. CRF appears to mediate the neuroendocrine, autonomic, immune and behavioral responses to stress; the CRF1 Receptor (CRF1R) plays a central role in the stress response, while CRF2R exerts a modulating effect on the CRF1R. The CRF hypothesis of depression suggests that CRF is hypersecreted in depressed subjects and persistently elevated CSF CRF may serve as a marker for depressive vulnerability and early relapse. Pharmacological data support the view that chronic antidepressant treatment may decrease CRF sensitivity to stress. Our group's findings, and others', on the nexus of childhood trauma, depression and HPA axis disruption are explored; data are highly suggestive of far-reaching CNS changes associated with a history of childhood trauma that may underlie increased vulnerability to future depression. A distinct biological subtype of depression with a history of childhood trauma is proposed for future investigation. Gender differences in response to the triad of early life trauma, depression and HPA axis disruption are reviewed, as are gene studies for the CRF1R, CRHBP and FKBP5. A variant of the CRF1R gene may exert a protective effect in men. Studies of CRF1R antagonists as novel antidepressants have been inconclusive, yet the studies haven't sub-typed the depressed patients with a history of childhood trauma. Mefipristone and other glucocorticoid receptor antagonists may be effective in the treatment of psychotic depression.

Keywords: hypothalamic-pituitary-adrenal (HPA) axis, corticotropin-releasing factor (CRF), adrenocorticotropic hormone (ACTH), paraventricular nucleus (PVN) of hypothalamus, childhood trauma, stress response, psychotic and atypical depression, antidepressant drugs, alcohol dependence and withdrawal.

1. INTRODUCTION

As investigators have sought to elucidate the manifold functions of the Hypothalamus-Pituitary-Adrenal (HPA) axis over time, a compelling picture of its role in psychiatric illness has emerged, in particular the interaction of the Hypothalamus-Pituitary-Adrenal (HPA) axis and mood and anxiety disorders. Here, we shall review the major findings of the HPA axis and depression. This chapter will focus on the dysregulation of the CRF-HPA axis in depression, the pathogenesis of depression in relation to HPA axis disruption and the intriguing interplay between the two.

1.1. OVERVIEW OF HPA AXIS ORGANIZATION AND MECHANISMS

Activation of the HPA axis originates with corticotropin-releasing factor (CRF) in the parvocellular cells of the paraventricular nucleus (PVN) of the hypothalamus. Neurons of the hypothalamic

***Address correspondence to Christopher L. la Riche:** University of Miami Miller School of Medicine, Miami, Florida, USA; E-mail: LaRicheMD@gmail.com

Bruno P Guiard and Eliyahu Dremencov (Eds)

PVN project to the median eminence, one of the brain's circumventricular organs, where CRF is secreted into the hypophyseal (pituitary) portal system [1] and is humorally transported to the anterior pituitary corticotrophs where it stimulates the release of ACTH. ACTH in turn acts on the adrenal cortex to stimulate glucocorticoid release. Cortisol, the main human glucocorticoid, accesses energy stores[2]. CRF not only regulates adrenal production of steroids, catecholamine synthesis and their adrenal release, regulating noradrenergic and adrenergic tone [3], but CRF neurons also project to the locus coeruleus, regulating and activating central noradrenergic circuits and the sympathetic nervous system [4]. The "Fight or Flight" response, controlled in large part by CRF modulation of limbic regions affecting fear, increased alertness, decreased libido and digestion and contributes to pathological states including mood and anxiety disorders [5]. CRF clearly plays a vital physiologic role in regulating the HPA axis and a pathophysiological one as well, as described below.

2. HPA AXIS DYSREGULATION IN DEPRESSION

Approximately 50 years ago, depressed patients were discovered to exhibit hypersecretion of cortisol [6,7] and its metabolites [8]. Since that seminal observation, a myriad of studies of cerebrospinal

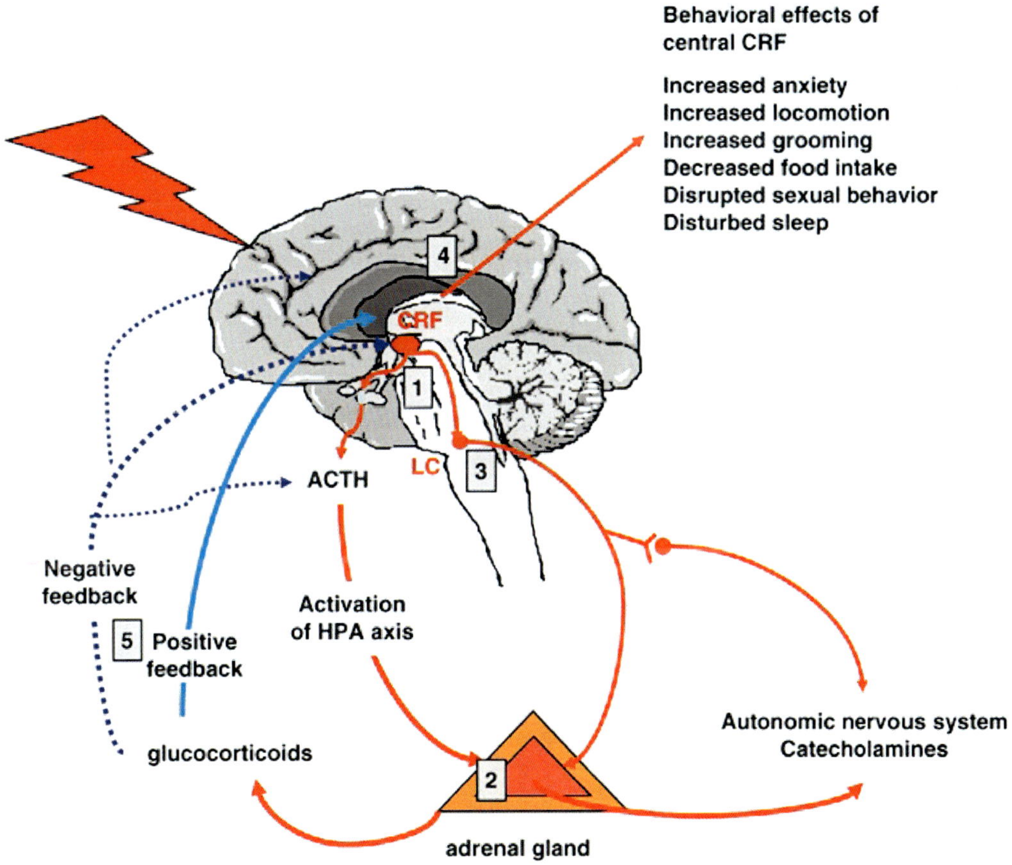

Figure 1: The actions of CRF at different levels of the stress response. 1. CRF nerve terminal in the median eminence release CRF into the hypothalamo-hypophyseal portal system and stimulate ACTH release from the anterior pituitary. 2. CRF directly stimulates cortisol and cathecholamine synthesis from the adrenal gland. 3. CRF stimulates noradrenergic neurons in the locus coeruleus (LC). 4. CRF mediates a series of behaviors through actions on cortical and limbic brain regions. 5. CRF transcription is negatively regulated by glucocorticoids in the hypothalamus, but positive regulation has been reported in limbic brain regions. (Reprinted from Binder EB, 2010) [28].

fluid (CSF), post-mortem tissue and blood have documented HPA axis hyperactivity. In addition, patients with Cushing's disease or Cushing's Syndrome—endocrine pathological states resulting in increased secretion of ACTH and/or cortisol—exhibited increased levels of anxiety and depression. These findings and results with the dexamethasone suppression test (DST) led to the diathesis-stress hypothesis of depression associated with high cortisol secretion [8].

2.1. CORTISOL, DEXAMETHASONE AND THE DEXAMETHASONE SUPPRESSION TEST

Dexamethasone is a synthetic glucocorticoid that similar to--though more potent than--cortisol. Dexamethasone suppresses anterior pituitary ACTH secretion, which, in turn, reduces the adrenocortical secretion of cortisol. The dexamethasone suppression test (DST) was designed to assess HPA axis activity by measuring anterior pituitary suppression of ACTH secretion, and subsequently, adrenal cortisol secretion by dexamethasone. The DST was originally developed for the diagnosis of Cushing's syndrome. In the DST, small doses (1 mg) of dexamethasone are administered orally at 11 p.m., and plasma cortisol concentrations are measured 2 or 3 times the following day. In the normal subject, dexamethasone reduces the secretion of ACTH, and consequently decreases plasma cortisol concentrations. Failure to suppress plasma cortisol concentration in the DST reflects impaired feedback regulation and hyperactivity of the HPA axis [8,9].

A multitude of studies using the DST documented high ratios of dexamethasone non-suppression in depressed patients [8-11]. These observations led to the hypothesis that DST non-suppression may be a biological marker for depression [12,13], a claim that has largely been refuted due to a clear lack of specificity [14-17].

2.2. CRF, CRF1 R, CRF2 R, UROCORTINS

In 1981, the major regulator of the HPA axis, corticotropin-releasing factor (CRF), was discovered [13,18]. CRF is a 41-amino acid peptide that plays a central role in modulation of the HPA axis. The CRF peptide, three structurally related peptides (urocortin 1, urocortin 2 and urocortin 3) and two major CRF receptors form a system of regulation of stress, anxiety and mood [19]. CRF has been found both in the CNS and peripherally; centrally, CRF is most highly expressed in the hypothalamus, amygdala, septum and peripherally, in skin, testes, ovaries, lung, blood vessels and placenta [20].

CRF has two identified receptor subtypes, CRF1 R and CRF2 R [19] which are expressed in different CNS and peripheral sites and seem to have differing functions and substrate affinities. CRF1 R is highly expressed in the CNS in hippocampus, amygdala, cerebellum, pituitary and the cerebral cortex, and peripherally--though less densely--in the ovaries, testes, skin and adrenal gland. CRF2 R is expressed subcortically, in the hypothalamus, amygdala, raphe nucleus, bed nucleus of the stria terminalis, and peripherally in the heart, ovaries, testes, lungs and adrenal gland. CRF and urocortin 1 show high affinities for CRF1 R while urocortins 1, 2 and 3 bind to the CRF2 R with high affinity [21]. The CRF1 R is believed to be the prime regulator of the stress response, while the CRF2 R modulates CRF1 R's effects.

The three identified urocortins (urocortin 1, 2 and 3) are CRF-like neuropeptides [22-25], each with differing CNS and peripheral distributions. Urocortin 1 is quite widespread, both centrally (Edigner-Westphal nucleus, hypothalamus) and peripherally (GI tract, pituitary, testes, kidney, and cardiac myocytes) [20,26,27]. Urocortins 2 and 3, also expressed both centrally and peripherally, exhibit differing patterns of distribution. Urocortin 2 is distributed in the hypothalamic paraventricular nucleus (PVN) and arcuate nucleus, the locus coeruleus (LC), spinal motor neurons and, perhaps significantly, its distribution coincides, partially, with that of CRF [24]. The distribution of urocortin

3 does not overlap with CRF and is confined largely to the bed nucleus of the stria terminalis, rostral perifornical area, median pre-optic area and medial nucleus of the amygdala [23].

Of importance, the three urocortins and CRF bind with high affinity to a circulating, soluble glycoprotein, the CRF-binding protein (CRFBP); its hypothesized function is detailed below [28]. CRFBP, circulating and soluble, is widely distributed itself, and partially co-localizes with CRF, commensurate with its role as a modulator of CRF neurotransmission [29].

2.2.1. CRF and CRF Hypothesis of Depression

CRF is the major CNS regulator of HPA axis functioning and has been hypothesized to play an important role in the pathology of mood and anxiety disorders [28]. A growing body of literature suggests that the HPA axis disruption in depression is at least partly due to CRF hypersecretion [64,84]. Depressed patients and suicide victims have been shown to exhibit elevated CSF CRF in several studies [30-33]. Successful treatment with ECT lowers CSF CRF concentrations [34] as does treatment with anti-depressants [28]. Animal studies have revealed that direct CNS administration of CRF produces symptoms of depression including decreased appetite, weight loss, disrupted sleep and decreased sexual behavior [35]. Additionally, persistently elevated CSF CRF concentrations are associated with early relapse of depression [31].

If CRF rises in depressed patients and later normalizes with resolution of depressive symptoms, this would suggest that elevated CRF and HPA axis disruption comprise a state phenomenon—a disease phase-specific phenomenon--rather than a constitutive, more enduring, trait phenomenon [8]. There is some evidence supporting the state hypothesis of HPA axis disruption which includes: plasma cortisol in depressed patients [36], DST non-suppression status [9], blunted ACTH response following CRF infusion [37], hypersecretion of CRF in depression [34] and adrenal hypertrophy [38]. All these HPA axis alterations have been reported to normalize following resolution of depressive symptoms. However, HPA axis disruption, and in particular, persistently elevated CSF CRF, may also serve as a marker for depressive vulnerability and early relapse of depression even following symptomatic improvement [31].

2.2.2. Psychotic Depression and Bipolar Mixed states

It has been suggested that psychotic depression represents a distinct and etiologically discrete subgroup within depressive disorders, and although outside the scope of this review, some of the HPA axis findings support this view. DST non-suppressors were more commonly found in the sub-group of psychotic depression and bipolar mixed states than other depressed groups and DST-NS predicted a more severe course of illness [9-11]. When the DST is used as a tool for predicting treatment response, baseline status on DST did not clearly predict a response to treatment, though post-treatment DST non-suppression is a significant risk factor for relapsing depression and poorer outcome [15,16]. A metanalysis supported the association of hypercortisolemia, psychotic depression and non-suppression of cortisol on the DST [17]. However, when used as a marker to detect suicidality, the power of the DST-NS status to predict suicide remains unclear [39,40].

2.2.3. Atypical Depression and the HPA Axis

It has been hypothesized the different subtypes of depression (*i.e.*, melancholic *vs.* atypical) imply a diversity in HPA activity. Gold and Chrousos (2002) suggest that patients with atypical depression exhibit a down-regulation of the HPA axis activity and a CRH deficiency when compared to melancholic depression [201] and recommend that each subtype be studied separately. Continuing in this vein, there is good evidence that CRH exerts diminished control over HPA axis output in atypical depression when compared to melancholic subtype but there is no convincing evidence that cortisol output, or overall HPA activity, is reduced in atypical depression [202]. O'Keane *et al* conjecture that

Table 1: Studies of CRF, ACTH, Cortisol and Depression		
Source	Methods	Findings
Nemeroff et al. [30]	Controlled study measuring CSF CRF immunoreactivity in depressed patients.	Patients with major depression had significantly elevated CSF concentrations of CRF-like immunoreactivity. In 11 out of the 23 depressed patients, the CRF immunoreactivity was elevated compared to controls.
Nemeroff et al. [60]	Controlled study assessing the number and affinity of CRF binding sites in 26 suicide victims compared with 29 controls.	Study found 23% reduction in the number of CRF binding sites in the frontal cortex of suicide victims compared with controls.
Holsboer-Trachsler et al. [70]	Controlled study assessing effect of h-CRH on cortisol response administered to 14 patients with major depression, after premedication with 1.5 mg dexamethasone.	Cortisol response was significantly elevated in depressed patients compared to controls. ACTH levels were also significantly higher than controls. After treatment with trimipramine (200mg/day) for 6 weeks, depression scores were significantly better than controls.
Ising et al. [72]	Controlled study assessing the effect of DEX/CRH test on depression at two time points (baseline and 2-3wks).	ACTH and cortisol were elevated for DEX/CRH at baseline in depressed subjects compared to controls. At 2-3wks, 36 out of 50 depressed patients showed attenuated cortisol response in the second DEX/CRH test, suggesting the DEX/CRH test may be a reliable biomarker to predict clinical outcome.

as depression develops over time, a "switch" occurs in HPA regulation from CRH- to AVP-control as stress becomes more sustained or repeated, and that this switch from CRH to AVP may explain the changing longitudinal profile of depression [203]. This remains an area of great interest to researchers and further studies are needed.

2.2.4. CRF Hypothesis and Pharmacologic Findings

There is significant evidence that antidepressants modulate activity of the CRF-containing neural circuits. Tan *et al* [41] found evidence of (serotonergic) dorsal raphe nuclei projections to the frontal cortex modulating GABAergic activity and found that CRF influences the serotonergic regulation of GABA transmission. Chronic but not acute administration of the TCA imipramine to rats increased CRF1 R binding sites in striatum, cerebellum, frontal cortex but not in the parietal or temporal cortex, hippocampus or anterior pituitary [42]. These increased CRF1 R binding densities are thought to be due to the antidepressant's effect on reducing CRFergic activity. Evidence that antidepressant administration decreases CRFergic activity is derived from clinical studies that demonstrated reductions in CSF CRF concentrations after treatment with desipramine [43] and fluoxetine [44].

The MAO inhibitor tranylcypromine and dual reuptake inhibitor venlafaxine, chronically administered to stressed rats, reduced hypothalamic CRF responsiveness to stress and reduced chronic variable stress-induced increases in CRF heteronuclear RNA expression in the PVN compared to controls. Venlafaxine blocked chronic variable stress-induced elevations in CRF mRNA expression in PVN with no changes in CRF or HPA baseline measures. These findings suggest that chronic antidepressant treatment decreases CRF neuronal sensitivity to stress [45]. The well-known depressogenic and antihypertensive reserpine causes monoamine depletion and, of note, reserpine causes CRF to increase in rats in the level of the median eminence [46] and the posterior pituitary [47]. The MAO inhibitors tranylcypromine and pargyline decrease CRF release [46]. All of these findings help us build a more nuanced model of antidepressant/CRF interactions. (For a fuller discussion of CRF 1 Receptor antagonists, see below).

In more general terms, the CRF1 R is the prime receptor regulating the stress response, while CRF2 R is hypothesized to be the main modulator of the CRF1R effects [48-50]. Intriguingly, studies by Kunzel and Zobel suggest that the CRF1 R antagonists exert their CRF-lowering effect and antidepressant effect at doses that do not persistently affect the HPA axis activation in subsequent CRH stimulation tests [51,52]. It is hypothesized that the antidepressant effect is largely extra-hypothalamic, an important point in developing new antidepressants.

2.2.5. CRF Stimulation Test and Findings

The CRF stimulation test is one of the most sensitive tests of HPA axis activity. In the CRF stimulation test, synthetic human or ovine CRF is administered IV (1 mg/kg or at 100 mg) and plasma ACTH and cortisol are measured at 30-minute intervals over a 2- to 3-hour period [53,54]. In healthy patients, a CRF infusion increases secretion of ACTH and cortisol; depressed patients exhibit a blunted ACTH response but a normal cortisol response [55-57]. Not surprisingly, depressed non-suppressors on the DST showed the most blunted ACTH response likely due to chronic CRF hypersecretion. Depressed patients with normal DST suppression generally show a normal ACTH response [58]. Post-mortem tissue studies have shown elevated CRF concentrations and CRF mRNA expression in the hypothalamus of depressed patients [59]. If CRF is hypersecreted in depressed patients, then secondary to receptor down-regulation, CRF binding sites should be reduced in density. Post-mortem studies of depressed patients who completed suicide have indeed revealed decreased density of CRF receptors [60] in the frontal cortex and decreased expression of CRF1R mRNA, increased CRF concentration in frontal cortex [61], and increased CSF CRF concentrations compared with controls [33]. Findings from the CRF stimulation test studies further support the hypothesis of CRF hypersecretion and CRF1 receptor downregulation in depression.

Table 2: Antidepressant Studies, the HPA Axis and Depression

Source	Methods	Findings
Grigoriadis et al. [42]	Rat model assessing antidepressants or benzodiazepines on CRF receptors in the brain and pituitary.	Chronic antidepressant therapy down-regulated expression of cortical 5-HT2 serotonin and beta-adrenergic receptors. After imipramine treatment, there were increases in CRF binding in the rat brain stem. After chronic benzodiazepine treatment, CRF receptor binding was significantly decreased in the frontal cerebral cortex and hippocampus.
Bellis et al. [44]	Study assessing the effect of CRF and arginine vasopressin concentrations in CSF before and after administration of fluoxetine in 9 depressed patients.	Depressed patients treated with fluoxetine showed significant decreases in CSF CRH, CSF arginine vasopressin, and Hamilton depression rating scores.
Veith et al. [43]	Placebo-controlled trial assessing the effect of desipramine on CRF concentrations in CSF.	A non-significant 6% reduction in CRF concentration in subjects who received 50mg of desipramine (DMI) was found, while those treated with 100 mg of DMI showed a significant decrease in CRF concentrations. DMI had no effect on CSF norepinephrine or plasma cortisol concentrations.
Stout et al. [45]	Assessed the effect of chronic antidepressant therapy on the availability of CRF, on CRF gene expression and peptide concentration.	4-week treatment with venlafaxine and tranylcypromine resulted in decreases in the acute stress-induced increase of CRF hnRNA in the PVN. Similar trends were found with fluoxetine and reboxetine. Basal CRF hnRNA and mRNA were not affected in any area of the brain studied. CRF receptor expression was unaffected by antidepressant administration.
Shule et al. [71]	5-week longitudinal study assessing the effect of either reboxetine (8mg/day; n=20) or mirtazapine (45mg/day; n=20) on the DEX/CRH test in depressed patients.	There were differential effects of reboxtine and mirtazapine on the DEX/CRH test. Reboxetine caused the most pronounced effects after 5 weeks of treatment. Mirtazapine significantly reduced cortisol and ACTH within 1 wk, suggesting differential effects of antidepressants on the HPA axis that may be time-dependent.

2.2.6. Extra-hypothalamic CRF and Depression

Differences in the effects of cortisol on CRF gene expression in the hypothalamus and in extra-hypothalamic areas have been reported. Glucocorticoids have been shown to decrease CRF mRNA expression *via* negative feedback in the hypothalamic PVN [27] and, in contrast, to increase CRF mRNA expression in limbic areas such as the amygdala and lateral septum [64]. In fact, a lentiviral vector study in rats showed that increased CRF expression in the central nucleus of the amygdala (CeA) was depressogenic, and HPA axis hyperactivity was shown to increase [62]. This increased CRF synthesis decreased glucocorticoid negative feedback, a phenomenon observed in depressed patients. CRF mRNA expression is hypothesized to be increased in depressed patients, with consequent CRF hypersecretion through the CNS. This hypersecretion of CRF in the CNS probably includes the locus coeruleus (LC), perhaps *via* the amygdalar/LC pathway, and there is a reciprocal noradrenergic projection from the LC to the amygdala that activates CRF-containing cells [63]. Central amygdalar (CeA) projections to cortical and brainstem regions have been hypothesized to increase noradrenergic neurotransmission of LC neurons. The hyperactivity of the CeA-LC projection might explain the finding of elevated locus coeruleus CRF in depressed patients [64]. In laboratory animals, CRF injected into specific extrahypothalamic brain regions produced behavioral changes suggestive of depression, including slow-wave sleep, increased anxiety, psychomotor changes, anhedonia, decreased libido and decreased appetite [65,66].

CRF appears to mediate the neuroendocrine, autonomic, immune and behavioral responses to stress [64]. CRF1 R seems to be largely responsible for the behavioral responses to stress, while CRF2 R exerts a modulating effect on the CRF1 R [48,67]. Activity of the limbic forebrain may be the key locus of depressogenic and anxiogenic activity. Knockout mice of CRF1R with CRF overexpression restricted to the forebrain expressed anxious and depressed phenotypes independent of HPA axis involvement [68,69] though the authors surmised, the depressogenic HPA endocrine effects may well contribute to depressive symptomatology.

2.2.7. The Dex-CRF Test and Antidepressant Response

Holsboer *et al* [69] devised a more sensitive variant of the CRF stimulation test called the dexamethasone-CRF Test. In this test, patients are pretreated with oral dexamethasone (1 mg) at 11 p.m. and given a 100 mg infusion of CRF the following day. Depressed patients show elevated (as opposed to blunted) secretion of ACTH and cortisol compared to normal controls [69,70]. The dexamethasone-CRF test is the most sensitive measure of HPA axis activity in depressed patients and abnormalities in the test can be shown in asymptomatic 1st degree relatives of depressed patients which are maintained over time [43] (see Gillespie 2005 for review). These findings suggest a heritable vulnerability to depression that is expressed as dysregulation of the HPA axis. The dex/CRF stimulation test holds promise as a biomarker for predicting a patient's response to antidepressant treatment as suggested by the finding that patients with symptomatic improvement without normalization on the dex/CRF Stim test showed a greater rate of relapse [71]. Depressed inpatients who showed improvement on the dex/CRF test after two weeks were associated with better outcomes and remission three weeks later [72]. In a 16-week study, the magnitude of decreased cortisol plasma concentration with the dex/CRF test from pre-treatment to 5 weeks post-treatment with citalopram predicted the magnitude of symptom improvement at the end of the study [73].

2.3 CRF, Alcohol Dependence and Alcohol Withdrawal

Depression and anxiety disorders are highly comorbid with alcohol dependence and abuse. Though beyond the scope of this review, the interrelationship of CRF and alcohol dependence, and in particular alcohol withdrawal, show compelling evidence in animal studies [74]. Acute alcohol withdrawal has been associated with increased CSF CRF concentrations [75,76] and benzodiazepine anxiolytics, in particular alprazolam, have been shown to decrease CRF-ergic activity [77].

3. CHILDHOOD TRAUMA AND DEPRESSION: HPA AXIS INVOLVEMENT

In the US alone, approximately 3 million child maltreatment reports are filed annually, and more than 1 million reports are substantiated. 60% of the cases involve neglect, 20% physical abuse and 10% sexual abuse [78]. Several epidemiology studies have estimated the trauma exposure in children to be from 25-45% [79,80] and other adult community samples estimated the prevalence of childhood maltreatment by self-report at 30% in women and 41% in men [81]. Emotional abuse and neglect are even more prevalent than sexual or physical abuse, and parental loss through separation or death is an early life trauma associated with increased psychopathology in adulthood [82].

The central hypothesis is that early life stress (ELS), also known as adverse childhood experiences (ACE), which, depending on the study, can include early life physical or sexual abuse, neglect, early parental loss or permanent separation, sensitizes the central stress response system, especially the CRF containing systems, enhancing the neuroendocrine, autonomic, behavioral, and immune responsiveness to stress in a persistent fashion [83]. Findings from ACE studies suggest that persistent changes occur in the function, structure and epigenetics of the HPA axis and associated neural circuits after ACEs. There is evidence to support a strong association between ACEs, changes in autonomic and endocrine control systems, regulation of arousal and vigilance, the integration of emotional and cognitive processing and the responsivity to stress and anhedonia [84-87].

The CDC performed a large study of 8776 HMO members and found a strong dose-response relationship between the number of ACEs experienced and adult mental health scores [88]. Including mood and addictive disorders, and more specifically the presence of a depressive episode in the past year, lifetime chronic depression and suicide risk [89] (see below). In a seminal study conducted in a cohort of 1900 women from 4 internal medicine practices, childhood physical or sexual abuse was associated with increased symptoms of depression and anxiety, though significantly, adult physical or sexual abuse did not show the same association [90]. These and a myriad of other epidemiological studies suggest that environmental influences early in life bring much to bear on a genetic diathesis that confers a depressive vulnerability to individuals later in their life [83].

Childhood trauma and neglect are non-specific risk factors for psychopathology. There is a strong link between ACEs and mood and anxiety disorders, bipolar depression, unipolar depression, generalized anxiety disorder, PTSD, panic disorder and phobias [91]. ACEs dramatically increase lifetime prevalence of suicide attempts. In a CDC study of 17,337 male and female primary care patients in San Diego, CA, the lifetime prevalence of suicide attempts in patients with no ACEs was 1.1% while it climbed to 3.8% in patients with a history of an ACE [92]. The study found that an adverse childhood experience of any category increased the risk of attempted suicide 2- to 5-fold and the odds ratio of ever attempting suicide among people with 7 or more adverse childhood events was 31.1.

ACEs impact the clinical course of anxiety and depression and make depression less likely to remit [93]. Multiple episodes of trauma exposure increase the risk of depression [94]. Not surprisingly, increased severity, frequency and duration of abuse result in an increased likelihood of depression [95], and ELS or neglect increased the risk of a current major depressive episode in young adulthood (OR: 1.51), and physical abuse and multiple types of abuse increased the lifetime prevalence of a depressive episode (OR 1.59 and 1.75 respectively) while childhood neglect increased later lifetime depression (OR 1.59) [96].

Parental loss through death or permanent separation has proven to be another identifiable risk factor for depression [97,99] as is the death of a mother or a lengthy separation from mother by the age of 11

[98,100]. Early parental loss due to death or permanent separation before 17 years of age increases the likelihood of adult depression (OR 3.8) and early parental loss is associated with an increased rate of bipolar disorder (OR 2.6) [82].

3.1. HPA AXIS AND RESPONSE TO PSYCHOSOCIAL STRESS

In our 2008 study of the link between childhood trauma and adult HPA axis disruption, the psychosocial stress protocol of public speaking and a mental arithmetic task in front of an audience, the so-called Trier Social Stress Test (TSST) was used; ACTH and cortisol concentrations were measured before, during and after the stress protocol. Four groups of subjects were studied: a) with no history of ELS and no psychopathology b) a history of ELS with no current depression c) a history of ELS with current depression and d) no ELS history but current depression. We found that in depressed abused women vs controls, the ACTH response was 6 times greater in response and the cortisol greater as well to the stress protocol. Of note, abused women without depression had a normal cortisol but increased ACTH response, suggesting a possible adrenal gland adaptation to chronic central sensitization, which could signify a marker of resilience to early life stress [83]. Significantly, depressed women without abuse had normal endocrine responses to the stressor. These findings suggest that hyperactivity of the HPA axis following childhood trauma, likely CRF hypersecretion, may persist into adulthood and contribute to a neuroendocrine diathesis of adult psychopathology [83].

In a multiple linear regression modeling study examining the relative role that ACEs had on producing neuroendocrine reactivity, child abuse proved to be the strongest predictor of ACTH responsiveness followed by the number of abusive events, then by adult trauma and depression [99]. ACTH reactivity was strongly predicted by childhood and adulthood trauma, and the authors hypothesized that childhood trauma may increase stress reactivity, a state which can be enhanced by additional adult trauma [99]. In examining the subgroups further, the authors found that in comparing never-depressed women with history of childhood trauma and depressed women with an ACE history, both groups exhibited similar ACTH responses. This surprising finding suggests that a history of childhood trauma represents a discrete biological risk for later depression, even in the absence of lifetime psychopathology [99].

3.2. CHILDHOOD TRAUMA FINDINGS FROM PROVOCATION TESTS

Further tests were performed to explore HPA axis disruption in women with ACE, including the CRF stimulation test and the ACTH1-24 stimulation test. Heim *et al* hypothesized that if women with ACE showed a difference in CRF responsiveness, this would reflect CRF receptor changes on pituitary corticotrophs secondary to changes in the "PVN-median eminence-CRF circuit". Moreover, high doses of ACTH1-24 would allow the adrenal cortex to be evaluated for maximal responsiveness [83]. A blunted ACTH response to CRF has been repeatedly demonstrated in depression [101,102]. In this study, increased ACTH responses to CRF were observed in ACE women without depression, similar to the same group's responses in the TSST. As previously hypothesized, depressed women, with and without ACE, showed a blunted ACTH response to CRF. In the ACTH1-24 stimulation test, the group of ACE women without depression exhibited less cortisol secretion than any of the other groups; both groups of depressed and non-depressed ACE women showed decreased basal levels of cortisol [57,83]. The findings suggest that childhood trauma may decrease the availability of cortisol, a state that facilitates the disinhibition of the central stress response. Those women may, upon further stress, hypersecrete CRF which may result in depressive symptoms through CRF effects in extra-hypothalamic regions [83].

Table 3: Adverse Childhood Events (ACE) Studies, the HPA Axis and Depression

Findings from studies of the HPA axis, ACE and depression suggest that:	Adrenal gland adaptation to chronic central sensitization is a possible biomarker of resilience to ACE [83]
	A history of ACE may represent a discrete biological risk for later depression [99]
	Estrogen may play a role in conferring vulnerability to HPA axis disruption [137-142]
Other findings from the studies of the HPA axis, ACE and depression show that:	ACE is the strongest predictor of ACTH responsiveness, followed by the number of abusive events [99]
	Men with ACE showed markedly increased ACTH and cortisol response compared to non-abused men [100]
	Hippocampal volumes decrease in rat brains after repeat CRF injections [117]
	Human subjects with history of ACE showed an 18% smaller hippocampal volume than in non-abused controls [83]
	Subjects with depression and ACE were two times more likely to achieve remission with psychotherapy alone than when compared to non-ACE group [134]

3.3. GLUCOCORTICOID INVOLVEMENT

Following childhood trauma, there is evidence of enhanced stress responsiveness, possibly promoted by changes in cortisol- (glucocorticoid-] mediated feedback control of the stimulated HPA axis. The dex/CRF test is generally considered the most sensitive measure of HPA axis activity [103] and may even identify familial risk in non-depressed first degree relatives of depressed subjects [104,105]. In studying depression and cortisol response in abused and non-abused men using the dex/CRF test, men with a history of childhood abuse showed markedly increased ACTH and cortisol response as compared to non-abused men. When sub-groups were examined, only depressed men with ACE exhibited an exaggerated cortisol response [83]. These findings suggest a disruption in the glucocorticoid-mediated feedback control of the HPA axis during stimulated conditions—cortisol was no longer effectively inhibiting the HPA axis in men with a history of childhood trauma [83].

3.4. CRF IN CSF FINDINGS IN DEPRESSION AND CHILDHOOD TRAUMA

Both a blunted ACTH response to CRF challenge and a disruption in glucocorticoid-mediated feedback would be consistent with hypersecretion of CNS CRF. CRF1 R antagonists or CRF1R knockout mice showed an attenuated response to stress [64] and post-mortem studies of patients with major depression have shown increased CRF content or increased mRNA expression in hypothalamic PVN, prefrontal cortex and locus coeruleus [106-109]. In comparing CSF CRF concentrations in women with and without a history of ACE and with or without depression, women who were physically abused had higher CSF CRF concentrations than non-physically abused women in childhood, and also, women who had been both physically and sexually abused showed higher CSF CRF concentrations than those with no abuse history or with sexual abuse alone [83]. CSF CRF concentrations were positively correlated with the severity of the physical abuse, the severity of the sexual abuse and the duration of the physical and sexual abuse [83]. Women who had been physically or sexually abused after the age of 6 exhibited higher CSF CRF concentrations than women who had experienced their abuse earlier in their childhood [83].

3.5. HIPPOCAMPAL CHANGES IN CHILDHOOD TRAUMA

The hippocampus is involved in fear learning and explicit memory as well as in the regulation of HPA axis activity. Adult rodent exhibited plasticity with new neuronal growth in the hippocampus. Hippocampal neurons exhibit sensitivity to stress and glucocorticoid exposure, especially in the CA3 region, with impaired dendritic branching, loss of dendritic spines and decreased neurogenesis [110,111]. The hippocampus has been reported to be decreased in volume in both PTSD and depression [112-114], and has been suggested to represent a trait-like marker for depression because patients with remitted depression continued to show decreased hippocampal volumes [117]. Rodents separated from their mothers showed a decrease in the density of mossy fibers and impaired hippocampal neurogenesis [115,116]. Brunson *et al* [117] showed that repeatedly injecting CRF into the brains of developing rats reduced hippocampal volumes significantly and reproduced the findings of ELS without requiring stress levels of glucocorticoids. Other studies have shown decreased hippocampal volume in patients with childhood trauma both with and without PTSD [118,119]. Our study compared hippocampal volumes in two groups of depressed women, one group with a history of prepubertal physical or sexual abuse and the other group without ACE but with depression alone, finding an 18% smaller hippocampal volume in the group with childhood abuse than the non-ACE, depressed group [83]. Of note, the hippocampal volumes in the depressed women without abuse were similar to those of the healthy comparison subjects [120]. Increased cortisol pulses and/or repeated bursts of CRF in response to stress in early life may lead to a decrease in hippocampal volume in depressed patients who have been exposed to childhood trauma [83].

3.6. CNS CHANGES IN CHILDHOOD TRAUMA

The relationship between childhood trauma, changes in neuroendocrine stress response and adult vulnerability to depression implicates a set of changes along a widely distributed neural circuit regulating and organizing the endocrine-stress response [64]. This neural circuit comprises behavioral, autonomic and neural components that include the prefrontal cortex, amygdala, hippocampus and brainstem regions [64,111,121] and there is evidence that discrete changes occur within this neural circuit as a result of childhood trauma/ELS [86,87,122,88,89,125]. These neural circuit changes have been revealed in human studies after childhood trauma, with functional CNS changes ranging from impaired recognition of facial expressions in children [123] to an abnormal right-ventro-lateral-prefrontal-cortex amygdalar activation in the emotional labeling of angry faces [124], though the latter study was in families characterized by "harsh parenting".

3.7. ENDOPHENOTYPES OF DEPRESSION BASED ON CHILDHOOD TRAUMA

The findings suggest that the neurobiological changes in response to childhood trauma underlie an increased vulnerability to future depression. This may point to the existence of a distinct biological subtype of depression, with significant implications for further investigation [83].

Not only are the implications for further research far-reaching, when looking at the results of previous studies in which these data were not collected--the effects of adverse childhood experience were not accounted for in previous studies--this could exert a considerable confounding effect on previous findings in depression and might account for discrepancies in past study outcomes [125]. Classifying a depressed population by history of childhood trauma leads to measurable differences in stress responsiveness, dex/CRF stimulation test and hippocampal volume findings as well as in treatment outcome [125] (see Figure **2** and Figure **3**).

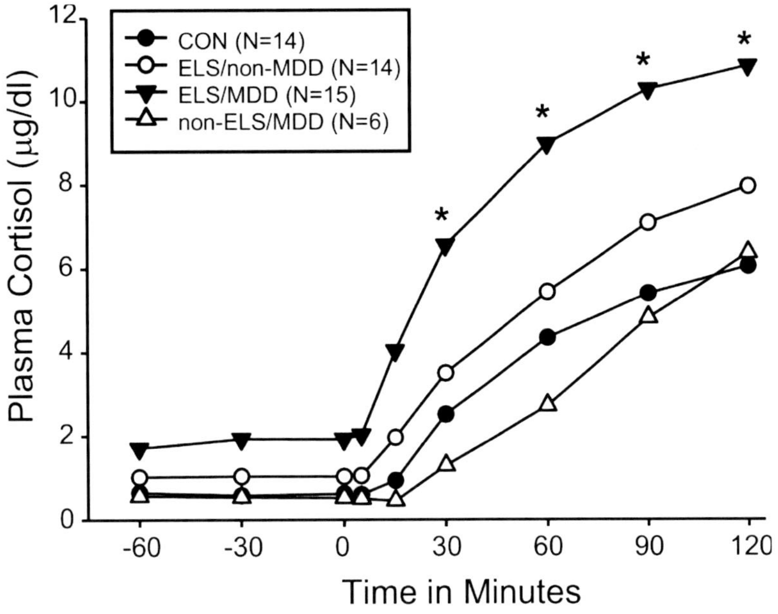

Figure 2: Mean plasma cortisol concentrations in the dexamethasone/CRF test in men without a history of significant early life stress (ELS) and no psychiatric disorder (CON; *n*=14), men with a history of childhood sexual or physical abuse without major depression (ELS/non-MDD; *n*=14), men with a history of childhood sexual or physical abuse and current major depression (ELS/MDD; *n*=15), and men without a history of significant early life stress and current major depression (non-ELS/MDD; *n*=6). *ELS/MDD versus control subjects and non-ELS/MDD: $p < .05$ (Reprinted from Heim *et al* 2008) [125].

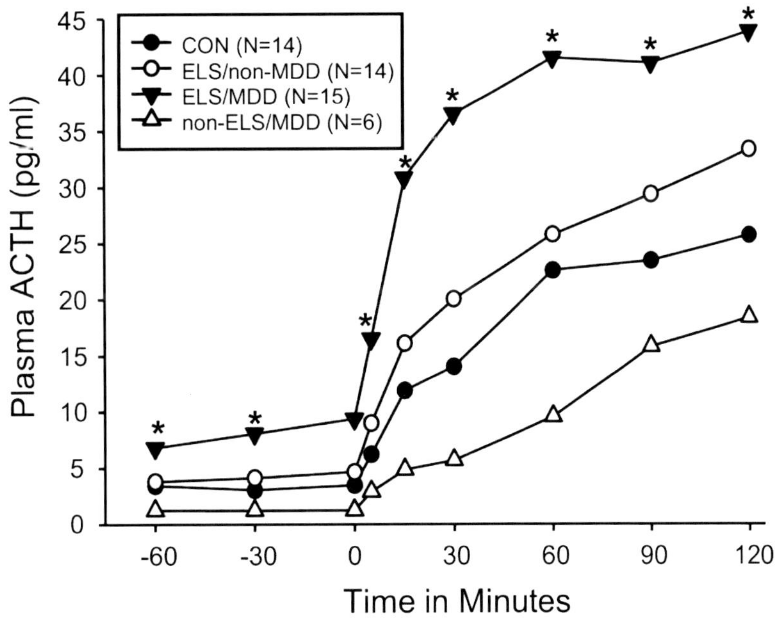

Figure 3: Mean plasma adrenocorticotropin (ACTH) concentrations in the dexamethasone/CRF test in men without a history of significant ELS and no psychiatric disorder (CON; *n*=14), men with a history of childhood sexual or physical abuse without major depression (ELS/non-MDD; *n*=14), men with a history of childhood sexual or physical abuse and current major depression (ELS/MDD; *n*=15), and men without a history of significant early life stress and current major depression (non-ELS/MDD; *n*=6). *ELS/MDD versus control subjects and non-ELS/MDD: $p < .05$ (Reprinted from Heim *et al* 2008) [125].

The presence of ELS appears to affect the course of later life depression in a number of ways: the presence of the early life trauma may predict the potency of a stressor necessary to provoke onset of depression later in life [126,127] and childhood abuse or trauma may influence the course of depression, hastening its onset [128-130]. The presence of ACE may predict the number of depressive episodes and the chronicity of depression [93,128,131,95,134].

3.8. CHILDHOOD TRAUMA, DEPRESSION AND TREATMENT RESPONSE

Some of the most surprising findings in the area of early life trauma (and neglect) come from the realm of treatment response. There are some data that ELS predict poor treatment response to pharmacotherapy [132,133]. Of note, Hayden and Klein's prospective study did not focus on major depression per se, but on the diagnosis of dysthymic disorder and—given its prospective design—included patients who later developed "double depression". Some findings about recurrence and cyclicity of the depression have also come to light: patients with ACE have a higher chance of relapse after initial remission [122].

A vital clinical question that bears on treatment is whether psychotherapy, pharmacotherapy or the combination show better outcome in patients with ELS and depression [134]. In a re-analysis of a large multisite treatment trial, the effectiveness of pharmacological treatment with the antidepressant nefazodone or treatment with the cognitive-behavioral analysis system of psychotherapy or both treatments was analyzed. The authors found that in their large sample size of 519 completing subjects, combination therapy was moderately more effective than either treatment alone [135]. Yet when the data were re-analyzed with subgroupings of ACE in mind, clear differences in treatment outcome emerged (see Figure **4**). In the chronically depressed subgroup with no ACE, combination therapy was most effective in retaining remission (nefazodone and psychotherapy) whereas in the chronically depressed with ACE, remission rates for psychotherapy alone were significantly higher (than the non-ACE depressed group) than in the combined therapy-nefazodone group [134]. And more specifically, depression with history of ACE was two times more likely to achieve remission with psychotherapy alone (compared to the non-ACE group). Also, patients with early parental loss were three times more likely to achieve remission with therapy alone than the non-ACE group [134].

These data suggest that psychotherapy alone may be the most important treatment modality for patients with a history of depression and early life trauma or parental loss. Furthermore, these findings are suggestive of different neuronal pathways in treatment response within a diagnosis of depression once stratified for the presence or absence of ELS, with pharmacotherapy and cognitive therapy exhibiting strong separation in treatment response. Future studies are urgently needed [83].

3.9. GENDER DIFFERENCES IN DEPRESSION AND HPA AXIS RESPONSIVENESS

Some considerations about variability of gender in stress response, depression and HPA axis disruption are important to explore. The differing response to ACE by gender may be an important factor in vulnerability to adult psychopathology.

Women are more likely to develop depression after childhood sexual abuse than men [136]. Also, females may exhibit a greater magnitude and duration of HPA axis change in response to stress challenge than males [137]. The effect of circulating estrogen on CRF neurons appears significant. Ovariectomized rats administered chronic estradiol showed an enhanced CRF mRNA expression and enhanced ACTH/corticosterone stress response [138,139]. This enhanced response suggests that estrogen (or estradiol) may play a role in conferring vulnerability to HPA axis disruption. In psychosocial stress studies,

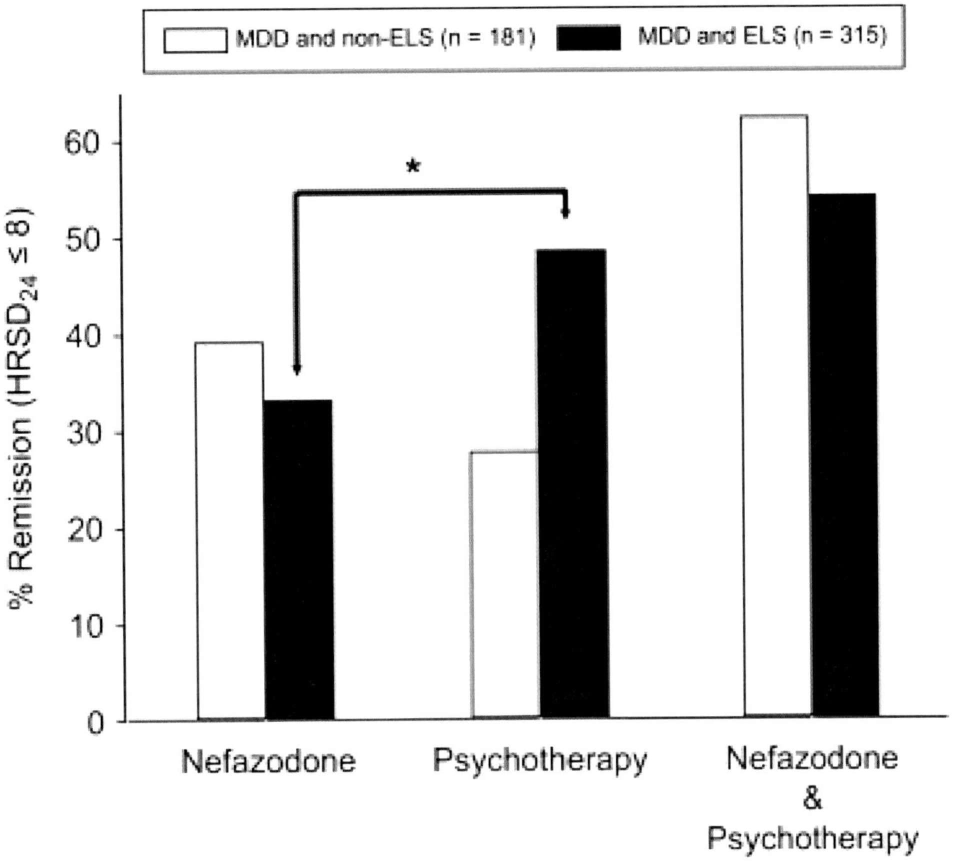

Figure 4: Remission rates as a function of treatment type and early adverse life events (ELS) in patients with chronic forms of major depression (Reprinted from Nemeroff *et al* 2003) [134].

male subjects were administered short-term estradiol transdermal patch *vs.* placebo patch; the estradiol group showed exaggerated peak ACTH and cortisol responses compared to the placebo control group and the norepinephrine response was greater in the estradiol group than in controls [100]. Estrogen receptor mRNA has been co-localized within the parvocellular CRF neurons of the PVN, and the human CRF gene may have a promoter region which is estrogen-responsive [140].

The life-long role that sex steroids play in neuroplasticity of hippocampal and amygdalar regions also suggests an influence on stress response [141] The role of hypothalamus-pituitary-gonadal axis and sex steroids has become an area of some interest and early life parental separation has been investigated in a primate model. Female rhesus monkeys [142] were separated from their mothers for 3 and 6 months. The separated female monkeys exhibited increased cortisol responsiveness to subsequent separation and flattened diurnal cortisol cycles. They also showed increased acoustic startle reactivity at later ages—changes not observed in male macaques [142].

There is considerable evidence that ELS casts a wider net of influence than only vulnerability to mood disorders by also increasing risk for anxiety disorders, schizophrenia and substance use disorders [128,143]. Here we arrive at the horns of a dilemma. Given depression's heterogeneity and variability of findings clinically (presentation, onset and course, treatment response) and neurobiologically, the existence of subtypes of depression seems highly plausible, or that "depression" is an umbrella term, representing various distinct etiological entities. For many years there prevailed a dichotomous

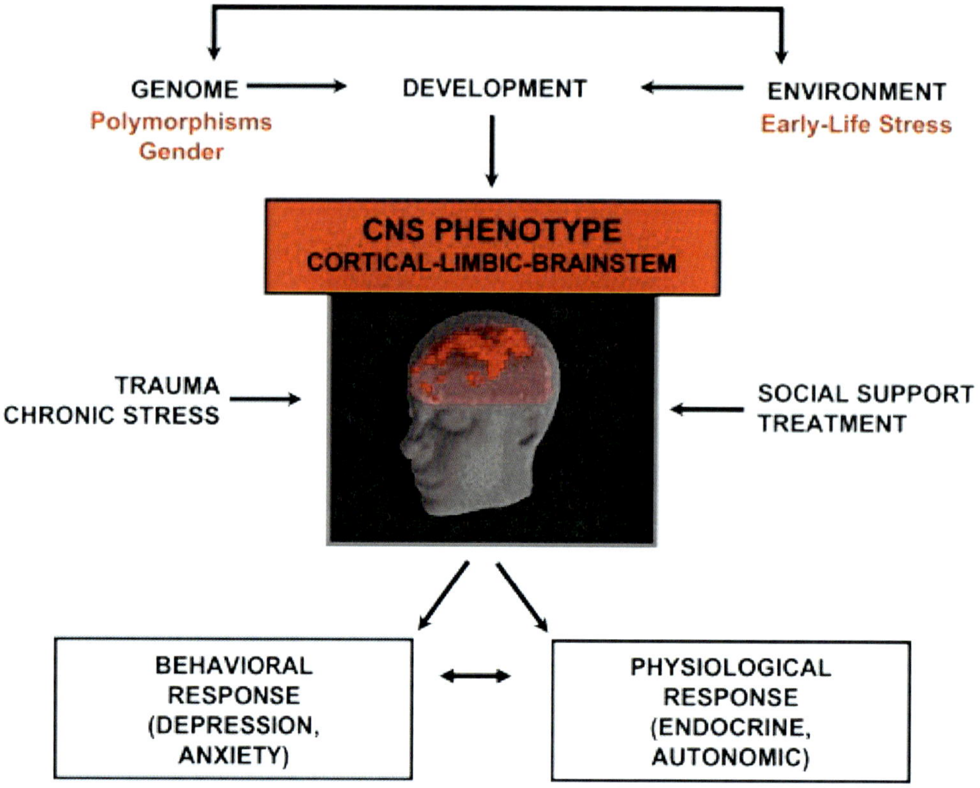

Figure 5: A working model. Genetic disposition and early-life stress (ELS) interact in shaping a vulnerable phenotype with changes in cortical-limbic-brainstem circuits. **Upon stress or trauma, maladaption in these circuits leads to increased endocrine-autonomic and behavioral-emotional responses.** Social support and successful treatments modify the stress responses system in different components (Reprinted from Heim *et al* 2008) [83].

conceptualization of depression, with endogenous and psychotic depression constituting one extreme group and neurotic or reactive depression representing another. Akiskal and McKinney [144] posited a single broad depressive spectrum, a psychobiological "common pathway", with all depressive presentations representing a spot on their continuum. The available evidence suggests that depression represents a great variability of subtypes, and the distinct paradigms should continue to be tested for differing course, treatment response and genetic origin [83,144]. Developmental factors such as ELS, genetic and epigenetic factors and neurobiological alterations should all be brought to bear on future classification and research efforts (see Figure **5**).

4. HPA AXIS GENETIC VARIABILITY, SEX DIFFERENCES AND DEPRESSION

The effects of both gene and environment contribute to the susceptibility to anxiety and mood disorders and the heritability of these disorders has been estimated to be between 30-60% [145-148]. Genome-wide association studies, candidate gene studies, and functional polymorphisms for the CRF (referred to in genetics as *CRH* gene) as well as the Urocortin and CRHBP findings are reviewed elsewhere [28]. Here we will look at findings of more immediate clinical import, namely the CRF 1 receptor and FKBP5.

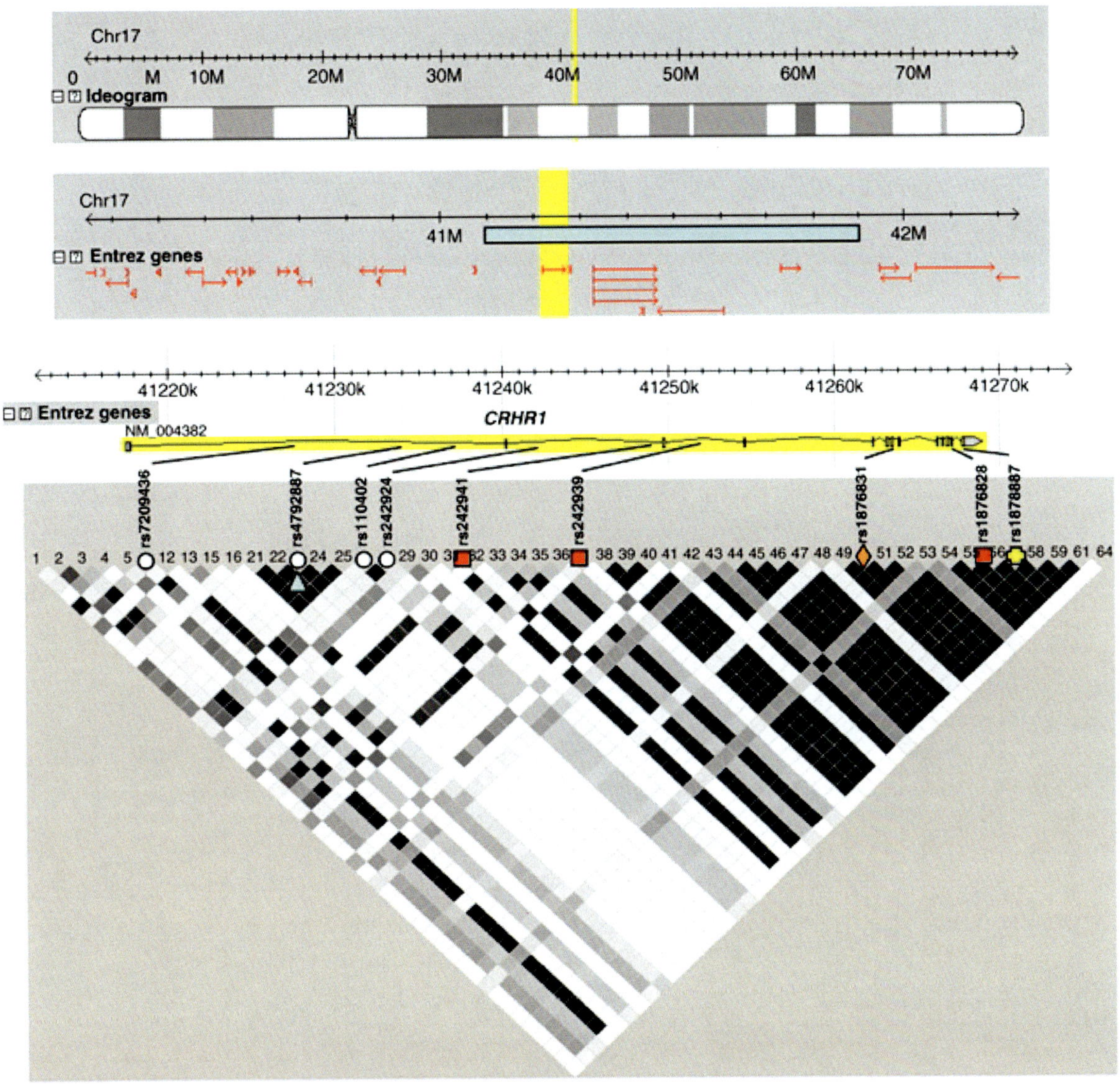

Figure 6: The genetic organization of the CRHR1 gene encoding CRF1. All representations have been derived from *http://www.hapmap.org*. The top panel shows the position of the CRHR1 gene (highlighted in yellow) with the position of the neighboring genes (red) and the position of the inversion polymorphism (light blue). The next panel shows the position of the exons and introns of the CRHR1 gene, with the 5' end of the gene on the left. Below are the SNPs available for this gene in the HapMap project with the linkage disequilibrium (LD) structure for the Caucasian CEU population, as most studies on the genetic of CRF-system genes have been performed on Caucasians. Only the names of the relevant SNPs are listed. LD is represented with the r-squared measure with black squares connecting SNPs in complete LD (r-squared=1) and white squares connecting SNPs with no LD (r-squared=0). Shades of gray represent r-squared values between 0 and 1. White circles denote the position of SNPs interacting with child abuse to **predict adult depressive symptoms** [157,158] or cortisol response in the combined dexamethasone/CRF test [3,159]. The light blue triangle denotes the SNPs interacting with life events to **predict suicide attempts** [156]. Red squares denote SNPs **predicting response to antidepressants in patients with anxious depression** [148,155]. The orange diamond denotes the SnP interacting with life stress to predict heavy drinking [161,199] and the yellow cross denotes the **SNP associated with panic disorders** together with an SNP in AVPR1B [200] (Reprinted from Bender EB & Nemeroff CB 2010) [28].

4.1. CRHR1 AND CRHBP GENE STUDIES

There is some evidence that the CRHR1 gene is involved in antidepressant response in depressed patients. In an association study of Han Chinese patients, a CRHR1 gene polymorphism was associated with good response to antidepressant treatment (fluoxetine) in MDD patients with high anxiety [148]. More specifically, the rs242941 G/G genotype and homozygous GAG haplotype of the three SNPs were associated with the therapeutic response to fluoxetine. Further CRHR1 studies have isolated 8 splice variants of the receptor ("a" through "h"), with CRHR1 alpha being the principal isoform [149-151]. When variants of the receptor were studied, they resulted in a change in the binding affinity or in signal transduction. Isoforms of the CRF1 R receptor have been localized to different parts of the body. The CRFR1-alpha splice variant is expressed both in the CNS and peripherally, while the e-h splice variants are expressed in skin and b-h isoforms in the myometrium [150,152,153]. A complete picture of how the polymorphisms affect the functioning of the CRF1 R receptor is not yet clear, but these polymorphisms may alter the ratio of isoforms and this altered expression may affect CRF1 R signaling [28]. (see Figure **6**)

The effects of CRH R1 SNPs on response to antidepressant treatment in MDD [148,154,155] have been investigated and one study [155] scrutinized the response to fluoxetine or desipramine in Mexican Americans. Intriguingly, this study was replicated in the Han Chinese population cited above [148] and both studies observed more pronounced CRHR1 haplotype effects in patients with anxious depression.

Gene x environment studies have examined interactions of CRH1 R SNPs and lifetime stress. One study [156] examined CRHR1 SNPs and stressful life events within different psychiatric phenotypes. 500 family trios with male suicide attempter offspring were studied and the rarer T-allele of the intronic CRHR1 SNP rs4792887 was found to be over-transmitted in these family trios; of note, data showed over-transmission of the T-allele in those family individuals with low stressful life events suggesting an interaction between the CRHR1 polymorphism and stressful life events on male suicide attempters in depression. These findings suggest a genetic susceptibility to suicide through altered HPA axis activity in males exposed to low levels of stress.

Another study [157] revealed the interaction of CRHR1 SNPs and child abuse in vulnerability to adult depression in an urban African-American population of over 400 subjects. Two three-SNP CRHR1 haplotypes were shown to exert protective effects. Subjects with higher levels of ELS who were homozygous for the protective haplotypes exhibited fewer depressive symptoms than subjects who carried other haplotype combinations. (see Figure **7**)

The above study's findings of gene x ELS interaction were replicated by Polanczyk *et al* in 2009 in a female cohort assessed for ELS and recurrent depression or depression in the past year. In the female ELS group, a TAT haplotype of the CRHR1 gene exerted a protective effect against adult depression. Using a questionnaire that elicited emotional memories, the authors surmised that the protective effect of the haplotypes may relate to the consolidation of emotionally arousing memories [158]. The protective effect of the gene's haplotype was further evidenced in other studies. The dex/CRF challenge test was used to study the functional protective effect of the same SNP haplotypes and found that the protective alleles were associated with a lower cortisol response in this test both in their interaction with adverse childhood events [159] or as a main genetic effect [3].

Ressler *et al* [160] found a significant interaction between gene x gene x environment in which the CRHR1 SNPs interacted with the 5-HTTLPR serotonin transporter-linked polymorphic region and

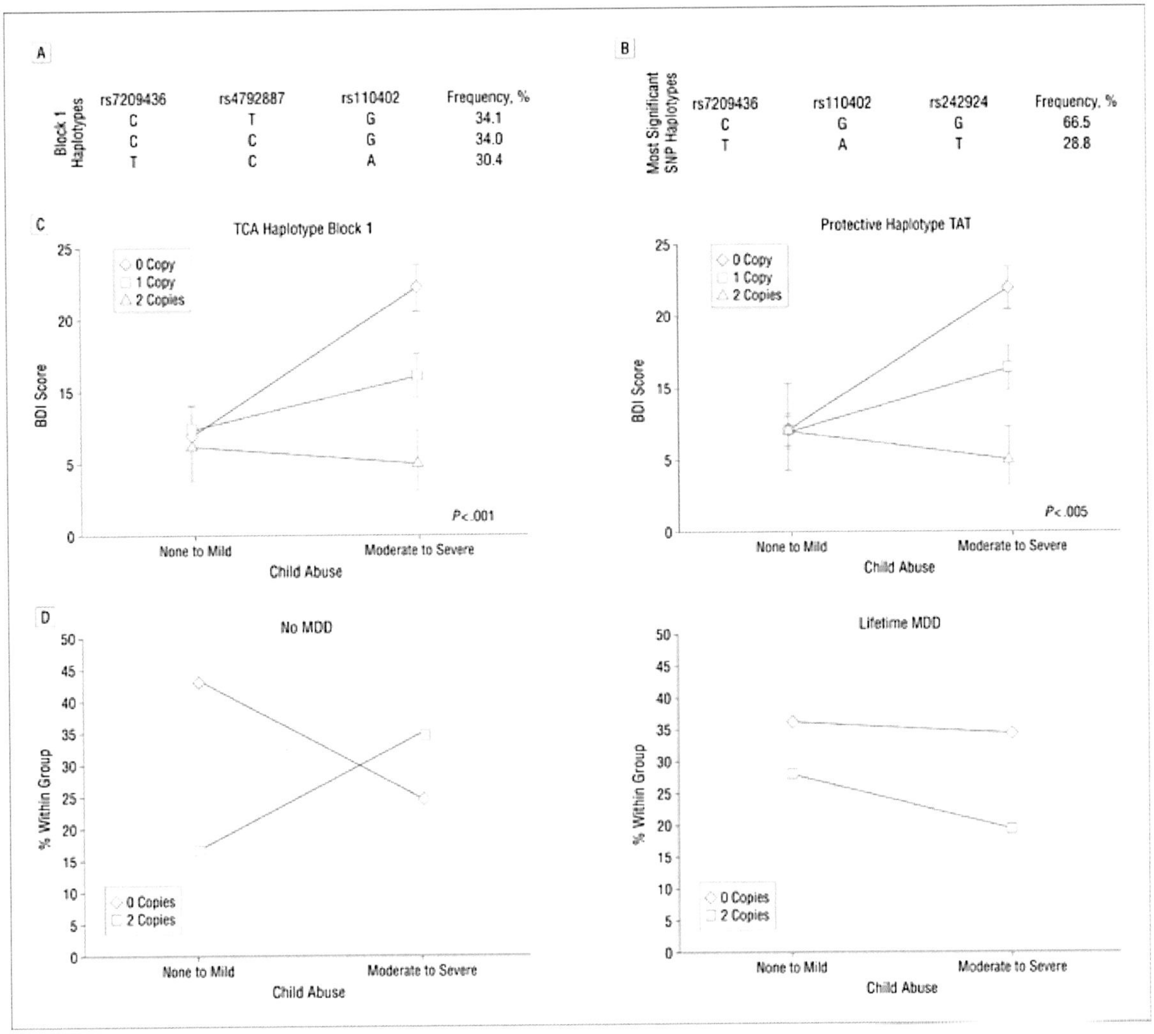

Figure 7: Effect of estimated CRHR1 haplotypes and child abuse on adult depressive symptoms. The frequencies of the estimated individual haplotypes within the first linkage disequilibrium block (A) and of the 3 most significant single-nucleotide polymorphisms (SNPs) (B). C, The effects of the estimated copy numbers of specific haplotypes on adult depression in the presence or absence of moderate to severe child abuse. Error bars indicate SEM. Only haplotypes with an estimation likelihood greater than 95.0% were included in the analysis. The sample sizes for no to mild child abuse and moderate to severe child abuse were as follows: TCA haplotype: 0 copies, 107 and 82, respectively; 1 copy, 109 and 60, respectively; 2 copies, 21 and 9, respectively; TAT haplotype: 0 copies, 118 and 91, respectively; 1 copy, 106 and 54, respectively; 2 copies, 19 and 9, respectively. *P* values of significance for the interaction effect of haplotype in the moderate to severe abuse group are shown. D, A graphical representation of the number of copies of the TAT haplotype in a smaller but ethnically and socioeconomically separate sample. In this separate sample, the best SNP haplotype frequencies were 41.6% for TAT and 56.0% for CGG. The frequencies of TAT haplotypes are shown within child abuse groups for those with no history of major depressive disorder (MDD) and those with a lifetime history of MDD. The protective alleles appear to be present at a higher rate in those with moderate to severe child abuse who have no lifetime MDD compared with those with a lifetime history of MDD. (Reprinted from Bradley *et al* 2008) [157].

child abuse to predict adult depression. The study's findings suggest that the effects of child abuse are moderated, in part, by interactions between the CRHR1 and 5-HTTLPR polymorphisms.

Another study of CRHR1 haplotypes focused on ELS and adolescent alcohol use. Adolescents with a large number of traumatic life events homozygous for a C allele showed twice as much heavy lifetime drinking as well as drinks per occasion than individuals homozygous for the T allele. This evidence suggests that the CRHR1 gene interacts with ELS to predict heavy alcohol use in adolescents [161].

CRF-binding protein (CRF- BP) is a circulating, soluble glycoprotein that binds centrally to CRF and is hypothesized to modulate CRF neurotransmission [28,162,163]. Though there have been few pharmacological trials to date investigating its efficacy in the treatment of mood disorders, one study of post-mortem tissue found CRF-BP mRNA levels were decreased in basolateral (BL) amygdala in men with bipolar disorder and schizophrenia and lateral (La) amygdala in men with bipolar disorder. This suggests that men with decreased BL and La amygdalar CRF-BP may be vulnerable to the effects of stress exposure in the development of and/or the maintenance of bipolar disorder or schizophrenia [164].

In patients studied within the Sequenced Treatment Alternatives to Relieve Depression (STAR*D) sample [165,165], genetic polymorphisms in genes encoding the CRF system were studied [154]. An SNP at the CRH-BP locus was significantly associated with reduction and remission of depressive symptoms with citalopram, and a T allele of the SNP was associated with increased HPA axis activity, especially in anxious depression in African American and Hispanic subsamples [154]. These data suggest that increased CRF-BP may modulate bioavailability of CRF and may decrease HPA axis hyperactivity [166].

4.1.1. Sex-Specific Genetic Studies

We have seen the role of CRFR1 polymorphisms in mediating the effects of ELS on the diathesis for anxiety and depression. Stratifying and subgrouping protective versus susceptible variants by their loci in future genetic and neuroendocrine studies should help inform how trauma affects neuronal circuitry and provide a better understanding of the compensatory mechanisms at play in stress-related psychopathology [23].

The association between childhood trauma and depression is well established [85,89,90,92,95], as are the protective effects of variants of the CRFR1 gene on developing adult depression after childhood trauma [157,158]. There is also strong evidence that women develop depression more frequently than men [168] and that women more frequently develop depression subsequent to ELS compared to men [136].

Heim *et al* [3] found that variants of the CRFR1 gene exerted protective effects in a sample of men but not women with childhood abuse, and that in men with ELS, the protective genotype exhibited less HPA axis hyperactivity than women with ELS, demonstrating the sex-specific protective effects of the A allele (of the rs110402 genotype) by, in one sense, diminishing the pathogenic power of early life trauma to produce later life depression. The CRFR1 gene and its protective variants seem to work, sex-specifically, to moderate the effect of childhood trauma on adult depression. The gene x sex x environment effects were observed on a neuroendocrine level, down to the level of decreased cortisol reactivity in men with the rs110402 A allele with a history of childhood trauma [3] and, significantly, this was observed in a specific type of abuse--namely physical abuse.

4.2. FKBP5 GENETIC STUDIES

There is increasing evidence showing that a binding protein of interest, FKBP5, is an important negative feedback protein in the regulation of GR stress-response. We will review some of the findings below.

FK506 Binding Protein 51 (FKBP5) functions with hsp90 within the cell as a co-chaperone to regulate glucocorticoid receptor (GR) sensitivity. Data has suggested that when bound to its receptor complex, cortisol will bind to the GR with lower affinity [169].

Briefly, when hormones bind to the GR, FKBP5 is replaced by FKBP4 and transport protein dynein is recruited to form a heterocomplex. This heterocomplex is translocated to the nucleus where it functions as a transcription factor and regulates expression of glucocorticoid response [170].

Evidence has emerged that FKBP5 expression is induced by glucocorticoids as part of an ultra-short negative feedback loop for glucocorticoid receptor activity [171] and that when human FKBP5 is overexpressed *in vitro*, it reduces hormone binding affinity [172]. Overexpression of FKBP5 occurs naturally in a primate (New World/spider monkeys) model, and it causes GR resistance with concomitant increased serum cortisol levels [172,173]. A study genotyping SNPs of FKBP5 in depressed subjects and matched controls showed a significant association of response to antidepressants and the recurrence of depressive episodes with SNPs of FKBP5 [174].

3 SNPs of FKBP5 were associated with an increase in FKBP5 expression, leading to less HPA-axis hyperactivity during depressive episodes in subjects carrying the associated genotypes [174]. The authors hypothesized that FKBP5 variant dependent alterations in HPA axis regulation could be related to a faster response to antidepressant drug treatment and the increased recurrence of depressive episodes observed in the subgroup of depressed subjects. Three homozygous genotypes of FKBP5 SNPs were associated with a greater expression of FKBP5 in human blood monocytes; there was also an association with stronger induction of FKBP5 mRNA by cortisol. These associations were accompanied by "less corticotropin release measured in patients who were depressed with the combined dex/CRH test" [174].

Koenen *et al* found an association of the same FKBP5 SNPs with increased peritraumatic dissociation in children after medical trauma [175].

Binder *et al* [176] have data suggesting an association between FKBP5 SNPs with ELS and risk of adult PTSD through altered sensitization of glucocorticoid signal transduction. These genotypes serve as possible predictors of risk and resilience for adult onset PTSD among survivors of early life stress.

5. TREATMENT IMPLICATIONS

Above, we reviewed the effects of well-established antidepressant agents and their modulating influence on CRF (see See section 2.2.3 for antidepressant findings). Here we review additional findings, including the data on CRF1 Receptor antagonists (referred to as CRF1 R antagonists).

The findings from benzodiazepine studies have been compelling, though not easily interpreted into a simple, unified hypothesis of therapeutic effect. Acute benzodiazepine administration (alprazolam/adinazolam) in rats decreases CRF concentrations in rat amygdala, locus coeruleus and cortical regions [177,204]. This finding was most likely due to decreased CRF secretion and was associated with a decrease in plasma ACTH concentrations. CRF levels in hypothalamus were elevated. The locus coeruleus and hypothalamus CRF findings were opposite to those seen after stress, suggesting a triazolobenzodiazepine anxiolytic effect.

Another study showed that chronic--but not acute--treatment with alprazolam decreased baseline HPA axis activity, CRF mRNA expression in the central nucleus of the amygdala and CRF1 mRNA and receptor binding in the basolateral amygdala [77]. Intriguingly and in marked contrast, increases were found in urocortin mRNA expression in the Edinger-Westphal nucleus and in CRF 2A receptor binding in the lateral septum and ventromedial hypothalamus, intimating an inverse relationship between CRF1 and CRF2A receptors. This suggests that the neuronal circuit of the CRF1R and CRF2RA receptors may comprise two distinct yet interrelated subsystems. Further findings suggest that the anxiolytic properties of alprazolam and other benzodiazepines might be mediated by normalizing the CRF circuit activity at the level of the LC [77].

The majority of the pharmacological development work has been directed at testing CRF1 R antagonists as novel antidepressants.

5.1. CRF-1 RECEPTOR ANTAGONISTS

It has long been hypothesized that by antagonizing the CRH1 Receptor, central CRF circuits and HPA axis tone can be reduced both at baseline and after stress exposure, thus impacting vulnerability to depression. To date most of the data supporting this hypothesis come from animal models in which knockout mice of the CRF-R1 receptor show decreases in ACTH, decreases in stress-induced glucocorticoid levels and less anxiety than controls [177-179]. The efforts to develop CRF1 receptor antagonists have not been successful. Most importantly, the target of the CRF receptor antagonists are extra-hypothalamic and extra-pituitary CRF receptor sites [180,181].

The first open label clinical trial of a CRF1 R antagonist (NBI-30775/R121919) was performed on patients in a dose-escalation study of up to 80 mg/day and the antidepressant effect was found to be equivalent to that of paroxetine [52]. Important in this and all subsequent CRF1 antagonist studies is that basal ACTH and cortisol levels were not affected, allaying concerns that over-suppression of the HPA axis might bring about an Addison-like hypoadrenocortisolism [182]. Larger and more recent studies have failed to show efficacy of CRF 1 receptor antagonists in the treatment of depression. Pfizer introduced CP-316.311, an antagonist tested in a placebo- and sertraline-controlled clinical trial [183]. The antagonist showed no efficacy whereas sertraline showed its usual antidepressant effect. Of note, the study did not sub-type its depressed patients and no subset of depressed patients with childhood abuse or neglect was considered. Clearly, a trial specifically designed to determine the efficacy of a CRF receptor antagonist in depressed patients with a history of ELS is sorely needed.

5.2. GLUCOCORTICOID RECEPTOR ANTAGONISTS

Patients with psychotic depression exhibited the highest rates of dexamethasone non-suppression compared to non-psychotic depressed and normal subjects [184]. High cortisol levels have been associated with hyperactivity of dopaminergic neurons, the foundation for the corticosteroid/dopamine hypothesis in psychotic depression [185]. There are two types of intracellular corticosteroid receptors: glucocorticoid receptors (GR) and mineralcorticoid receptors (MR).

One approach has been to antagonize cortisol. Cortisol, a glucocorticoid, is similar in structure to progesterone, a sex hormone with glucocorticoid effects. There is substantial evidence that mifepristone, a progesterone (and glucocorticoid) antagonist, is effective in the treatment of depression with psychotic features. Mifepristone antagonizes glucocorticoid receptors at high doses, but not mineralcorticoid receptors [167,186-190].

One hypothesis is that GR antagonists exert an upregulating effect on MR expression, which may, in turn, increase HPA axis feedback regulation and could account for the antidepressant effect of the GR antagonists [191]. Belanoff *et al* [192] studied mifepristone's antidepressant effect in psychotic depression in a small sample and found efficacy on both HAM-D and Brief Psychiatric Rating Scale (BPRS). Building on these findings in a larger study with higher doses of mefipristone (doses from 50-1,200mg/day), Belanoff *et al* found HAM-D and BPRS improvements again with psychotic major depression [193]. Larger clinical trials with psychotic major depression and bipolar disorder also confirmed the efficacy of mifepristone as an antidepressant on HAM-D, BPRS, Clinical Global Impressions Scale (CGI) and Montgomery-Asberg Depression Rating Scales [188,194,195]. Corcept sponsored three large, placebo-controlled mifepristone trials of 221, 258 and 443 patients with psychotic depression and all showed a positive effect on psychotic symptoms [167,187,196]. The data supporting the use of mifepristone in managing psychotic depression are promising and more studies are needed.

Mifepristone has a wide affinity for progesterone, and there is interest in pharmaceutical research in finding a more selective glucocorticoid receptor (GR) antagonist. Of several GR antagonists actively researched, two experimental compounds—RU-43044 and CORT-108297—are being actively investigated (for mood disorders and obesity) but have yet to show positive results in reducing symptoms of psychotic depression [197,198].

6. SUMMARY AND CONCLUSIONS

This chapter has presented an overview of the components of the HPA system, including some of its extra-hypothalamic elements and their interaction in the pathogenesis of depression. Considerable evidence for the CRF hypothesis of depression exists. Childhood trauma and early life adverse experience contribute to lasting changes in the stress response and a review of existing antidepressants, anxiolytic agents and novel agents such as CRF1 receptor antagonists has been summarized. The role of the HPA axis and its profound influence on depression will continue to be an area of rich interest to researchers in the basic sciences and clinicians treating patients with depression.

BIBLIOGRAPHIC REFERENCES

[1] Swanson LW, Sawchenko PE, Rivier J, Vale WW. Organization of ovine corticotropin-releasing factor immunoreactive cells and fibers in the rat brain: an immunohistochemical study. Neuroendocrinology 1983, 36:165-186.

[2] Martin EI NC. The role of corticotropin-releasing factor in the pathophysiology of depression: Implications for antidepressant mechanisms of action. Psychiat Annals 2008 April 2008, 38:260-266.

[3] Heim C, Bradley B, Mletzko TC, Deveau TC, Musselman DL, Nemeroff CB, *et al.* Effect of Childhood Trauma on Adult Depression and Neuroendocrine Function: Sex-Specific Moderation by CRH Receptor 1 Gene. Front Behav Neurosci 2009, 3:41.

[4] Valentino RJ, Foote SL, Aston-Jones G. Corticotropin-releasing factor activates noradrenergic neurons of the locus coeruleus. Brain Res 1983, 270:363-367.

[5] Nemeroff CB. The corticotropin-releasing factor (CRF) hypothesis of depression: new findings and new directions. Mol Psychiatry 1996, 1:336-342.

[6] GIBBONS JL, McHUGH PR. Plasma cortisol in depressive illness. J Psychiatr Res 1962 Sep, 1:162-171.

[7] Carpenter WT,Jr, Bunney WE,Jr. Adrenal cortical activity in depressive illness. Am J Psychiatry 1971, 128:31-40.

[8] Gillespie CF, Nemeroff CB. Hypercortisolemia and depression. Psychosom Med 2005, 1:S26-8.

[9] Arana GW, Baldessarini RJ, Ornsteen M. The dexamethasone suppression test for diagnosis and prognosis in psychiatry. Commentary and review. Arch Gen Psychiatry 1985, 42:1193-1204.

[10] Evans DL, Nemeroff CB. The dexamethasone suppression test in mixed bipolar disorder. Am J Psychiatry 1983, 140:615-617.

[11] Schatzberg AF, Rothschild AJ, Bond TC, Cole JO. The DST in psychotic depression: diagnostic and pathophysiologic implications. Psychopharmacol Bull 1984, 20:362-364.

[12] Carroll BJ, Martin FI, Davies B. Pituitary-adrenal function in depression. Lancet 1968, 1:1373-1374.

[13] Carroll BJ. Use of the dexamethasone suppression test in depression. J Clin Psychiatry 1982, 43:44-50.

[14] Ribeiro SC, Tandon R, Grunhaus L, Greden JF. The DST as a predictor of outcome in depression: a meta-analysis. Am J Psychiatry 1993, 150:1618-1629.

[15] Greden JF, Albala AA, Haskett RF, James NM, Goodman L, Steiner M, *et al.* Normalization of dexamethasone suppression test: a laboratory index of recovery from endogenous depression. Biol Psychiatry 1980, 15:449-458.

[16] Nemeroff CB, Evans DL. Correlation between the dexamethasone suppression test in depressed patients and clinical response. Am J Psychiatry 1984, 141:247-249.

[17] Nelson JC, Davis JM. DST studies in psychotic depression: a meta-analysis. Am J Psychiatry 1997, 154:1497-1503.

[18] Vale W, Spiess J, Rivier C, Rivier J. Characterization of a 41-residue ovine hypothalamic peptide that stimulates secretion of corticotropin and beta-endorphin. Science 1981, 213:1394-1397.

[19] Hauger RL, Grigoriadis DE, Dallman MF, Plotsky PM, Vale WW, Dautzenberg FM. International Union of Pharmacology. XXXVI. Current status of the nomenclature for receptors for corticotropin-releasing factor and their ligands. Pharmacol Rev 2003, 55:21-26.

[20] Boorse GC, Denver RJ. Widespread tissue distribution and diverse functions of corticotropin-releasing factor and related peptides. Gen Comp Endocrinol 2006, 146:9-18.

[21] Potter E, Sutton S, Donaldson C, Chen R, Perrin M, Lewis K, *et al.* Distribution of corticotropin-releasing factor receptor mRNA expression in the rat brain and pituitary. Proc Natl Acad Sci U S A 1994, 91:8777-8781.

[22] Donaldson CJ, Sutton SW, Perrin MH, Corrigan AZ, Lewis KA, Rivier JE, *et al.* Cloning and characterization of human urocortin. Endocrinology 1996, 137:3896.

[23] Lewis K, Li C, Perrin MH, Blount A, Kunitake K, Donaldson C, *et al.* Identification of urocortin III, an additional member of the corticotropin-releasing factor (CRF) family with high affinity for the CRF2 receptor. Proc Natl Acad Sci U S A 2001, 98:7570-7575.

[24] Reyes TM, Lewis K, Perrin MH, Kunitake KS, Vaughan J, Arias CA, *et al.* Urocortin II: a member of the corticotropin-releasing factor (CRF) neuropeptide family that is selectively bound by type 2 CRF receptors. Proc Natl Acad Sci U S A 2001, 98:2843-2848.

[25] Vaughan J, Donaldson C, Bittencourt J, Perrin MH, Lewis K, Sutton S, *et al.* Urocortin, a mammalian neuropeptide related to fish urotensin I and to corticotropin-releasing factor. Nature 1995, 378:287-292.

[26] Wong ML, al-Shekhlee A, Bongiorno PB, Esposito A, Khatri P, Sternberg EM, *et al.* Localization of urocortin messenger RNA in rat brain and pituitary. Mol Psychiatry 1996, 1:307-312.

[27] Kageyama K, Suda T. Regulatory mechanisms underlying corticotropin-releasing factor gene expression in the hypothalamus. Endocr J 2009, 56:335-344.

[28] Binder EB, Nemeroff CB. The CRF system, stress, depression and anxiety-insights from human genetic studies. Mol Psychiatry 2010, 15:574-588.

[29] Potter E, Behan DP, Linton EA, Lowry PJ, Sawchenko PE, Vale WW. The central distribution of a corticotropin-releasing factor (CRF)-binding protein predicts multiple sites and modes of interaction with CRF. Proc Natl Acad Sci U S A 1992, 89:4192-4196.

[30] Nemeroff CB, Widerlov E, Bissette G, Walleus H, Karlsson I, Eklund K, *et al.* Elevated concentrations of CSF corticotropin-releasing factor-like immunoreactivity in depressed patients. Science 1984, 226:1342-1344.

[31] Banki CM, Karmacsi L, Bissette G, Nemeroff CB. CSF corticotropin-releasing hormone and somatostatin in major depression: response to antidepressant treatment and relapse. Eur Neuropsychopharmacol 1992, 2:107-113.

[32] Hartline KM, Owens MJ, Nemeroff CB. Postmortem and cerebrospinal fluid studies of corticotropin-releasing factor in humans. Ann N Y Acad Sci 1996, 780:96-105.

[33] Arato M, Banki CM, Bissette G, Nemeroff CB. Elevated CSF CRF in suicide victims. Biol Psychiatry 1989, 25:355-359.

[34] Nemeroff CB, Bissette G, Akil H, Fink M. Neuropeptide concentrations in the cerebrospinal fluid of depressed patients treated with electroconvulsive therapy. Corticotrophin-releasing factor, beta-endorphin and somatostatin. Br J Psychiatry 1991, 158:59-63.

[35] Heinrichs SC, Menzaghi F, Merlo Pich E, Britton KT, Koob GF. The role of CRF in behavioral aspects of stress. Ann N Y Acad Sci 1995, 771:92-104.

[36] Sachar EJ, Hellman L, Fukushima DK, Gallagher TF. Cortisol production in depressive illness. A clinical and biochemical clarification. Arch Gen Psychiatry 1970, 23:289-298.

[37] Amsterdam JD, Maislin G, Winokur A, Berwish N, Kling M, Gold P. The oCRH stimulation test before and after clinical recovery from depression. J Affect Disord 1988, 14:213-222.

[38] Rubin RT, Phillips JJ, Sadow TF, McCracken JT. Adrenal gland volume in major depression. Increase during the depressive episode and decrease with successful treatment. Arch Gen Psychiatry 1995, 52:213-218.

[39] Coryell W, Schlesser M. The dexamethasone suppression test and suicide prediction. Am J Psychiatry 2001, 158:748-753.

[40] Black DW, Monahan PO, Winokur G. The relationship between DST results and suicidal behavior. Ann Clin Psychiatry 2002, 14:83-88.

[41] Tan H, Zhong P, Yan Z. Corticotropin-releasing factor and acute stress prolongs serotonergic regulation of GABA transmission in prefrontal cortical pyramidal neurons. J Neurosci 2004, 24:5000-5008.

[42] Grigoriadis DE, Pearsall D, De Souza EB. Effects of chronic antidepressant and benzodiazepine treatment on corticotropin-releasing-factor receptors in rat brain and pituitary. Neuropsychopharmacology 1989, 2:53-60.

[43] Veith RC, Lewis N, Langohr JI, Murburg MM, Ashleigh EA, Castillo S, *et al.* Effect of desipramine on cerebrospinal fluid concentrations of corticotropin-releasing factor in human subjects. Psychiatry Res 1993, 46:1-8.

[44] De Bellis MD, Gold PW, Geracioti TD,Jr, Listwak SJ, Kling MA. Association of fluoxetine treatment with reductions in CSF concentrations of corticotropin-releasing hormone and arginine vasopressin in patients with major depression. Am J Psychiatry 1993, 150:656-657.

[45] Stout SC, Owens MJ, Nemeroff CB. Regulation of corticotropin-releasing factor neuronal systems and hypothalamic-pituitary-adrenal axis activity by stress and chronic antidepressant treatment. J Pharmacol Exp Ther 2002, 300:1085-1092.

[46] Bugnon C, Hadjiyiassemis M, Fellmann D, Cardot J. Reserpine-induced depletion of corticoliberin (CRF)-like immunoreactivity in the zona externa of the rat median eminence. Brain Res 1983, 275:198-201.

[47] Tizabi Y, Skofitsch G, Jacobowitz DM. Effect of chronic reserpine and desmethylimipramine treatment on CRF-like immunoreactivity of discrete brain areas of rat. Brain Res 1985, 335:389-391.

[48] Reul JM, Holsboer F. Corticotropin-releasing factor receptors 1 and 2 in anxiety and depression. Curr Opin Pharmacol 2002, 2:23-33.

[49] Nemeroff CB, Vale WW. The neurobiology of depression: inroads to treatment and new drug discovery. J Clin Psychiatry 2005, 7:5-13.

[50] Hauger RL, Risbrough V, Brauns O, Dautzenberg FM. Corticotropin releasing factor (CRF) receptor signaling in the central nervous system: new molecular targets. CNS Neurol Disord Drug Targets 2006, 5:453-479.

[51] Kunzel HE, Zobel AW, Nickel T, Ackl N, Uhr M, Sonntag A, *et al*. Treatment of depression with the CRH-1-receptor antagonist R121919: endocrine changes and side effects. J Psychiatr Res 2003, 37:525-533.

[52] Zobel AW, Nickel T, Kunzel HE, Ackl N, Sonntag A, Ising M, *et al*. Effects of the high-affinity corticotropin-releasing hormone receptor 1 antagonist R121919 in major depression: the first 20 patients treated. J Psychiatr Res 2000, 34:171-181.

[53] Hermus AR, Pieters GF, Smals AG, Benraad TJ, Kloppenborg PW. Plasma adrenocorticotropin, cortisol, and aldosterone responses to corticotropin-releasing factor: modulatory effect of basal cortisol levels. J Clin Endocrinol Metab 1984, 58:187-191.

[54] Watson SJ, Lopez JF, Young EA, Vale W, Rivier J, Akil H. Effects of low dose ovine corticotropin-releasing hormone in humans: endocrine relationships and beta-endorphin/beta-lipotropin responses. J Clin Endocrinol Metab 1988, 66:10-15.

[55] Gold PW, Loriaux DL, Roy A, Kling MA, Calabrese JR, Kellner CH, *et al*. Responses to corticotropin-releasing hormone in the hypercortisolism of depression and Cushing's disease. Pathophysiologic and diagnostic implications. N Engl J Med 1986, 314:1329-1335.

[56] Kathol RG, Jaeckle RS, Lopez JF, Meller WH. Consistent reduction of ACTH responses to stimulation with CRH, vasopressin and hypoglycaemia in patients with major depression. Br J Psychiatry 1989, 155:468-478.

[57] Heim C, Newport DJ, Bonsall R, Miller AH, Nemeroff CB. Altered pituitary-adrenal axis responses to provocative challenge tests in adult survivors of childhood abuse. Am J Psychiatry 2001, 158:575-581.

[58] Krishnan KRR, Rayasam K, Reed D, Smith M, Chapell P, Saunders WB, Ritchie JC, Carroll BJ, Nemeroff CB. The corticotropin releasing factor stimulation test in patients with major depression: Relationship to dexamethasone suppression test results. Depression 1993, 1:133-133-136.

[59] Mitchell AJ. The role of corticotropin releasing factor in depressive illness: a critical review. Neurosci Biobehav Rev 1998, 22:635-651.

[60] Nemeroff CB, Owens MJ, Bissette G, Andorn AC, Stanley M. Reduced corticotropin releasing factor binding sites in the frontal cortex of suicide victims. Arch Gen Psychiatry 1988, 45:577-579.

[61] Merali Z, Du L, Hrdina P, Palkovits M, Faludi G, Poulter MO, *et al*. Dysregulation in the suicide brain: mRNA expression of corticotropin-releasing hormone receptors and GABA (A) receptor subunits in frontal cortical brain region. J Neurosci 2004, 24:1478-1485.

[62] Keen-Rhinehart E, Michopoulos V, Toufexis DJ, Martin EI, Nair H, Ressler KJ, *et al*. Continuous expression of corticotropin-releasing factor in the central nucleus of the amygdala emulates the dysregulation of the stress and reproductive axes. Mol Psychiatry 2009, 14:37-50.

[63] Nutt DJ. Neurobiological mechanisms in generalized anxiety disorder. J Clin Psychiatry 2001, 11:22-7, discussion 28.

[64] Arborelius L, Owens MJ, Plotsky PM, Nemeroff CB. The role of corticotropin-releasing factor in depression and anxiety disorders. J Endocrinol 1999, 160:1-12.

[65] Dunn AJ, Berridge CW. Physiological and behavioral responses to corticotropin-releasing factor administration: is CRF a mediator of anxiety or stress responses? Brain Res Brain Res Rev 1990, 15:71-100.

[66] Keck ME. Corticotropin-releasing factor, vasopressin and receptor systems in depression and anxiety. Amino Acids 2006, 31:241-250.

[67] Keck ME, Holsboer F, Muller MB. Mouse mutants for the study of corticotropin-releasing hormone receptor function: development of novel treatment strategies for mood disorders. Ann N Y Acad Sci 2004, 1018:445-457.

[68] Lu A, Steiner MA, Whittle N, Vogl AM, Walser SM, Ableitner M, *et al.* Conditional mouse mutants highlight mechanisms of corticotropin-releasing hormone effects on stress-coping behavior. Mol Psychiatry 2008, 13:1028-1042.

[69] Holsboer F, von Bardeleben U, Wiedemann K, Muller OA, Stalla GK. Serial assessment of corticotropin-releasing hormone response after dexamethasone in depression. Implications for pathophysiology of DST nonsuppression. Biol Psychiatry 1987, 22:228-234.

[70] Holsboer-Trachsler E, Stohler R, Hatzinger M. Repeated administration of the combined dexamethasone-human corticotropin releasing hormone stimulation test during treatment of depression. Psychiatry Res 1991, 38:163-171.

[71] Schule C, Baghai TC, Eser D, Zwanzger P, Jordan M, Buechs R, *et al.* Time course of hypothalamic-pituitary-adrenocortical axis activity during treatment with reboxetine and mirtazapine in depressed patients. Psychopharmacology (Berl) 2006, 186:601-611.

[72] Ising M, Horstmann S, Kloiber S, Lucae S, Binder EB, Kern N, *et al.* Combined dexamethasone/ corticotropin releasing hormone test predicts treatment response in major depression - a potential biomarker? Biol Psychiatry 2007, 62:47-54.

[73] Nikisch G, Mathe AA, Czernik A, Thiele J, Bohner J, Eap CB, *et al.* Long-term citalopram administration reduces responsiveness of HPA axis in patients with major depression: relationship with S-citalopram concentrations in plasma and cerebrospinal fluid (CSF) and clinical response. Psychopharmacology (Berl) 2005, 181:751-760.

[74] Valdez GR, Koob GF. Allostasis and dysregulation of corticotropin-releasing factor and neuropeptide Y systems: implications for the development of alcoholism. Pharmacol Biochem Behav 2004, 79:671-689.

[75] Adinoff B, Anton R, Linnoila M, Guidotti A, Nemeroff CB, Bissette G. Cerebrospinal fluid concentrations of corticotropin-releasing hormone (CRH) and diazepam-binding inhibitor (DBI) during alcohol withdrawal and abstinence. Neuropsychopharmacology 1996, 15:288-295.

[76] Hawley RJ, Nemeroff CB, Bissette G, Guidotti A, Rawlings R, Linnoila M. Neurochemical correlates of sympathetic activation during severe alcohol withdrawal. Alcohol Clin Exp Res 1994, 18:1312-1316.

[77] Skelton KH, Nemeroff CB, Knight DL, Owens MJ. Chronic administration of the triazolobenzodiazepine alprazolam produces opposite effects on corticotropin-releasing factor and urocortin neuronal systems. J Neurosci 2000, 20:1240-1248.

[78] Children's Bureau, Administration of Children, Youth, and Families. U.S. Department of Health and Human Services. *Child Maltreatment 2004*. 2006 (Washington, DC: U.S. Government Printing Office).

[79] Costello EJ, Angold A. Developmental psychopathology and public health: past, present, and future. Dev Psychopathol 2000, 12:599-618.

[80] McCloskey LA, Walker M. Posttraumatic stress in children exposed to family violence and single-event trauma. J Am Acad Child Adolesc Psychiatry 2000, 39:108-115.

[81] Scher CD, Forde DR, McQuaid JR, Stein MB. Prevalence and demographic correlates of childhood maltreatment in an adult community sample. Child Abuse Negl 2004, 28:167-180.

[82] Agid O, Shapira B, Zislin J, Ritsner M, Hanin B, Murad H, *et al*. Environment and vulnerability to major psychiatric illness: a case control study of early parental loss in major depression, bipolar disorder and schizophrenia. Mol Psychiatry 1999, 4:163-172.

[83] Heim C, Newport DJ, Mletzko T, Miller AH, Nemeroff CB. The link between childhood trauma and depression: insights from HPA axis studies in humans. Psychoneuroendocrinology 2008, 33 :693-710.

[84] Plotsky PM, Owens MJ, Nemeroff CB. Psychoneuroendocrinology of depression. Hypothalamic-pituitary-adrenal axis. Psychiatr Clin North Am 1998, 21:293-307.

[85] Ladd CO, Huot RL, Thrivikraman KV, Nemeroff CB, Meaney MJ, Plotsky PM. Long-term behavioral and neuroendocrine adaptations to adverse early experience. Prog Brain Res 2000, 122:81-103.

[86] Meaney MJ, Szyf M. Environmental programming of stress responses through DNA methylation: life at the interface between a dynamic environment and a fixed genome. Dialogues Clin Neurosci 2005, 7:103-123.

[87] Sanchez MM, Ladd CO, Plotsky PM. Early adverse experience as a developmental risk factor for later psychopathology: evidence from rodent and primate models. Dev Psychopathol 2001 Summer, 13:419-449.

[88] Edwards VJ, Holden GW, Felitti VJ, Anda RF. Relationship between multiple forms of childhood maltreatment and adult mental health in community respondents: results from the adverse childhood experiences study. Am J Psychiatry 2003 Aug, 160:1453-1460.

[89] Chapman DP, Whitfield CL, Felitti VJ, Dube SR, Edwards VJ, Anda RF. Adverse childhood experiences and the risk of depressive disorders in adulthood. J Affect Disord 2004, 82:217-225.

[90] McCauley J, Kern DE, Kolodner K, Dill L, Schroeder AF, DeChant HK, *et al*. Clinical characteristics of women with a history of childhood abuse: unhealed wounds. JAMA 1997, 277:1362-1368.

[91] Heim C, Shugart M, Craighead WE, Nemeroff CB. Neurobiological and psychiatric consequences of child abuse and neglect. Dev Psychobiol 2010, 52:671-690.

[92] Dube SR, Anda RF, Felitti VJ, Chapman DP, Williamson DF, Giles WH. Childhood abuse, household dysfunction, and the risk of attempted suicide throughout the life span: findings from the Adverse Childhood Experiences Study. JAMA 2001, 286:3089-3096.

[93] Zlotnick C, Mattia J, Zimmerman M. Clinical features of survivors of sexual abuse with major depression. Child Abuse Negl 2001, 25:357-367.

[94] Mcquaid JR, Pedrelli P, McCahill ME, Stein MB. Reported trauma, post-traumatic stress disorder and major depression among primary care patients. Psychol Med 2001, 31:1249-1257.

[95] Bifulco A, Brown GW, Adler Z. Early sexual abuse and clinical depression in adult life. Br J Psychiatry 1991, 159:115-122.

[96] Widom CS, DuMont K, Czaja SJ. A prospective investigation of major depressive disorder and comorbidity in abused and neglected children grown up. Arch Gen Psychiatry 2007, 64:49-56.

[97] Weller RA, Weller EB, Fristad MA, Bowes JM. Depression in recently bereaved prepubertal children. Am J Psychiatry 1991, 148:1536-1540.

[98] Brown GW, Moran P. Clinical and psychosocial origins of chronic depressive episodes. I: A community survey. Br J Psychiatry 1994, 165:447-456.

[99] Heim C, Newport DJ, Wagner D, Wilcox MM, Miller AH, Nemeroff CB. The role of early adverse experience and adulthood stress in the prediction of neuroendocrine stress reactivity in women: a multiple regression analysis. Depress Anxiety 2002, 15:117-125.

[100] Kirschbaum C, Schommer N, Federenko I, Gaab J, Neumann O, Oellers M, *et al.* Short-term estradiol treatment enhances pituitary-adrenal axis and sympathetic responses to psychosocial stress in healthy young men. J Clin Endocrinol Metab 1996, 81:3639-3643.

[101] Holsboer F, Von Bardeleben U, Gerken A, Stalla GK, Muller OA. Blunted corticotropin and normal cortisol response to human corticotropin-releasing factor in depression. N Engl J Med 1984, 311:1127.

[102] Gold PW, Chrousos G, Kellner C, Post R, Roy A, Augerinos P, *et al.* Psychiatric implications of basic and clinical studies with corticotropin-releasing factor. Am J Psychiatry 1984, 141:619-627.

[103] Heuser I, Yassouridis A, Holsboer F. The combined dexamethasone/CRH test: a refined laboratory test for psychiatric disorders. J Psychiatr Res 1994, 28:341-356.

[104] Modell S, Lauer CJ, Schreiber W, Huber J, Krieg JC, Holsboer F. Hormonal response pattern in the combined DEX-CRH test is stable over time in subjects at high familial risk for affective disorders. Neuropsychopharmacology 1998, 18:253-262.

[105] Holsboer F, Lauer CJ, Schreiber W, Krieg JC. Altered hypothalamic-pituitary-adrenocortical regulation in healthy subjects at high familial risk for affective disorders. Neuroendocrinology 1995, 62:340-347.

[106] Bissette G, Klimek V, Pan J, Stockmeier C, Ordway G. Elevated concentrations of CRF in the locus coeruleus of depressed subjects. Neuropsychopharmacology 2003, 28:1328-1335.

[107] Merali Z, Kent P, Du L, Hrdina P, Palkovits M, Faludi G, *et al.* Corticotropin-releasing hormone, arginine vasopressin, gastrin-releasing peptide, and neuromedin B alterations in stress-relevant brain regions of suicides and control subjects. Biol Psychiatry 2006, 59:594-602.

[108] Raadsheer FC, Hoogendijk WJ, Stam FC, Tilders FJ, Swaab DF. Increased numbers of corticotropin-releasing hormone expressing neurons in the hypothalamic paraventricular nucleus of depressed patients. Neuroendocrinology 1994, 60:436-444.

[109] Raadsheer FC, van Heerikhuize JJ, Lucassen PJ, Hoogendijk WJ, Tilders FJ, Swaab DF. Corticotropin-releasing hormone mRNA levels in the paraventricular nucleus of patients with Alzheimer's disease and depression. Am J Psychiatry 1995, 152:1372-1376.

[110] Fuchs E, Gould E. Mini-review: *in vivo* neurogenesis in the adult brain: regulation and functional implications. Eur J Neurosci 2000, 12:2211-2214.

[111] Nestler EJ, Barrot M, DiLeone RJ, Eisch AJ, Gold SJ, Monteggia LM. Neurobiology of depression. Neuron 2002, 34:13-25.

[112] Sheline YI, Wang PW, Gado MH, Csernansky JG, Vannier MW. Hippocampal atrophy in recurrent major depression. Proc Natl Acad Sci U S A 1996, 93:3908-3913.

[113] Bremner JD, Narayan M, Anderson ER, Staib LH, Miller HL, Charney DS. Hippocampal volume reduction in major depression. Am J Psychiatry 2000, 157:115-118.

[114] Frodl T, Meisenzahl EM, Zetzsche T, Born C, Groll C, Jager M, *et al.* Hippocampal changes in patients with a first episode of major depression. Am J Psychiatry 2002, 159:1112-1118.

[115] Huot RL, Plotsky PM, Lenox RH, McNamara RK. Neonatal maternal separation reduces hippocampal mossy fiber density in adult Long Evans rats. Brain Res 2002, 950:52-63.

[116] Mirescu C, Peters JD, Gould E. Early life experience alters response of adult neurogenesis to stress. Nat Neurosci 2004, 7:841-846.

[117] Brunson KL, Eghbal-Ahmadi M, Bender R, Chen Y, Baram TZ. Long-term, progressive hippocampal cell loss and dysfunction induced by early-life administration of corticotropin-releasing hormone reproduce the effects of early-life stress. Proc Natl Acad Sci U S A 2001, 98:8856-8861.

[118] Bremner JD, Randall P, Vermetten E, Staib L, Bronen RA, Mazure C, *et al.* Magnetic resonance imaging-based measurement of hippocampal volume in posttraumatic stress disorder related to childhood physical and sexual abuse--a preliminary report. Biol Psychiatry 1997, 41:23-32.

[119] Stein MB, Koverola C, Hanna C, Torchia MG, McClarty B. Hippocampal volume in women victimized by childhood sexual abuse. Psychol Med 1997, 27:951-959.

[120] Vythilingam M, Heim C, Newport J, Miller AH, Anderson E, Bronen R, *et al.* Childhood trauma associated with smaller hippocampal volume in women with major depression. Am J Psychiatry 2002, 159:2072-2080.

[121] Feldman S, Conforti N, Weidenfeld J. Limbic pathways and hypothalamic neurotransmitters mediating adrenocortical responses to neural stimuli. Neurosci Biobehav Rev 1995, 19:235-240.

[122] Lara ME, Klein DN, Kasch KL. Psychosocial predictors of the short-term course and outcome of major depression: a longitudinal study of a nonclinical sample with recent-onset episodes. J Abnorm Psychol 2000, 109:644-650.

[123] Pollak SD, Kistler DJ. Early experience is associated with the development of categorical representations for facial expressions of emotion. Proc Natl Acad Sci U S A 2002, 99:9072-9076.

[124] Taylor SE, Eisenberger NI, Saxbe D, Lehman BJ, Lieberman MD. Neural responses to emotional stimuli are associated with childhood family stress. Biol Psychiatry 2006 Aug 1, 60:296-301.

[125] Heim C, Mletzko T, Purselle D, Musselman DL, Nemeroff CB. The dexamethasone/corticotropin-releasing factor test in men with major depression: role of childhood trauma. Biol Psychiatry 2008, 63:398-405.

[126] Dougherty LR, Klein DN, Davila J. A growth curve analysis of the course of dysthymic disorder: the effects of chronic stress and moderation by adverse parent-child relationships and family history. J Consult Clin Psychol 2004, 72:1012-1021.

[127] Hammen C, Henry R, Daley SE. Depression and sensitization to stressors among young women as a function of childhood adversity. J Consult Clin Psychol 2000, 68:782-787.

[128] Bernet CZ, Stein MB. Relationship of childhood maltreatment to the onset and course of major depression in adulthood. Depress Anxiety 1999, 9:169-174.

[129] Gladstone GL, Parker GB, Mitchell PB, Malhi GS, Wilhelm K, Austin MP. Implications of childhood trauma for depressed women: an analysis of pathways from childhood sexual abuse to deliberate self-harm and revictimization. Am J Psychiatry 2004, 161:1417-1425.

[130] Young EA, Abelson JL, Curtis GC, Nesse RM. Childhood adversity and vulnerability to mood and anxiety disorders. Depress Anxiety 1997, 5:66-72.

[131] Zlotnick C, Ryan CE, Miller IW, Keitner GI. Childhood abuse and recovery from major depression. Child Abuse Negl 1995, 19:1513-1516.

[132] Hayden EP, Klein DN. Outcome of dysthymic disorder at 5-year follow-up: the effect of familial psychopathology, early adversity, personality, comorbidity, and chronic stress. Am J Psychiatry 2001, 158:1864-1870.

[133] Kaplan MJ, Klinetob NA. Childhood emotional trauma and chronic posttraumatic stress disorder in adult outpatients with treatment-resistant depression. J Nerv Ment Dis 2000, 188:596-601.

[134] Nemeroff CB, Heim CM, Thase ME, Klein DN, Rush AJ, Schatzberg AF, *et al.* Differential responses to psychotherapy versus pharmacotherapy in patients with chronic forms of major depression and childhood trauma. Proc Natl Acad Sci U S A 2003, 100:14293-14296.

[135] Keller MB, McCullough JP, Klein DN, Arnow B, Dunner DL, Gelenberg AJ, *et al.* A comparison of nefazodone, the cognitive behavioral-analysis system of psychotherapy, and their combination for the treatment of chronic depression. N Engl J Med 2000, 342:1462-1470.

[136] Weiss EL, Longhurst JG, Mazure CM. Childhood sexual abuse as a risk factor for depression in women: psychosocial and neurobiological correlates. Am J Psychiatry 1999, 156:816-828.

[137] Rhodes ME, Rubin RT. Functional sex differences ('sexual diergism') of central nervous system cholinergic systems, vasopressin, and hypothalamic-pituitary-adrenal axis activity in mammals: a selective review. Brain Res Brain Res Rev 1999, 30:135-152.

[138] Swanson LW, Simmons DM. Differential steroid hormone and neural influences on peptide mRNA levels in CRH cells of the paraventricular nucleus: a hybridization histochemical study in the rat. J Comp Neurol 1989, 285:413-435.

[139] Burgess LH, Handa RJ. Chronic estrogen-induced alterations in adrenocorticotropin and corticosterone secretion, and glucocorticoid receptor-mediated functions in female rats. Endocrinology 1992, 131:1261-1269.

[140] Vamvakopoulos NC, Chrousos GP. Evidence of direct estrogenic regulation of human corticotropin-releasing hormone gene expression. Potential implications for the sexual dimophism of the stress response and immune/inflammatory reaction. J Clin Invest 1993, 92:1896-1902.

[141] McEwen BS. Invited review: Estrogens effects on the brain: multiple sites and molecular mechanisms. J Appl Physiol 2001, 91:2785-2801.

[142] Sanchez MM, Noble PM, Lyon CK, Plotsky PM, Davis M, Nemeroff CB, *et al.* Alterations in diurnal cortisol rhythm and acoustic startle response in nonhuman primates with adverse rearing. Biol Psychiatry 2005, 57:373-381.

[143] Molnar BE, Buka SL, Kessler RC. Child sexual abuse and subsequent psychopathology: results from the National Comorbidity Survey. Am J Public Health 2001, 91:753-760.

[144] Akiskal HS, McKinney WT,Jr. Depressive disorders: toward a unified hypothesis. Science 1973, 182:20-29.

[145] Kendler KS. Genetic epidemiology in psychiatry. Taking both genes and environment seriously. Arch Gen Psychiatry 1995, 52:895-899.

[146] Hettema JM, Neale MC, Kendler KS. A review and meta-analysis of the genetic epidemiology of anxiety disorders. Am J Psychiatry 2001, 158:1568-1578.

[147] Kendler KS, Gatz M, Gardner CO, Pedersen NL. A Swedish national twin study of lifetime major depression. Am J Psychiatry 2006 Jan, 163:109-114.

[148] Liu Z, Zhu F, Wang G, Xiao Z, Tang J, Liu W, *et al.* Association study of corticotropin-releasing hormone receptor1 gene polymorphisms and antidepressant response in major depressive disorders. Neurosci Lett 2007, 414:155-158.

[149] Pisarchik A, Slominski A. Molecular and functional characterization of novel CRFR1 isoforms from the skin. Eur J Biochem 2004, 271:2821-2830.

[150] Grammatopoulos DK, Chrousos GP. Functional characteristics of CRH receptors and potential clinical applications of CRH-receptor antagonists. Trends Endocrinol Metab 2002, 13:436-444.

[151] Ross PC, Kostas CM, Ramabhadran TV. A variant of the human corticotropin-releasing factor (CRF) receptor: cloning, expression and pharmacology. Biochem Biophys Res Commun 1994 30, 205:1836-1842.

[152] Pisarchik A, Slominski AT. Alternative splicing of CRH-R1 receptors in human and mouse skin: identification of new variants and their differential expression. FASEB J 2001, 15:2754-2756.

[153] Jin D, He P, You X, Zhu X, Dai L, He Q, *et al.* Expression of corticotropin-releasing hormone receptor type 1 and type 2 in human pregnant myometrium. Reprod Sci 2007, 14:568-577.

[154] Binder EB, Owens MJ, Liu W, Deveau TC, Rush AJ, Trivedi MH, *et al.* Association of polymorphisms in genes regulating the corticotropin-releasing factor system with antidepressant treatment response. Arch Gen Psychiatry 2010, 67:369-379.

[155] Licinio J, O'Kirwan F, Irizarry K, Merriman B, Thakur S, Jepson R, *et al.* Association of a corticotropin-releasing hormone receptor 1 haplotype and antidepressant treatment response in Mexican-Americans. Mol Psychiatry 2004, 9:1075-1082.

[156] Wasserman D, Sokolowski M, Rozanov V, Wasserman J. The CRHR1 gene: a marker for suicidality in depressed males exposed to low stress. Genes Brain Behav 2008, 7:14-19.

[157] Bradley RG, Binder EB, Epstein MP, Tang Y, Nair HP, Liu W, *et al.* Influence of child abuse on adult depression: moderation by the corticotropin-releasing hormone receptor gene. Arch Gen Psychiatry 2008, 65:190-200.

[158] Polanczyk G, Caspi A, Williams B, Price TS, Danese A, Sugden K, *et al.* Protective effect of CRHR1 gene variants on the development of adult depression following childhood maltreatment: replication and extension. Arch Gen Psychiatry 2009, 66:978-985.

[159] Tyrka AR, Price LH, Gelernter J, Schepker C, Anderson GM, Carpenter LL. Interaction of childhood maltreatment with the corticotropin-releasing hormone receptor gene: effects on hypothalamic-pituitary-adrenal axis reactivity. Biol Psychiatry 2009, 66:681-685.

[160] Ressler KJ, Bradley B, Mercer KB, Deveau TC, Smith AK, Gillespie CF, *et al.* Polymorphisms in CRHR1 and the serotonin transporter loci: gene x gene x environment interactions on depressive symptoms. Am J Med Genet B Neuropsychiatr Genet 2010, 153B:812-824.

[161] Blomeyer D, Treutlein J, Esser G, Schmidt MH, Schumann G, Laucht M. Interaction between CRHR1 gene and stressful life events predicts adolescent heavy alcohol use. Biol Psychiatry 2008, 63:146-151.

[162] Orth DN, Mount CD. Specific high-affinity binding protein for human corticotropin-releasing hormone in normal human plasma. Biochem Biophys Res Commun 1987, 143:411-417.

[163] Potter E, Behan DP, Fischer WH, Linton EA, Lowry PJ, Vale WW. Cloning and characterization of the cDNAs for human and rat corticotropin releasing factor-binding proteins. Nature 1991, 349:423-426.

[164] Herringa RJ, Roseboom PH, Kalin NH. Decreased amygdala CRF-binding protein mRNA in post-mortem tissue from male but not female bipolar and schizophrenic subjects. Neuropsychopharmacology 2006, 31:1822-1831.

[165] Rush AJ, Fava M, Wisniewski SR, Lavori PW, Trivedi MH, Sackeim HA, *et al.* Sequenced treatment alternatives to relieve depression (STAR*D): rationale and design. Control Clin Trials 2004, 25:119-142.

[166] Herringa RJ, Nanda SA, Hsu DT, Roseboom PH, Kalin NH. The effects of acute stress on the regulation of central and basolateral amygdala CRF-binding protein gene expression. Brain Res Mol Brain Res 2004, 131:17-25.

[167] Blasey CM, Block TS, Belanoff JK, Roe RL. Efficacy and safety of mifepristone for the treatment of psychotic depression. J Clin Psychopharmacol 2011, 31:436-440.

[168] Kessler RC, McGonagle KA, Swartz M, Blazer DG, Nelson CB. Sex and depression in the National Comorbidity Survey. I: Lifetime prevalence, chronicity and recurrence. J Affect Disord 1993, 29:85-96.

[169] Binder EB. The role of FKBP5, a co-chaperone of the glucocorticoid receptor in the pathogenesis and therapy of affective and anxiety disorders. Psychoneuroendocrinology 2009, 34:S186-95.

[170] Davies TH, Ning YM, Sanchez ER. A new first step in activation of steroid receptors: hormone-induced switching of FKBP51 and FKBP52 immunophilins. J Biol Chem 2002, 277:4597-4600.

[171] Vermeer H, Hendriks-Stegeman BI, van der Burg B, van Buul-Offers SC, Jansen M. Glucocorticoid-induced increase in lymphocytic FKBP51 messenger ribonucleic acid expression: a potential marker for glucocorticoid sensitivity, potency, and bioavailability. J Clin Endocrinol Metab 2003, 88:277-284.

[172] Denny WB, Prapapanich V, Smith DF, Scammell JG. Structure-function analysis of squirrel monkey FK506-binding protein 51, a potent inhibitor of glucocorticoid receptor activity. Endocrinology 2005, 146:3194-3201.

[173] Scammell JG, Denny WB, Valentine DL, Smith DF. Overexpression of the FK506-binding immunophilin FKBP51 is the common cause of glucocorticoid resistance in three New World primates. Gen Comp Endocrinol 2001, 124:152-165.

[174] Binder EB, Salyakina D, Lichtner P, Wochnik GM, Ising M, Putz B, *et al.* Polymorphisms in FKBP5 are associated with increased recurrence of depressive episodes and rapid response to antidepressant treatment. Nat Genet 2004, 36:1319-1325.

[175] Koenen KC, Saxe G, Purcell S, Smoller JW, Bartholomew D, Miller A, *et al.* Polymorphisms in FKBP5 are associated with peritraumatic dissociation in medically injured children. Mol Psychiatry 2005, 10:1058-1059.

[176] Binder EB, Bradley RG, Liu W, Epstein MP, Deveau TC, Mercer KB, *et al.* Association of FKBP5 polymorphisms and childhood abuse with risk of posttraumatic stress disorder symptoms in adults. JAMA 2008, 299:1291-1305.

[177] Kehne JH, Cain CK. Therapeutic utility of non-peptidic CRF1 receptor antagonists in anxiety, depression, and stress-related disorders: evidence from animal models. Pharmacol Ther 2010, 128:460-487.

[178] Timpl P, Spanagel R, Sillaber I, Kresse A, Reul JM, Stalla GK, *et al.* Impaired stress response and reduced anxiety in mice lacking a functional corticotropin-releasing hormone receptor 1. Nat Genet 1998, 19:162-166.

[179] Gutman DA, Owens MJ, Thrivikraman KV, Nemeroff CB. Persistent anxiolytic affects after chronic administration of the CRF receptor antagonist R121919 in rats. Neuropharmacology 2011, 60:1135-1141.

[180] Britton DR, Koob GF, Rivier J, Vale W. Intraventricular corticotropin-releasing factor enhances behavioral effects of novelty. Life Sci 1982, 31:363-367.

[181] Eaves M, Thatcher-Britton K, Rivier J, Vale W, Koob GF. Effects of corticotropin releasing factor on locomotor activity in hypophysectomized rats. Peptides 1985, 6:923-926.

[182] Ising M, Zimmermann US, Kunzel HE, Uhr M, Foster AC, Learned-Coughlin SM, *et al.* High-affinity CRF1 receptor antagonist NBI-34041: preclinical and clinical data suggest safety and efficacy in attenuating elevated stress response. Neuropsychopharmacology 2007, 32:1941-1949.

[183] Binneman B, Feltner D, Kolluri S, Shi Y, Qiu R, Stiger T. A 6-week randomized, placebo-controlled trial of CP-316,311 (a selective CRH1 antagonist) in the treatment of major depression. Am J Psychiatry 2008, 165:617-620.

[184] Evans DL, Burnett GB, Nemeroff CB. The dexamethasone suppression test in the clinical setting. Am J Psychiatry 1983, 140:586-589.

[185] Schatzberg AF, Rothschild AJ, Langlais PJ, Bird ED, Cole JO. A corticosteroid/dopamine hypothesis for psychotic depression and related states. J Psychiatr Res 1985, 19:57-64.

[186] Murphy BE, Filipini D, Ghadirian AM. Possible use of glucocorticoid receptor antagonists in the treatment of major depression: preliminary results using RU 486. J Psychiatry Neurosci 1993, 18:209-213.

[187] DeBattista C, Belanoff J, Glass S, Khan A, Horne RL, Blasey C, *et al.* Mifepristone versus placebo in the treatment of psychosis in patients with psychotic major depression. Biol Psychiatry 2006, 60:1343-1349.

[188] Young AH, Gallagher P, Watson S, Del-Estal D, Owen BM, Ferrier IN. Improvements in neurocognitive function and mood following adjunctive treatment with mifepristone (RU-486) in bipolar disorder. Neuropsychopharmacology 2004, 29:1538-1545.

[189] Nemeroff CB. New directions in the development of antidepressants: the interface of neurobiology and psychiatry. Hum Psychopharmacol 2002, 17:S13-6.

[190] Krishnan KR, Reed D, Wilson WH, Saunders WB, Ritchie JC, Nemeroff CB, *et al.* RU486 in depression. Prog Neuropsychopharmacol Biol Psychiatry 1992, 16:913-920.

[191] Bachmann CG, Linthorst AC, Holsboer F, Reul JM. Effect of chronic administration of selective glucocorticoid receptor antagonists on the rat hypothalamic-pituitary-adrenocortical axis. Neuropsychopharmacology 2003, 28:1056-1067.

[192] Belanoff JK, Flores BH, Kalezhan M, Sund B, Schatzberg AF. Rapid reversal of psychotic depression using mifepristone. J Clin Psychopharmacol 2001, 21:516-521.

[193] Belanoff JK, Rothschild AJ, Cassidy F, DeBattista C, Baulieu EE, Schold C, *et al.* An open label trial of C-1073 (mifepristone) for psychotic major depression. Biol Psychiatry 2002, 52:386-392.

[194] Simpson GM, El Sheshai A, Loza N, Kingsbury SJ, Fayek M, Rady A, *et al.* An 8-week open-label trial of a 6-day course of mifepristone for the treatment of psychotic depression. J Clin Psychiatry 2005, 66:598-602.

[195] Flores BH, Kenna H, Keller J, Solvason HB, Schatzberg AF. Clinical and biological effects of mifepristone treatment for psychotic depression. Neuropsychopharmacology 2006, 31:628-636.

[196] Blasey CM, Debattista C, Roe R, Block T, Belanoff JK. A multisite trial of mifepristone for the treatment of psychotic depression: a site-by-treatment interaction. Contemp Clin Trials 2009, 30:284-288.

[197] Ago Y, Arikawa S, Yata M, Yano K, Abe M, Takuma K, *et al.* Antidepressant-like effects of the glucocorticoid receptor antagonist RU-43044 are associated with changes in prefrontal dopamine in mouse models of depression. Neuropharmacology 2008, 55:1355-1363.

[198] Asagami T, Belanoff JK, Azuma J, Blasey CM, Clark RD, Tsao PS. Selective Glucocorticoid Receptor (GR-II) Antagonist Reduces Body Weight Gain in Mice. J Nutr Metab 2011, 2011:235389.

[199] Schmid B, Blomeyer D, Treutlein J, Zimmermann US, Buchmann AF, Schmidt MH, *et al*: Interacting effects of CRHR1 gene and stressful life events on drinking initiation and progression among 19-year-olds. Int J Neuropsychopharmacol 2010, 13:703-714.

[200] Keck ME, Kern N, Erhardt A, Unschuld PG, Ising M, Salyakina D, *et al.* Combined effects of exonic polymorphisms in CRHR1 and AVPR1B genes in a case/control study for panic disorder. Am J Med Genet B Neuropsychiatr Genet 2008, 147B:1196-1204.

[201] Gold PW, Chrousos GP. Organization of the stress system and its dysregulation in melancholic and atypical depression: high vs low CRH/NE states. Mol. Psychiatry 2002, 7 (3), 245-275.

[202] Stetler C, Miller GE. Depression and hypothalamic-pituitary-adrenal activation: a quantitative summary of four decades of research. Psychosom. Med 2011 73 (2), 114-125.

[203] O'Keane V, Frodl T, Dinan TG. A review of Atypical depression in relation to the course of depression and changes in HPA axis organization. Psychoneuroendocrinology 2012.

[204] Owens MJ, Bissette G, Nemeroff SB. Acute effects of alprazolam and adinazolam on the concentrations of corticotropin – releasing factor in the rat brain. Synapse 1989 4(3): 196-202.

Neurobiology of Mood Disorders, 2014, 210-233

CHAPTER 9

ROLE OF HIPPOCAMPAL NEUROGENESIS IN THE PATHOPHYSIOLOGY AND TREATMENT OF DEPRESSION

BENJAMIN ADAM SAMUELS, INDIRA DAVID, QUENTIN RAINER, ALAIN MICHEL GARDIER, RENÉ HEN, DENIS JOSEPH DAVID*

Faculty of Pharmacy, University Paris South IV, Paris, France

Abstract: Depression and anxiety are psychiatric illnesses that are major burdens on society and affect as much as 7% of the world's population. Here we review common approaches used to model depression in rodents such as chronic mild stress (CMS), social defeat, and chronic corticosterone treatment. We discuss the pros and cons of these different approaches. Furthermore, we provide a detailed review of adult hippocampal neurogenesis, including the distinct phases that a cell passes through when transitioning from precursor to neuron. Finally, we discuss at length the experiments that have related adult hippocampal neurogenesis to treatments of depression and anxiety, and why neurogenesis might be necessary for these treatments. We end by revisiting the neurogenesis hypothesis of depression and by providing suggestions for future research directions.

Keywords: Subventricular (SVZ) and subgranular zone (SGZ) of dentate gyrus (DG) of hippocampus, doublecortin (DCX) expressing cells, adult neurogenesis, cell differentiation, depression, antidepressant drugs, animal models.

1. INTRODUCTION

Depressive and anxiety disorders are a major burden on society. Mood disorders affect 7% of the world's population, while severe forms of depression impact 2-5% of the US population [1, 2]. Furthermore, approximately 32-35 million adults in the US population [16%] experience an episode of major depression in their lifetime [3]. The heterogeneous nature of depression suggests an involvement of multiple distinct brain regions, which may be responsible for the diverse symptoms. Human imaging and post-mortem studies have supported this hypothesis, implicating brain areas including the prefrontal and cingulate cortex, hippocampus, striatum, amygdala, and thalamus [4]. Together, these brain regions operate a series of highly interacting circuits that forms a neural circuitry involved in depression [5]. The hippocampus is one of several limbic structures that have been extensively studied in individuals with psychiatric and neurologic disorders in the last decade [5, 6]. Besides its critical role in learning and memory, the hippocampus is one of only two areas in mammalian brain where adult neurogenesis occurs [6]. Adult hippocampal neurogenesis is therefore defined as the progression from neural stem cell to mature dentate granule neuron.

Moreover, while many classes of drugs with antidepressant activity have been developed and approved [7], many patients do not respond to treatment [8]. Therefore it is critical for basic research to develop animal models that present behavioral, neurochemical and brain morphological phenotypes reminiscent of depression and anxiety. Given that anxiety and depression have a high comorbidity

***Address correspondence to Denis J. David:** Faculty of Pharmacy, University Paris South IV, Paris, France; E-mail: denis.david@u-psud.fr

Bruno P Guiard and Eliyahu Dremencov (Eds)

with co-occurrence rates up to 60% in patients [9, 10], animal models that present signs of both diseases could potentially be the most useful.

To fully understand the pathophysiology and treatment of depression, it is essential to delineate molecular, cellular and circuit-level determinants of chronic antidepressant action in addition to behavioral models. Of the current leading hypotheses of the pathophysiology and treatment of depression, the Neurogenesis Hypothesis of Depression deserves particular attention because it allows the characterization because changes in neurogenesis are only seen after chronic, but not acute, antidepressant treatment. This review revisits the role of adult hippocampal neurogenesis in the pathophysiology of mood disorders, especially anxiety/depression, and also in the antidepressant responses, especially in non-stressed and stressed rodents.

2. HIPPOCAMPAL NEUROGENESIS

Neurogenesis refers to the production of new neurons in the brain. Originally, it was only described during development. The dogma of Ramon y Cajal (1913) that the adult brain was unable of generating new neurons was first questioned by the work of Altman in the 1960s, who revealed the genesis of new cells in the brain of adult rat and cat by autoradiography with tritiated thymidine [11]. Unfortunately, it was uncertain whether the new cells were actually neuronal cells. The work of Kaplan and Hinds (1977) [12] confirmed this by using an ultrastructural analysis of the labeled cells. Many years later, a combination of specific neuronal markers and an analogue of thyminidine, 5-bromo-2'-deoxy-uridine (BrdU), confirmed the neuronal phenotype [13]. The process of adult neurogenesis is located in two discrete brain regions: the subventricular zone (SVZ) and subgranular zone (SGZ) of dentate gyrus of the hippocampus. In this chapter, only the hippocampal neurogenesis and its involvement in depression will be presented.

2.1. PRODUCTION OF NEW NEURONS IN THE SGZ

Hippocampal neurogenesis is possible in the SGZ of the dentate gyrus of the hippocampus because of to the presence of stem cells. These stem cells evolve into neural progenitor cells that can produce multiple cell types in the central nervous system such as neurons, astrocytes, oligodendrocytes, or microglial cells [14]. In rodents, the duration of the mitotic cycle of proliferating precursors is approximately 12 to 24 hours, leading to the production of about 8,000 to 10,000 new neurons per day [15] Given that the dentate gyrus consists of approximately one million granule cells, this phenomenon is capable of generating a little less than 1% of total granule cells each day. However, the proportion of new neurons that survive beyond one month is less than 50%, and the production of new cells is offset by the daily loss of mature granule cells. The surviving cells are predominantly a neuronal phenotype (75%), mainly glutamatergic granule cells, but also some are GABAergic interneuron basket cells. A smaller proportion of cells differentiate into astrocytes (15%), oligodendrocytes or microglia [16].

2.2. NEUROGENIC NICHE

Adult hippocampal neurogenesis, therefore, mainly refers to the production of a single neuronal type: the granule cells of the dentate gyrus. These cells are the principal excitatory neurons of the dentate gyrus (DG), receiving connections from the entorhinal cortex and sending projections along mossy fibers into the CA3 subfield of the hippocampus, where they terminate in structures rich in synapses and interneurons. Several projections are also sent into the hilus. The precursors are located between the hilus and the granular zone, in a niche called the subgranular zone (SGZ). The SGZ provides a microenvironment that promotes neuronal development. This neurogenic niche includes precursors, immature neurons, glial and endothelial cells, microglia and some immune cells. The niche is surrounded by a basement membrane. Because of the important role of vascularization in this region, this niche is also called a vascular niche [17]. In all cases, the niche provides a unique environment for neuronal development. Studies suggest that astrocytes have a local key role in neurogenesis. *In vivo*, the development of cells has a preferred spatial relationship with astrocytes. *Ex vivo*, astrocytes and astrocyte-derived factors are potent inducers of hippocampal neurogenesis for the precursors [18]. The SGZ is also special because it receives connections from several brain regions: dopamine fibers in the ventral tegmental area, projections of serotonergic raphe nuclei, septum acetylcholine connections, and connections of GABAergic local interneurons. Manipulations of these neurotransmitter systems has also demonstrated regulatory effects on neurogenesis [19] [20]. The fact that these neurotransmitter systems regulate neurogenesis is of particular interest because antidepressants mainly act by changing monoamine levels [see later section entitled ANTIDEPRESSANTS AND ADULT HIPPOCAMPAL NEUROGENESIS]. A prominent example is that mice deficient in the Serotonin 1A receptor do not show a neurogenic response to chronic fluoxetine treatment [21].

2.3. CELLULAR STAGES OF HIPPOCAMPAL NEUROGENESIS

Neurogenesis can be divided into four phases: a step in which precursor cells are dividing, then surviving, a post mitotic maturation phase, and a late phase of survival.

2.3.1. The stage of precursor cell

The precursors have properties reminiscent of glial cells, including the morphology of radial glia. The cell body is located in the subgranular zone and the dendrites extend into the molecular layer. The nature of hippocampal astrocyte precursors was first revealed by [22]. Type 1 precursor cells yield intermediate progenitor cells, or type-2 cells, with a high proliferation activity. A subset of these cells continue to express glial markers, but lack the morphological characteristics of radial cells (type-2a). The type-2 cells that express nestin filaments (such as cell type-1) also express markers such as NEUROD1 and Prox1. This particular phenotype is used to classify cells as type-2b [16, 23]. Prox1 is specific to the development of granule cells. In type 2 cells, the developing cells receive GABAergic innervation [24], and are more sensitive to GABAergic stimulation. Similarly, type-1 cells respond to these stimuli by increasing cell proliferation [25]. Among the early expressed neuronal markers, doublecortin (DCX) is expressed on the type-2b cells. The expression of DCX extends from the proliferation phase to post mitotic maturation, which lasts about 2-3 weeks [26].

2.3.2. The phase of survival

Soon after the release of the cell cycle, new neurons express markers, such NeuN ["Specific neuronal nuclear protein"] and the transient marker calretinin [27]. A majority of cells fail to establish connections with the molecular layer and die. In contrast, cells that establish stable connections develop a stable dendritic arborization that extends in a specific way in time. In the days following the exit of the cell cycle, new cells emanate their axons to their target region CA3 to form appropriate synapses. This period is marked by the expression of a protein mediator, such as TOAD-64 or TUC-4, implicated in axon guidance. The first GABAergic innervations are excitatory and then become inhibitory when glutamatergic connections are established [24]. The GABAergic action leads cells to mature into glutamatergic cells and to develop synaptic integration [28] Most regulatory elements and processes occur at the stage of neuronal development, and rarely during the expansion phase [27, 29].

2.3.3. The maturation step; from early to late stage

Doublecortin is expressed in granule cells that range from 1 day to about 4 weeks of age, with 20% of its total population being proliferating neuroblasts and the rest being post-mitotic neurons [30].

Another marker of maturation, called calretinin, is also used as a marker for immature GCs at the early postmitotic stage. The period of expression of calretinin (3-4 weeks), is closely linked to dendritic maturation. However, using a lentiviral approach expressing the Green Fluorescent protein, it has been shown that the axonal growth to CA3 precedes the development of dendritic arborization [14]. After full integration to existing circuits, the new cells move from the calcium-binding protein calretinin to calbindin [27]. It is several weeks before the cells are no longer distinguishable electrophysiologically from mature neurons of the granule cells [31]. It has been postulated that the time needed to complete the functionality of these young neurons is related to the formation and storage of new elements of memory [32]. Finally, calbindin-like immunoreactivity has been described as a marker for mature granule cells.

2.4. QUANTITATIVE ANALYSIS OF PROLIFERATION, SURVIVAL, MATURATION AND DIFFERENTIATION, NEWBORN CELLS.

For a full characterization of the neurogenic effects of new compounds, all the steps of neurogenesis, including proliferation, survival, maturation, and differentiation have to be completed. So far, no specific and exclusive marker has been identified that would allow for prospective studies of neurogenesis. As a result, detection of neurogenic steps depends on a combination of labeling approaches. Thus, proliferation, differentiation and survival steps each require a specific protocol using the administration of a synthetic thymidine analogue, "5-bromo-3'-deoxyuridine" (BrdU) that substitutes for thymidine incorporation into DNA synthesized during the S phase of the cycle. Quantitative analysis of proliferation, differentiation, and survival of newborn cells is made by varying the time interval between the pulse administration of BrdU and the sacrifice of animals [33].

2.4.1. Main methods for a Detection of cell proliferation

For the quantification of rate of cell division, animals are administered BrdU [between 50 to 150 mg/kg 2h before sacrifice [34]. Proliferation is quantified by counting BrdU-positive cells. To simplify the experiment, quantification of BrdU-positive clusters can also be performed to measure proliferation since a positive correlation exists between BrdU-positive clusters and BrdU-positive cells. Since the quantification of BrdU-positive clusters is much less time consuming than counting BrdU-positive cells, this method can be used as a rapid indicator of the neurogenic effect of drugs or other manipulations [33]. This is important also because BrdU immunostaining has been used not only to test whether new drugs affect adult hippocampal neurogenesis, but also whether the anxiety/ depressive-like state has been related to changes in hippocampal neurogenesis.

2.4.2. Endogenous markers of cell proliferation

Endogenous cell cycle proteins are expressed at different stages of cell cycle progression. For exemple the "Proliferating Cell Nuclear Antigen, PCNA" is expressed throughout the cell cycle and provide low temporal resolution. Ki-67 closely corresponds to BrdU as it is expressed both during S phase and through the remainder of the cell cycle (Figure **1**).

2.4.3. Survival and fate of the newly generated cells

Usually, for the quantification of rate of cell survival, animals are administered BrdU (100 to 150 mg/ kg) twice a day during three days, 3 to 4 weeks before sacrifice [35]. The reason to wait for sacrifice is that the fate of the newly generated cells can only be determined three to four weeks later, once neuronal migration has occurred [13, 36]. Once progenitor cells reach maturity they begin expressing neuronal markers such as neurofilaments, NeuN, and Calcium-binding proteins or astrocyte markers such as glial fibrillary acidic protein (GFAP). Calcium-binding proteins such as calbindin are produced when cells become electrophysiological active. It is not until 4 weeks after birth that newly generated granule cells have acquired the typical features of mature granule cells and cease to express immature neuronal markers.

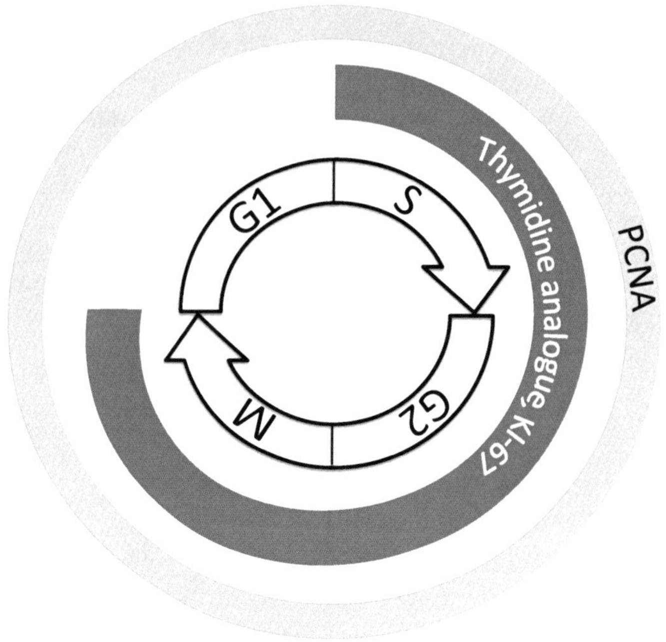

Figure 1: Schema representing the endogenous or exogenous markers used to study adult neurogenesis

2.4.4. *Markers of maturation*

Several markers have been used to assess maturation such as microtubule-associated protein [doublecortin]. In the adult dentate gyrus, DCX is exclusively expressed in immature neurons [26, 37], and thus has been widely used as an immature neuronal marker that reliably reflects the level of neurogenesis and its modulation [26]. To assess the impact of antidepressants on dendritic maturation, the morphology of cells that express doublecortin (DCX) are examined. DCX-positive cells with tertiary dendrites, which display more complex dendritic arborization, can be distinguished from others DCX cells. The ratio of DCX-positive cells with tertiary dendrites over total DCX-positive cells is informative of the rate of maturation. The polysialylated form of the neural cell adhesion molecule (PSA-NCAM) also has a transient expression pattern that marks neuronal progenitors. However, it should be noted that, in contrary to DCX, PSA-NCAM has also been detected in glial cells.

2.5. METHODS USED TO ABLATE OR INCREASE NEUROGENESIS

The analysis of the causal relationship between neurogenesis and behavior came from the removal of progenitor cells. Several methods to date have been developed to reduce or abolish neurogenesis (Table **1**):

An X-irradiation of either the whole brain or locally in the hippocampus [21];

A systemic treatment with an anti-mitotic agent such as methylazoxymethanol acetate [MAM] [38];

By genetic manipulation, such as GFAP-TK mice, in which the GFAP + progenitor cells die following treatment with ganciclovir [39].

In a contrary experiment, Sahay and colleagues [40] developed a genetic gain-of-function strategy to inducibly augment the survival of adult-born neurons in a cell-autonomous manner [40]. Because

Pharmacological manipulation	Cranial Irradiation	Genetic manipulation
5-fluorouracil [5-Fu], methylazoxymethanol [MAM], temozolomide [TMZ] cytosine arabinoside [Ara-C]	X-irradiation, gamma-rays	GFAP-TK, Nestin-TK, Nestin-Bax, $TrkB^{lox/lox\text{-}Cre\ ERT2}$ Cyclin D2 transgenic
[38] [96] [115]	[21, 39, 52, 69, 73, 97, 116-118]	[6, 51, 100, 101, 114, 119];

Table 1: Methods used to ablate or increase neurogenesis

60–80% of young adult-born neurons undergo programmed cell death, for which the pro-apoptotic gene Bax is required, they used a transgenic mouse line in which the tamoxifen (TAM)-regulatable recombinase CreERT2 is expressed under the control of a 5.26-kilobase fragment of the rat nestin (Nes) gene promoter [41] together with a floxed Bax mouse line to ablate Bax selectively in neural stem cells in the adult brain and promote survival.

3. HIPPOCAMPAL NEUROGENESIS AND MAJOR DEPRESSION AND ITS TREATMENT

3.1. THE ANXIETY / DEPRESSION STATE AND HIPPOCAMPAL NEUROGENESIS

The neurogenic hypothesis of depression postulates that decreased production of new granule cells in the dentate gyrus of the hippocampus is linked to the pathophysiology of depression and that the increase in hippocampal neurogenesis is required for the behavioral effects of antidepressant treatment [42]. The few studies of hippocampal neurogenesis in depressed patients published to date have mainly relied on histological examinations of post-mortem brain tissue and studies of magnetic resonance imaging. Thus, a reduction in hippocampal volume in depressed patients is somewhat established, and the contribution of two meta-analysis confirmed this reduction in hippocampal volume in patients with depression [43]. The frequency of depressive episodes and the period during which they are not treated coincide with the severity of the decline in hippocampal volume. However, pathophysiological studies on post-mortem brain tissue indicates that the change in the number of neuropil and glial cells may be responsible for reducing the volume of the hippocampus [44]. It is highly unlikely that loss of hippocampal neurogenesis can account for the decreased volume. These imaging results, involving hippocampal neurogenesis in the pathophysiology of major depressive episodes, have been challenged by a recent histology study [45]. This study did not actually detect the difference in stem cell proliferation [by Ki-67] in the hippocampus between patients with depression and healthy volunteers. The results of this study are limited, however, since the patients were on antidepressant medication at the time of death, which could mask the specific effects of depression on cell proliferation. In addition, in the absence of toxicology studies, it is not clear that the patients observed treatment. Moreover, given the diversity in the stages of neurogenesis, it is difficult to conclude any involvement of neurogenesis after only observation of cell proliferation. In contrast, a more recent study actually showed a 50% decrease in proliferation [by Ki-67] in patients with depression than in controls [46, 47]. However, this difference did not reach statistical significance.

Preclinical studies are useful to prove causal links between hippocampal neurogenesis and behavior. Using exposure to different types of stress, like chronic stress or social submission, causes a decrease in cell proliferation in the hippocampus. It is important to keep in mind the disadvantages of these methods, such as non-specific effects of ablation that can involve structures other than the hippocampus, and therefore other functions. Dysfunction of hippocampal neurogenesis is only hypothesized to be part of the pathogenesis of major depressive disorders [48], [23]. In reality, the suppression of hippocampal neurogenesis in mice does not alter anxiety behavior in the open field or the light/dark paradigms, the elevated plus maze, or novelty suppressed feeding [49], [21], [39]. Thus, the X-irradiation in the hippocampus has no effect in the previously mentioned paradigms, suggesting that the loss of hippocampal neurogenesis is not sufficient for a behavioral phenotype of anxiety/ depression, and does not exacerbate those induced by stress. Similarly, ablation of neurogenesis by MAM, a pharmacological agent, is not sufficient to induce an anhedonic behavior in rats [38]. Airan *et al* [50] explored in more detail the link between depression and hippocampal neurogenesis. It is clear from their study that chronic stress in rats is not associated with a decrease in neurogenesis, and that the removal of neurogenesis does not induce a depressive-like behavior [50]. However, other studies suggest that the mechanisms are more complex. Recently it was shown that adult hippocampal neurogenesis plays an important role in the regulation of affective states [51]. Indeed, transgenic mice that overexpress the protein Bax in apoptotic progenitor cells and thus have a deficit in neurogenesis, have an anxiety phenotype. In sum, there is evidence indicating that neurogenesis is not a major factor in the development of depression, but may be necessary for the behavioral effects of antidepressants [2].

4. ANTIDEPRESSANTS AND ADULT HIPPOCAMPAL NEUROGENESIS

4.1. IN PHYSIOLOGICAL CONDITIONS.

To study the effects of antidepressants in unstressed animals, the choice of the strain is essential. It should be noted that 129SvEv mice express a low basal level of proliferating cells in the SGZ, and therefore are more relevant to study an induced increase in antidepressant treatment in conditions without stress than BALB / cJ or C57Bl / 6 mice, which express a higher cell proliferation [52]. Instead, the study of the impact of stress on hippocampal neurogenesis is more relevant in these last two strains.

Effects of antidepressants on the proliferation and cell survival. In addition to the effects of fluoxetine [18 mg/kg] in increasing cell proliferation in 129/SvEvTAc mice [21] [Table **2**], it also increases the survival of postmitotic granule cells. These effects of SSRIs on proliferation and cell survival were also found in rats [53, 54]. It is important to note that the neurogenic effects of antidepressants are only seen with chronic treatment [21, 49, 54-56]. In addition, other treatments such as the atypical antidepressant tianeptine, electroconvulsive therapy, mood stabilizers such as lithium, and new antidepressants such as agomelatine, increase proliferation and cell survival in the adult hippocampus [57]. Furthermore, agomelatine selectively alters neurogenesis in the ventral hippocampus, a region more involved in the emotional response [58]. Therefore, it seems that proliferation and survival are regulated by distinct mechanisms. For example, an enriched environment increases the survival of immature cells without affecting proliferation [59]. In contrast, voluntary exercise increases the proliferation and survival, without affecting the maturation [30] or dendritic morphology of newborn neurons [60]. Finally, a recent study showed that fluoxetine targets a class of neural progenitor cells by directly increasing symmetric divisions [53]. Effects of antidepressants on the maturation. Until recently, it was not clear that SSRIs also targeted immature neurons by affecting their maturation and functional integration to the network. Wang and colleagues [2008] demonstrated that chronic treatment with fluoxetine stimulates maturation of young neurons [56]. Indeed, they have a dendritic

Table 2: Effects of chronic antidepressant treatment on hippocampal neurogenesis in rodents

Antidepressant	Specie	Dose (mg/kg)	Length of Treatment	Prolif.	Diff.	Survival	References
			25 days	=	ø	=	(120)
			21 days	↑	ø	ø	(121)
			7 days	=	ø	ø	
	Sprague Dawley Rat	5	1 day	=	ø	ø	(54)
			5 days	=	ø	ø	
			14 days	↑	ø	ø	
			28 days	↑	ø	ø	
		0.6	28 days	↑	ø	ø	(122)
	Wistar Rat	10	28 days	↑	↑	ø	(123)
	Lister Rat	7	14 days	↑	↑	ø	(124)
	(BALB/c * DBA/2) mice	10	21 days	↑	ø	ø	(125)
			10 days	↑	ø	ø	
			5 days	=	ø	ø	
Fluoxetine		?	?	↑			(126)
	S129 SvEv mice	10	5 days	=	ø	ø	(21)
			11 days	↑	ø	ø	
			28 days	↑	ø	↑	
		18	5 days	=	=	=	(56)
			28 days	↑	↑	↑	
	129Sl mice	18	21 days	↑	ø	ø	(127)
	A/J mice	18	21 days	=	ø	ø	
		18	28 days	=	=	ø	(52)
	BALB/cJ mice	10	28 days	=	=	=	(68)
		16	24 days	=	=	=	(128)
	C57BL/6 mice	16	24 days	=	=	=	
	CD1 mice	10	28 days	↑	=	↑	(129)
	DBA/2 mice	18	21 days	↑	ø	ø	(127)
	SWR/J mice	18	21 days	=	ø	ø	
			21 days	↑	↓	↑	
Agomelatine	Wistar Rat	40	7 days	=	ø	ø	(57)
			1 day	=	ø	ø	
AMPA	Rodents	?	?	↑	ø	ø	(130)
Glutamatergic antagonist	Rodents	?	?	↑	ø	ø	(131)
Interleukine beta 1receptor antagonist	Rodents	?	?	↑	ø	ø	(132)
Citalopram	Wistar Rat	10	28 days	=	=	=	(133)
ECT	Wistar Rat	1 fois par jour	5 days	↑	↑	ø	(134)

Legend : ↑, increase; ↓, decrease; =, no change; ø, not study

Antidepressant	Species	Dose (mg/kg)	Length of Treatment	Prolif.	Diff.	Survival	References
Fluoxéeine/adolescent	BALB/cJ mice	16	24 days	↑	=	=	(128)
	C57BL/6 mice	16	24 days	↑	↑	↑	
Imipramine	Wistar Rat	5	56 days	↑	ø	ø	(135)
	(BALB/c * DBA/2) mice	30	21 days	↑	ø	↑	(125)
	129 SvEv mice	20	28 days	↑	ø	↑	(21)
Lithium	Wistar Rat	2,5	14 days	↑	↑	↑	(136)
	C57BL/6 mice	2.4 g/kg	28 days	↑	=	↑	(137)
Olanzapine	Sprague Dawley Rat	2	21 days	↑	ø	ø	(121)
		2	7 days	=	ø	ø	
Reboxétine	Rat Sprague Dawley	20 (2/day)	21 days	↑	ø	ø	(54)
Riluzole	Rodents	?	?	↑	ø	ø	(138)
Rolipram	129 SvEv mice	?	?	↑		ø	(139)
Tesofensine	Wistar Rat	3	5 days	=	ø	=	(140)
		3	14 days	↑	ø	↑	
Tianeptine	Tree Shrews	50	28 days	=	ø	ø	(141)
Tranylcypromine	Sprague Dawley Rat	7.5, then 10 (14 last days)	21 days	↑	ø	ø	(142)
Venlafaxine	Wistar Rat	10	14 days	=	ø	ø	(143)
		40		↑	ø	ø	

Legend : ↑, increase; ↓, decrease; =, no change; ø, not study

arborization more complex than those present in untreated animals, suggesting an accelerating effect of fluoxetine on hippocampal neuronal maturation [56]. The duration of onset of fluoxetine effects on maturation also coincides with the time required for the onset of behavioral effects of this treatment in mice. Similarly, electroconvulsive therapy (ECT), which provides a very rapid therapeutic effect, stimulates neurogenesis faster than fluoxetine [61]. In addition, ECT stimulates dendritic development and maturation [62]. After ECT, young neurons express an increase in dendritic growth, and begin to receive glutamatergic synaptic connections early. These results suggest that molecules that increase the maturation of new neurons are targets for the development of future treatments.

4.1. EFFECTS OF ANTIDEPRESSANTS ON THE DIFFERENTIATION

Four weeks after birth, progenitor cells acquire properties of mature granule cells. For example, the new cells no longer express the immature neuronal markers DCX or PSA-NCAM, and receive the same GABAergic and glutamatergic afferents as mature granule cells of the dentate gyrus [14, 63, 64]. However, these new cells continue to mature morphologically and physiologically. The dendritic spines of a neuron at four weeks old are more associated with multiple synaptic boutons that older neurons and the density continues to increase even after 8 weeks [63]. In addition, neurons aged 2 to 4 weeks exhibit an increase in excitability and a lower threshold for induction of long-term potentiation (LTP), while at 4 to 6 weeks, new neurons exhibit greater LTP amplitude [65]. In addition, a specific form of LTP (ACSF-LTP) requires the hippocampal neurogenesis, as this form of LTP is blocked after ablation of neurogenesis [39]. This critical period in young neurons coincides with the development of receptor expression of NMDA NR2B [28].

At any given time following differentiation, young neurons can be found across stages of development and with distinct morphological and physiological characteristics. Similar to new neurons in the developing brain, the newborn granule cells depolarize in response to GABA because of their high intracellular concentration of chloride ions [66]. Somewhere between 2 to 4 weeks after birth the response to GABA changes from depolarization to hyperpolarization as the young cells develop their dendritic spines and receive glutamatergic connections. In addition, new granule cells begin to make connections with the hilus and CA3 region while synaptic complexity is similar to that of mature neurons [67].

4.2. DEPENDENT AND INDEPENDENT NEUROGENIC EFFECTS IN THE ACTION OF ANTIDEPRESSANTS

Recently Boldrini and colleagues [46] suggested that future studies in humans should determine at which level antidepressants should affect neurogenesis to maximize the response [46]. Preclinical studies in rodents, using approaches that override functional neurogenesis, are used to establish the relationship between neuronal activity and the contribution of hippocampal neurogenesis in the behavioral effects of antidepressants in animals that are either stressed or not. The study by Santarelli and colleagues [21] has raised many questions about the contribution of hippocampal neurogenesis in the behavioral improvement induced by antidepressants, unstressed mice [21]. From this study it was shown that the behavioral effect of SSRIs is dependent on the presence of hippocampal neurogenesis [56]. However, in BALB / cJ mice, abolishing neurogenesis by x-ray does not block the behavioral response induced by SSRIs in different behavioral paradigms related to anxiety / depression, especially the NSF [52]. Furthermore, chronic treatment with fluoxetine did not increase hippocampal neurogenesis [52, 68]. Likewise, the beneficial contributions of an enriched environment, physical exercise, or learning behavior related to anxiety appear to be independent of increased neurogenesis in adult mice [69].

To examine whether the increase induced by antidepressant treatment may simply be an epiphenomenon, the study of animal models of anxiety / depression in which hippocampal neurogenesis is reduced appears to be a good alternative.

5. ANIMAL MODELS OF DEPRESSIVE PHENOTYPES

Since no genetic variants with high penetrance that cause depression are known, animal models have mainly relied on different means of chronically exposing rodents to stressful experiences, or sensory tract lesions such as in olfactory bulbectomy, to induce behavioral states that present depression-like signs and are responsive to chronic antidepressant treatment.

The oldest most commonly used paradigm to induce a depression-like state is chronic mild stress (CMS). Initial observations suggested that animals subjected to multiple stressors over a prolonged period of time reduced their intake of saccharine or sucrose, a potential behavioral model of anhedonia [70]. Furthermore, this effect was selectively reversed by chronic treatment with the TCA imipramine [70]. Further work was able to repeat this result using more mild stressors, such as periods of food and water deprivation, small temperature reductions and changes of cage mates [71, 72]. Following these studies the CMS procedure, and modified versions such as chronic unpredictable stress (CUS or UCMS), became commonly used and much work demonstrated that other depression-like changes were induced in animals, such as decreased sexual and aggressive behavior, decreased self-care, and altered sleep patterns [71]. Furthermore these behaviors are all reversible by chronic, but not acute, treatment using multiple classes of antidepressants [73]. While historically potential pitfalls of the CMS procedure are that it is notoriously labor intensive, and that there has been some difficulty in getting the procedure established and the results replicated across laboratories [74], the modified versions of the CMS have proven more useful.

Recently, there have been some reports using CMS or variants to model treatment resistance in rodents. In one study, CMS significantly decreased sucrose consumption and the proliferation of adult hippocampal neural progenitors [75]. Following chronic treatment with a SSRI (escitalopram), the subjects were retested for sucrose consumption. A bimodal distribution was found where one group recovered [increased sucrose consumption] while another refracted treatment [no increase in sucrose consumption]. Interestingly, there was a correlation between the animals in the group that recovered with a reversal of the decreased proliferation that was absent in the group resistant to treatment [75]. More recently, follow-up work has taken a proteomic approach in an attempt to find molecular differences in the ventral hippocampus between responders and non-responders [76]. Another study demonstrated that if animals are on a high fat diet during multiple UCMS procedures they become resistant to treatment with a SSRI (fluoxetine) [77].

A distinct procedure that has gained traction is the usage of a social defeat model. In this paradigm a mouse is forced into the territory of a mouse from a larger, more aggressive strain leading to an interaction resulting in intruder subordination. Repeated defeats over 10 days can result in a long lasting reduced social interaction, sexual dysfunction, sleep dysregulation, anxiety, metabolic deficits and anhedonia [78-81]. Interestingly, following the social defeat procedure there remains a large variance in behavior outcomes in spite of using an inbred mouse strain (C57BL/6). Some animals display a resistance to social defeat (resilience) while others are susceptible (determined by interaction with a social target relative to an empty enclosure). If animals are separated based on this measure, susceptible mice demonstrate decreased sucrose intake, a blunted circadian rhythm, and conditioned place preference to cocaine [80]. Furthermore, phenotypes induced by social defeat in susceptible mice can be reversed by antidepressant treatment [79]. Given that molecular mechanisms for resilience to the stressful procedure are now being worked out [80, 82], it would be intriguing to see if similar pathways are necessary for mediating response to antidepressants.

A third procedure for inducing a depression-like state in animals is administration of chronic glucocorticoids in order to mimic the effects of chronic stress. A significant proportion of depressed patients display altered activity of the HPA axis, and stress generally leads to hypersecretion of corticosteroids, which imposes an increased risk for depression [10, 37, 83-88]. Chronic treatment of rodents with corticosterone effectively induces multiple anxiety- and depression-like changes in behavior, neurochemistry and brain morphology [89-92]. Behaviorally, depression-related changes include suppression of sucrose intake and decreased self-care [90, 93], while anxiety-related changes include increased latency to emerge into the light compartment in the light/dark test, decreased time, entries and percent distance in the center of an open field and increased latency to take a bite of food in the novelty suppressed feeding (NSF) test [90, 91].

6. ADULT HIPPOCAMPAL NEUROGENESIS IN PATHOLOGICAL CONDITIONS

One of the main findings of the role of adult hippocampal neurogenesis in depression is the observation that antidepressants confer behavioral effects by stimulating neurogenesis in rodents and humans. A recent study showed for the first time in the dentate gyrus in humans that there are more nestin-expressing progenitor cells, and increased dividing cells after treatment with an SSRI antidepressant (sertraline, fluoxetine) or tricyclic (nortriptyline, clomipramine) in patients with depression compared to untreated patients [46]. Another study also showed that antidepressants increase human hippocampal neurogenesis by activating the glucocortiocoid receptor [94]. In nonhuman primates, repeated separation stress resulted in depression-like behaviors [anhedonia and subordinance] accompanied by reduced hippocampal neurogenesis [95]. Treatment of the nonhuman primates with fluoxetine stimulated neurogenesis and prevented the emergence of depression-like behaviors. Furthermore, ablation of neurogenesis with irradiation of the nonhuman primates abolished the therapeutic effects of fluoxetine.

To address whether altered neurogenesis is important for the treatment of depression, Deisseroth's group used voltage sensitive dye imaging to probe hippocampal activity in the CMS in Rat and specifically the role of neurogenesis in depression-relevant neurophysiology and behavior [50]. Using irradiation to ablate neurogenesis, Airan and colleagues also found that antidepressant behavioral efficacy in the Forced Swim Test in Rat required intact neurogenesis. Overall, antidepressant treatment was sufficient to transiently increase neurogenesis and exert behavioral effects long after drug clearance from the system, and this effect was absent in animals lacking neurogenesis (X-Ray). Recently, an elegant study in Rat confirmed Deisseroth's study by showing that antidepressants retain some but not all their therapeutic efficacy in reducing measured indices of anxiety/depression-like behavior when hippocampal neurogenesis was blocked by a cytostatic agent [96]. Indeed, using CMS and the antimitotic agent MAM, authors showed that the various antidepressants ameliorated CMS-induced behavioral signs of depression to the same extent in vehicle and MAM-treated animals. Conversely, using the NSF paradigm, they found that the antidepressant drugs studied (imipramine, fluoxetine) reduced the hyperanxious state observed in CMS-exposed rats even though neurogeneis was blocked. Overall, authors concluded that antidepressants re-established neuronal plasticity in hippocampus. In the "CORT model", using X-irradiated mice, in which hippocampal neurogenesis was abolished, we demonstrated that antidepressant treatment still elicits some anxiolytic/antidepressant-like effects. Specifically we found that antidepressant effects in the Open Field and Forced Swim Test were neurogenesis independent, while effects in the Novelty Suppressed Feeding Test or on coat state were neurogenesis dependent. As such, our study reveals that the behavioral effects of fluoxetine are mediated through both neurogenesis-dependent and -independent actions [97]. Previously, Surget and colleagues [73] presented important evidence for both neurogenesis-dependent and -independent mechanisms for the reversal of stress-induced behaviors by antidepressant drugs, including fluoxetine [73]. Our paper, using a different model of stress, extends this study by utilizing a mechanistic approach to propose a neurogenesis-independent pathways for mediating the effects of SSRIs, namely the β-arrestin signaling pathway.

7. ADULT HIPPOCAMPAL NEUROGENESIS IN DIFFERENT GENDERS

Taking into consideration that depression is twice as common in women as in men, it is important to also consider sex differences in the effects of depression models and antidepressants on adult neurogenesis. In MRL/MpJ mice treated with fluoxetine (10 mg/kg b.i.d.) for 21 days, cell proliferation was increased in both genders, but females produced more new cells than males [95]. Furthermore, while fluoxetine did not alter survival in males, 10 mg/kg reduced survival in females. Another study showed that while acute stress reduced cell proliferation in males, it did not affect proliferation in the female hippocampus [98]. Repeated training with controllable stress did not influence proliferation in females and under all conditions, males were more likely than females to express helplessness behavior. This was true even for males that were not previously stressed. Another study also showed that female rats learn trace memories better than male rats and consequently retain a greater proportion of new neurons in their hippocampi [99]. Therefore, it is critical to also consider gender when planning experiments to study adult neurogenesis.

8. POTENTIAL MECHANISMS UNDERLYING THE REQUIREMENT OF NEUROGENESIS IN MEDIATING THE ANTIDEPRESSANT RESPONSE

While much work has been done that has laid a foundation for the understanding of how antidepressants increase neurogenesis, much less is known about why the increase in neurogenesis is required for the antidepressant response [2]. One likely mechanism would be negative feedback regulation of the HPA axis and the stress response. Consistent with this hypothesis, recent studies demonstrated that in mice with ablation of neurogenesis there was an increased HPA axis response to an acute stress [100, 101]. Since stimulation of the subiculum, CA3 or DG can yield an inhibitory effect on the HPA axis [102, 103] through well-described circuitry [103-105], it is possible that young neurons may contribute to hippocampal-dependent negative feedback of the HPA axis. One recent study even suggests that chronic stress severely impairs HPA axis activity and the ability of the hippocampus to modulate downstream brain areas involved in the stress response [73]. Chronic antidepressant treatment can restore the relationship between the hippocampus and the HPA axis, but only in the presence of an intact neurogenic niche. Another study also demonstrates that adult-born hippocampal neurons are required for normal expression of the endocrine and behavioral components of the stress response [106]. Future studies will need to use genetic methods to more directly determine if young neurons impact the negative feedback circuit to the HPA axis.

Another hypothesis, which is not mutually exclusive, that has gained traction is whether neurogenesis in different areas of the SGZ play distinct roles in the regulation of mood. Due to participation in different circuitry, it has been suggested that the dorsal and ventral hippocampus may be distinct structures [58]. In the hippocampus, the dorsal dentate gyrus receives inputs from lateral and caudomedial entorhinal cortex and medially located cells of the medial septal nucleus [107]. Outputs of the dorsal hippocampus are to the mammillary complex, dorsal lateral septum and lateral entorhinal cortex. In contrast ventral dentate gyrus receives inputs from the rostromedial entorhinal cortex and laterally located cells of the medial septal nucleus while ventral hippocampus outputs are to the prefrontal cortex, amygdala, nucleus accumbens, hypothalamus, medial entorhinal cortex, bed nucleus of stria terminalis and rostral and ventral lateral septum [108]. This different circuitry may suggest that the dorsal hippocampus is more important for learning and memory while the ventral hippocampus is more involved in emotion [58, 108]. Some lesion studies have supported this hypothesis [109, 110]. Based on this work, it has been proposed that neurogenesis along the dorsal-ventral axis may also play distinct roles in learning and mood [108]. In this idea, the main effect of neurogenesis in the antidepressant response would be on circuitry through ventral structures. Genetic models and ablation techniques that are restricted to dorsal or ventral SGZ need to be developed in order to test this hypothesis.

Much work has been done to advance the understanding of the synaptic and physiological properties of the young neurons and these unique properties allow for distinguishing young neurons from their mature granule neuron counterparts [111, 112]. Of particular relevance to antidepressant treatment is a form of long-term potentiation derived from a weak stimulation paradigm in the absence of GABA blockers [ACSF-LTP] that is sensitive to manipulations that block hippocampal neurogenesis [39, 56]. After chronic, but not acute, fluoxetine treatment, ACSF-LTP is enhanced in sham animals and completely blocked in animals subjected to X-irradiation [56], suggesting an effect of fluoxetine on the electrophysiological properties of young neurons that have integrated into the hippocampal circuitry.

Relatively little work has addressed the function of young neurons in an intact hippocampal circuit *in vivo*. In hippocampal slice work, it has been demonstrated that fluoxetine treatment enhances activity of the dentate gyrus relative to CA1 in a neurogenesis-dependent manner [50], suggesting a network effect of the young neurons. Furthermore, one very recent study used multiple methods to ablate adult neurogenesis *in vivo* and assessed hippocampal activity [113]. In anesthetized mice after X-irradiation or thymidine kinase mediated pharmacogenetic ablation, perforant-path evoked responses were reduced in magnitude. In striking contrast, there was an increase in the amplitude of spontaneous gamma-frequency bursts in the dentate gyrus and hilus, as well as increased synchronization of dentate neuron firing to these bursts. This striking result may suggest that the young neurons can serve to modulate activity in the much larger population of mature granule cells rather than acting solely as independent encoding units [113]. One could imagine that antidepressant treatment may modulate hippocampal circuitry by enhancing this effect of the young neurons on the mature granule neurons, but this possibility remains to be tested.

9. REVISITING THE NEUROGENESIS HYPOTHESIS OF DEPRESSION

The neurogenesis hypothesis of depression postulated that a decrease in the production of newborn granule cells in the dentate gyrus is related to the pathophysiology of depression while enhanced hippocampal neurogenesis is required for the beneficial effects of antidepressant treatment. With few exceptions [51, 114], in most studies ablation of hippocampal neurogenesis alone is not sufficient to induce a phenotype reminiscent of either anxiety or depression [14, 21, 39, 50, 52, 69, 73, 107]. It is also unlikely that decreased neurogenesis could account for the volumetric decreases seen in the hippocampus of depressed patients, as X-irradiation of mouse hippocampus does not yield a significant reduction [21]. Whether specific manipulations that increase hippocampal neurogenesis alone result in a "non-depressed" phenotype remains to be tested. However, evidence is strong that neurogenesis is required for at least some of the beneficial effects of antidepressant treatment. It will be critical for future work to determine how the addition of new units to the dentate is involved in mediating the effects of antidepressants.

It will also be critical for future work to validate the importance of antidepressant-induced neurogenesis in translational studies in humans. It will be important to test if biomarkers (such as CBV and MRS) are increased in patients treated with antidepressants. Furthermore, it may be interesting to correlate rates of neurogenesis as measured by these biomarkers with improvement of depressive signs and symptoms.

REFERENCES

[1] Murray CJ, Lopez AD. Evidence-based health policy--lessons from the Global Burden of Disease Study. Science 1996, 274:740-3.

[2] Samuels BA, Hen R. Neurogenesis and affective disorders. Eur J Neurosci. 2011, 33:1152-9. Epub 2011/03/15.

[3] Kessler RC, Berglund P, Demler O, Jin R, Koretz D, Merikangas KR, *et al.* The epidemiology of major depressive disorder: results from the National Comorbidity Survey Replication (NCS-R). JAMA 2003, 289:3095-105.

[4] Drevets WC, Bogers W, Raichle ME. Functional anatomical correlates of antidepressant drug treatment assessed using PET measures of regional glucose metabolism. Eur Neuropsychopharmacol 2002, 12:527-44.

[5] Nestler EJ, Barrot M, DiLeone RJ, Eisch AJ, Gold SJ, Monteggia LM. Neurobiology of depression. Neuron 2002, 34:13-25.

[6] Eisch AJ, Cameron HA, Encinas JM, Meltzer LA, Ming GL, Overstreet-Wadiche LS. Adult neurogenesis, mental health, and mental illness: hope or hype? J Neurosci 2008, 28:11785-91.

[7] Wong EH, Tarazi FI, Shahid M. The effectiveness of multi-target agents in schizophrenia and mood disorders: Relevance of receptor signature to clinical action. Pharmacol Ther 2010, 126:173-85.

[8] Trivedi MH, Rush AJ, Wisniewski SR, Nierenberg AA, Warden D, Ritz L, *et al*. Evaluation of outcomes with citalopram for depression using measurement-based care in STAR*D: implications for clinical practice. Am J Psychiatry 2006, 163:28-40.

[9] Gorman JM. Comorbid depression and anxiety spectrum disorders. Depress Anxiety 1996, 4:160-8.

[10] Leonardo ED, Hen R. Genetics of affective and anxiety disorders. Annu Rev Psychol 2006, 57:117-37.

[11] Altman A, Gilmartin TD, Katz DH. Differentiation of murine bone marrow stem cells *in vitro*: long-term growth promoted by a lymphocyte-derived mediator. Science 1981, 211:65-7.

[12] Kaplan MS, Hinds JW. Neurogenesis in the adult rat: electron microscopic analysis of light radioautographs. Science 1977, 197:1092-4.

[13] Cameron HA, Gould E. Adult neurogenesis is regulated by adrenal steroids in the dentate gyrus. Neuroscience 1994, 6:203-9.

[14] Zhao S, Cunha C, Zhang F, Liu Q, Gloss B, Deisseroth K, *et al*. Improved expression of halorhodopsin for light-induced silencing of neuronal activity. Brain cell biology 2008, 36:141-54.

[15] McDonald HY, Wojtowicz JM. Dynamics of neurogenesis in the dentate gyrus of adult rats. Neurosci Lett 2005, 385: 70-5.

[16] Steiner B, Klempin F, Wang L, Kott M, Kettenmann H, Kempermann G. Type-2 cells as link between glial and neuronal lineage in adult hippocampal neurogenesis. Glia 2006, 54:805-14.

[17] Palmer TD, Willhoite AR, Gage FH. Vascular niche for adult hippocampal neurogenesis. The Journal of comparative neurology 2000, 425:479-94.

[18] Barkho BZ, Song H, Aimone JB, Smrt RD, Kuwabara T, Nakashima K, *et al*. Identification of astrocyte-expressed factors that modulate neural stem/progenitor cell differentiation. Stem Cells Dev 2006,15:407-21.

[19] Cooper-Kuhn CM, Winkler J, Kuhn HG. Decreased neurogenesis after cholinergic forebrain lesion in the adult rat. Journal of neuroscience research 2004, 77:155-65.

[20] Dominguez-Escriba L, Hernandez-Rabaza V, Soriano-Navarro M, Barcia JA, Romero FJ, Garcia-Verdugo JM, *et al.* Chronic cocaine exposure impairs progenitor proliferation but spares survival and maturation of neural precursors in adult rat dentate gyrus. The European journal of neuroscience 2006, 24:586-94.

[21] Santarelli L, Saxe M, Gross C, Surget A, Battaglia F, Dulawa S, *et al.* Requirement of hippocampal neurogenesis for the behavioral effects of antidepressants. Science 2003, 301:805-9.

[22] Seri B, Garcia-Verdugo JM, McEwen BS, Alvarez-Buylla A. Astrocytes give rise to new neurons in the adult mammalian hippocampus. The Journal of neuroscience : the official journal of the Society for Neuroscience 2001, 21:7153-60.

[23] Kempermann G, Kronenberg G. Depressed new neurons--adult hippocampal neurogenesis and a cellular plasticity hypothesis of major depression. Biological Psychiatry 2003, 54:499-503.

[24] Tozuka Y, Fukuda S, Namba T, Seki T, Hisatsune T. GABAergic excitation promotes neuronal differentiation in adult hippocampal progenitor cells. Neuron 2005, 47:803-15.

[25] Huttmann K, Sadgrove M, Wallraff A, Hinterkeuser S, Kirchhoff F, Steinhauser C, *et al.* Seizures preferentially stimulate proliferation of radial glia-like astrocytes in the adult dentate gyrus: functional and immunocytochemical analysis. The European journal of neuroscience 2003, 18:2769-78.

[26] Couillard-Despres S, Winner B, Schaubeck S, Aigner R, Vroemen M, Weidner N, *et al.* Doublecortin expression levels in adult brain reflect neurogenesis. The European journal of neuroscience 2005, 21:1-14.

[27] Brandt MD, Jessberger S, Steiner B, Kronenberg G, Reuter K, Bick-Sander A, *et al.* Transient calretinin expression defines early postmitotic step of neuronal differentiation in adult hippocampal neurogenesis of mice. Mol Cell Neurosci. 2003, 24:603-13.

[28] Ge S, Sailor KA, Ming GL, Song H. Synaptic integration and plasticity of new neurons in the adult hippocampus. J Physiol 2008, 586:3759-65.

[29] Kempermann G, Gast D, Kronenberg G, Yamaguchi M, Gage FH. Early determination and long-term persistence of adult-generated new neurons in the hippocampus of mice. Development 2003,130:391-9.

[30] Plumpe T, Ehninger D, Steiner B, Klempin F, Jessberger S, Brandt M, *et al.* Variability of doublecortin-associated dendrite maturation in adult hippocampal neurogenesis is independent of the regulation of precursor cell proliferation. BMC Neurosci 2006, 7:77.

[31] van Praag H, Schinder AF, Christie BR, Toni N, Palmer TD, Gage FH. Functional neurogenesis in the adult hippocampus. Nature 2002, 415:1030-4.

[32] Aimone JB, Wiles J, Gage FH. Potential role for adult neurogenesis in the encoding of time in new memories. Nat Neurosci 2006, 9:723-7.

[33] David DJ, Wang J, Samuels BA, Rainer Q, David I, Gardier AM, *et al.* Implications of the functional integration of adult-born hippocampal neurons in anxiety-depression disorders. Neuroscientist 2010, 16:578-91.

[34] Taupin D. What value reassurance? J Gastroenterol Hepatol 2007, 22:2052-3.

[35] Taupin P. BrdU immunohistochemistry for studying adult neurogenesis: paradigms, pitfalls, limitations, and validation. Brain Res Rev 2007, 53:198-214.

[36] Paizanis E, Hamon M, Lanfumey L. Hippocampal neurogenesis, depressive disorders, and antidepressant therapy. Neural Plast 2007, 2007:73754.

[37] Brown ES, Varghese FP, McEwen BS. Association of depression with medical illness: does cortisol play a role? Biol Psychiatry 2004, 55:1-9.

[38] Jayatissa MN, Henningsen K, West MJ, Wiborg O. Decreased cell proliferation in the dentate gyrus does not associate with development of anhedonic-like symptoms in rats. Brain Res 2009, 1290:133-41.

[39] Saxe MD, Battaglia F, Wang JW, Malleret G, David DJ, Monckton JE, *et al.* Ablation of hippocampal neurogenesis impairs contextual fear conditioning and synaptic plasticity in the dentate gyrus. Proceedings of the National Academy of Sciences of the United States of America 2006,103:17501-6.

[40] Sahay A, Scobie KN, Hill AS, O'Carroll CM, Kheirbek MA, Burghardt NS, *et al.* Increasing adult hippocampal neurogenesis is sufficient to improve pattern separation. Nature 2011, 472:466-70.

[41] Dranovsky A, Picchini AM, Moadel T, Sisti AC, Yamada A, Kimura S, *et al.* Experience dictates stem cell fate in the adult hippocampus. Neuron 2011, 70:908-23.

[42] Sheline YI. Hippocampal atrophy in major depression: a result of depression-induced neurotoxicity? Mol Psychiatry 1996, 1:298-9.

[43] Videbech P, Ravnkilde B. Hippocampal volume and depression: a meta-analysis of MRI studies. The American journal of psychiatry 2004, 161:1957-66.

[44] Czeh B, Lucassen PJ. What causes the hippocampal volume decrease in depression? Are neurogenesis, glial changes and apoptosis implicated? Eur Arch Psychiatry Clin Neurosci 2007, 257:250-60.

[45] Reif A, Fritzen S, Finger M, Strobel A, Lauer M, Schmitt A, *et al.* Neural stem cell proliferation is decreased in schizophrenia, but not in depression. Mol Psychiatry 2006, 11:514-22.

[46] Boldrini M, Underwood MD, Hen R, Rosoklija GB, Dwork AJ, John Mann J, *et al.* Antidepressants increase neural progenitor cells in the human hippocampus. Neuropsychopharmacology. 2009, 34:2376-89.

[47] Boldrini M, Hen R, Underwood MD, Rosoklija GB, Dwork AJ, Mann JJ, *et al.* Hippocampal Angiogenesis and Progenitor Cell Proliferation Are Increased with Antidepressant Use in Major Depression. Biological Psychiatry 2012, 72:562-71.

[48] Duman RS, Malberg J, Nakagawa S, D'Sa C. Neuronal plasticity and survival in mood disorders. Biological Psychiatry 2000, 48:732-9.

[49] David DJ, Klemenhagen KC, Holick KA, Saxe MD, Mendez I, Santarelli L, *et al.* Efficacy of the MCHR1 antagonist N-[3-[1-{[4-[3,4-difluorophenoxy]phenyl]methyl}[4-piperidyl]]-4-methylphenyl]-2-methylpropanamide [SNAP 94847] in mouse models of anxiety and depression following acute and chronic administration is independent of hippocampal neurogenesis. J Pharmacol Exp Ther. 2007;321[1]:237-48.

[50] Airan RD, Meltzer LA, Roy M, Gong Y, Chen H, Deisseroth K. High-speed imaging reveals neurophysiological links to behavior in an animal model of depression. Science 2007, 317:819-23.

[51] Revest JM, Dupret D, Koehl M, Funk-Reiter C, Grosjean N, Piazza PV, *et al.* Adult hippocampal neurogenesis is involved in anxiety-related behaviors. Mol Psychiatry 2009, 14:959-67.

[52] Holick KA, Lee DC, Hen R, Dulawa SC. Behavioral effects of chronic fluoxetine in BALB/cJ mice do not require adult hippocampal neurogenesis or the serotonin 1A receptor. Neuropsychopharmacology 2008, 33:406-17.

[53] Encinas JM, Vaahtokari A, Enikolopov G. Fluoxetine targets early progenitor cells in the adult brain. Proc Natl Acad Sci U S A 2006, 103:8233-8.

[54] Malberg JE, Eisch AJ, Nestler EJ, Duman RS. Chronic antidepressant treatment increases neurogenesis in adult rat hippocampus. J Neurosci 2000, 20:9104-10.

[55] Duman RS, Malberg J, Nakagawa S. Regulation of adult neurogenesis by psychotropic drugs and stress. J Pharmacol Exp Ther 2001, 299:401-7.

[56] Wang P, Lushnikova T, Odvody J, Greiner TC, Jones SN, Eischen CM. Elevated Mdm2 expression induces chromosomal instability and confers a survival and growth advantage to B cells. Oncogene 2008, 27:1590-8.

[57] Banasr M, Soumier A, Hery M, Mocaer E, Daszuta A. Agomelatine, a new antidepressant, induces regional changes in hippocampal neurogenesis. Biol Psychiatry 2006, 59:1087-96.

[58] Fanselow MS, Dong HW. Are the dorsal and ventral hippocampus functionally distinct structures? Neuron 2010, 65:7-19.

[59] Kempermann G, Kuhn HG, Gage FH. Genetic influence on neurogenesis in the dentate gyrus of adult mice. Proc Natl Acad Sci U S A 1997, 94:10409-14.

[60] van Praag H, Shubert T, Zhao C, Gage FH. Exercise enhances learning and hippocampal neurogenesis in aged mice. J Neurosci 2005, 25:8680-5.

[61] Warner-Schmidt JL, Duman RS. Hippocampal neurogenesis: opposing effects of stress and antidepressant treatment. Hippocampus 2006, 16: 239-49.

[62] Overstreet-Wadiche LS, Bromberg DA, Bensen AL, Westbrook GL. Seizures accelerate functional integration of adult-generated granule cells. J Neurosci 2006, 26:4095-103.

[63] Laplagne DA, Esposito MS, Piatti VC, Morgenstern NA, Zhao C, van Praag H, *et al.* Functional convergence of neurons generated in the developing and adult hippocampus. PLoS biology 2006, 4:409.

[64] Toni N, Teng EM, Bushong EA, Aimone JB, Zhao C, Consiglio A, *et al.* Synapse formation on neurons born in the adult hippocampus. Nat Neurosci 2007, 10:727-34. Epub 2007/05/09.

[65] Schmidt-Hieber C, Jonas P, Bischofberger J. Enhanced synaptic plasticity in newly generated granule cells of the adult hippocampus. Nature 2004, 429:184-7.

[66] Ge S, Yang CH, Hsu KS, Ming GL, Song H. A critical period for enhanced synaptic plasticity in newly generated neurons of the adult brain. Neuron 2007, 54:559-66.

[67] Faulkner RL, Jang MH, Liu XB, Duan X, Sailor KA, Kim JY, *et al.* Development of hippocampal mossy fiber synaptic outputs by new neurons in the adult brain. Proc Natl Acad Sci U S A 2008, 105:14157-62.

[68] Huang GJ, Bannerman D, Flint J. Chronic fluoxetine treatment alters behavior, but not adult hippocampal neurogenesis, in BALB/cJ mice. Mol Psychiatry 2008, 13:119-21.

[69] Meshi D, Drew MR, Saxe M, Ansorge MS, David D, Santarelli L, *et al.* Hippocampal neurogenesis is not required for behavioral effects of environmental enrichment. Nature neuroscience 2006, 9:729-31.

[70] Katz RJ. Animal model of depression: pharmacological sensitivity of a hedonic deficit. Pharmacol Biochem Behav 1982, 16:965-8.

[71] Willner P. Chronic mild stress [CMS] revisited: consistency and behavioural-neurobiological concordance in the effects of CMS. Neuropsychobiology 2005, 52:90-110.

[72] Willner P, Towell A, Sampson D, Sophokleous S, Muscat R. Reduction of sucrose preference by chronic unpredictable mild stress, and its restoration by a tricyclic antidepressant. Psychopharmacology (Berl) 1987, 93:358-64.

[73] Surget A, Saxe M, Leman S, Ibarguen-Vargas Y, Chalon S, Griebel G, *et al.* Drug-dependent requirement of hippocampal neurogenesis in a model of depression and of antidepressant reversal. Biological Psychiatry 2008, 64:293-301.

[74] Nestler EJ, Gould E, Manji H, Buncan M, Duman RS, Greshenfeld HK, *et al.* Preclinical models: status of basic research in depression. Biological Psychiatry 2002, 52:503-28.

[75] Jayatissa MN, Bisgaard C, Tingstrom A, Papp M, Wiborg O. Hippocampal cytogenesis correlates to escitalopram-mediated recovery in a chronic mild stress rat model of depression. Neuropsychopharmacology 2006, 31:2395-404.

[76] Bisgaard CF, Jayatissa MN, Enghild JJ, Sanchez C, Artemychyn R, Wiborg O. Proteomic investigation of the ventral rat hippocampus links DRP-2 to escitalopram treatment resistance and SNAP to stress resilience in the chronic mild stress model of depression. J Mol Neurosci 2007, 32:132-44.

[77] Isingrini E, Camus V, Le Guisquet AM, Pingaud M, Devers S, Belzung C. Association between repeated unpredictable chronic mild stress (UCMS) procedures with a high fat diet: a model of fluoxetine resistance in mice. PLoS ONE 2010, 5:10404.

[78] Berton O, McClung CA, Dileone RJ, Krishnan V, Renthal W, Russo SJ, *et al.* Essential role of BDNF in the mesolimbic dopamine pathway in social defeat stress. Science 2006, 311:864-8.

[79] Tsankova NM, Berton O, Renthal W, Kumar A, Neve RL, Nestler EJ. Sustained hippocampal chromatin regulation in a mouse model of depression and antidepressant action. Nat Neurosci 2006, 9:519-25.

[80] Krishnan V, Han MH, Graham DL, Berton O, Renthal W, Russo SJ, *et al.* Molecular adaptations underlying susceptibility and resistance to social defeat in brain reward regions. Cell 2007, 131:391-404.

[81] Krishnan V, Nestler EJ. The molecular neurobiology of depression. Nature 2008, 455:894-902.

[82] Vialou V, Robison AJ, Laplant QC, Covington HE, 3rd, Dietz DM, Ohnishi YN, *et al.* DeltaFosB in brain reward circuits mediates resilience to stress and antidepressant responses. Nat Neurosci 2010, 13:745-52.

[83] de Kloet ER, Joels M, Holsboer F. Stress and the brain: from adaptation to disease. Nat Rev Neurosci 2005, 6:463-75.

[84] Antonijevic IA. Depressive disorders -- is it time to endorse different pathophysiologies? Psychoneuroendocrinology 2006, 31:1-15.

[85] Carroll BJ, Feinberg M, Greden JF, Tarika J, Albala AA, Haskett RF, *et al.* A specific laboratory test for the diagnosis of melancholia. Standardization, validation, and clinical utility. Arch Gen Psychiatry 1981, 38:15-22.

[86] Nemeroff CB, Widerlov E, Bissette G, Walleus H, Karlsson I, Eklund K, *et al.* Elevated concentrations of CSF corticotropin-releasing factor-like immunoreactivity in depressed patients. Science 1984, 226:1342-4.

[87] Sachar EJ, Hellman L, Fukushima DK, Gallagher TF. Cortisol production in depressive illness. A clinical and biochemical clarification. Arch Gen Psychiatry 1970, 23:289-98.

[88] Strohle A, Holsboer F. Stress responsive neurohormones in depression and anxiety. Pharmacopsychiatry 2003, 36:S207-14.

[89] Murray F, Smith DW, Hutson PH. Chronic low dose corticosterone exposure decreased hippocampal cell proliferation, volume and induced anxiety and depression like behaviours in mice. Eur J Pharmacol 2008, 583:115-27.

[90] David DJ, Samuels BA, Rainer Q, Wang J-W, Marsteller D, Mendez I, *et al.* Neurogenesis-dependent and -independent effects of fluoxetine in an animal model of anxiety/depression. Neuron 2009, 62:479-93.

[91] Ardayfio P, Kim K-S. Anxiogenic-like effect of chronic corticosterone in the light-dark emergence task in mice. Behav Neurosci 2006, 120:249-56.

[92] Gourley SL, Wu FJ, Kiraly DD, Ploski JE, Kedves AT, Duman RS, *et al.* Regionally specific regulation of ERK MAP kinase in a model of antidepressant-sensitive chronic depression. Biological Psychiatry 2008, 63:353-9.

[93] Gourley SL, Wu FJ, Taylor JR. Corticosterone regulates pERK1/2 map kinase in a chronic depression model. Ann N Y Acad Sci 2008, 1148:509-14.

[94] Anacker C, Zunszain PA, Cattaneo A, Carvalho LA, Garabedian MJ, Thuret S, *et al.* Antidepressants increase human hippocampal neurogenesis by activating the glucocorticoid receptor. Mol Psychiatry 2011, 16:738-50.

[95] Perera TD, Dwork AJ, Keegan KA, Thirumangalakudi L, Lipira CM, Joyce N, *et al.* Necessity of hippocampal neurogenesis for the therapeutic action of antidepressants in adult nonhuman primates. PloS one 2011, 6:17600.

[96] Bessa JM, Ferreira D, Melo I, Marques F, Cerqueira JJ, Palha JA, *et al.* The mood-improving actions of antidepressants do not depend on neurogenesis but are associated with neuronal remodeling. Mol Psychiatry 2009, 14:764-73.

[97] David DJ, Samuels BA, Rainer Q, Wang JW, Marsteller D, Mendez I, *et al.* Neurogenesis-dependent and -independent effects of fluoxetine in an animal model of anxiety/depression. Neuron 2009, 62:479-93.

[98] Shors TJ, Leuner B. Estrogen-mediated effects on depression and memory formation in females. Journal of affective disorders 2003, 74:85-96.

[99] Dalla C, Papachristos EB, Whetstone AS, Shors TJ. Female rats learn trace memories better than male rats and consequently retain a greater proportion of new neurons in their hippocampi. Proc Natl Acad Sci U S A 2009, 106:2927-32.

[100] Schloesser RJ, Manji HK, Martinowich K. Suppression of adult neurogenesis leads to an increased hypothalamo-pituitary-adrenal axis response. Neuroreport 2009, 20:553-7.

[101] Snyder JS, Soumier A, Brewer M, Pickel J, Cameron HA. Adult hippocampal neurogenesis buffers stress responses and depressive behaviour. Nature 2011, 476:458-61.

[102] Dunn JD, Orr SE. Differential plasma corticosterone responses to hippocampal stimulation. Experimental brain research Experimentelle Hirnforschung Experimentation cerebrale 1984, 54:1-6.

[103] Herman JP, Figueiredo H, Mueller NK, Ulrich-Lai Y, Ostrander MM, Choi DC, *et al.* Central mechanisms of stress integration: hierarchical circuitry controlling hypothalamo-pituitary-adrenocortical responsiveness. Frontiers in neuroendocrinology 2003, 24:151-80.

[104] Herman JP, Ostrander MM, Mueller NK, Figueiredo H. Limbic system mechanisms of stress regulation: hypothalamo-pituitary-adrenocortical axis. Progress in neuro-psychopharmacology & biological psychiatry 2005, 29:1201-13.

[105] Jankord R, Herman JP. Limbic regulation of hypothalamo-pituitary-adrenocortical function during acute and chronic stress. Annals of the New York Academy of Sciences 2008, 1148:64-73.

[106] Snyder JS, Ramchand P, Rabbett S, Radik R, Wojtowicz JM, Cameron HA. Septo-temporal gradients of neurogenesis and activity in 13-month-old rats. Neurobiol Aging 2011, 32:1149-56.

[107] Sahay A, Drew MR, Hen R. Dentate gyrus neurogenesis and depression. Prog Brain Res 2007, 163:697-722.

[108] Sahay A, Hen R. Adult hippocampal neurogenesis in depression. Nat Neurosci 2007, 10:1110-5.

[109] Moser E, Moser MB, Andersen P. Synaptic potentiation in the rat dentate gyrus during exploratory learning. Neuroreport 1993, 5:317-20.

[110] Bannerman DM, Rawlins JN, McHugh SB, Deacon RM, Yee BK, Bast T, *et al.* Regional dissociations within the hippocampus--memory and anxiety. Neuroscience and biobehavioral reviews 2004, 28:273-83.

[111] Ming GL, Song H. Adult neurogenesis in the mammalian central nervous system. Annual review of neuroscience 2005, 28:223-50.

[112] Li Y, Mu Y, Gage FH. Development of neural circuits in the adult hippocampus. Current topics in developmental biology 2009, 87:149-74.

[113] Lacefield CO, Itskov V, Reardon T, Hen R, Gordon JA. Effects of adult-generated granule cells on coordinated network activity in the dentate gyrus. Hippocampus 2012, 22:106-16.

[114] Bergami M, Rimondini R, Santi S, Blum R, Gotz M, Canossa M. Deletion of TrkB in adult progenitors alters newborn neuron integration into hippocampal circuits and increases anxiety-like behavior. Proc Natl Acad Sci U S A 2008, 105:15570-5.

[115] Shors TJ, Townsend DA, Zhao M, Kozorovitskiy Y, Gould E. Neurogenesis may relate to some but not all types of hippocampal-dependent learning. Hippocampus 2002, 12:578-84.

[116] Noonan MA, Bulin SE, Fuller DC, Eisch AJ. Reduction of adult hippocampal neurogenesis confers vulnerability in an animal model of cocaine addiction. J Neurosci 2010, 30:304-15.

[117] Surget A, Tanti A, Leonardo ED, Laugeray A, Rainer Q, Touma C, *et al.* Antidepressants recruit new neurons to improve stress response regulation. Mol Psychiatry 2011, 16:1177-88.

[118] Jiang W, Zhang Y, Xiao L, Van Cleemput J, Ji SP, Bai G, *et al.* Cannabinoids promote embryonic and adult hippocampus neurogenesis and produce anxiolytic- and antidepressant-like effects. The Journal of clinical investigation 2005, 115:3104-16.

[119] Jaholkowski P, Kiryk A, Jedynak P, Ben Abdallah NM, Knapska E, Kowalczyk A, *et al.* New hippocampal neurons are not obligatory for memory formation; cyclin D2 knockout mice with no adult brain neurogenesis show learning. Learn Mem 2009, 16:439-51.

[120] Cowen DS, Takase LF, Fornal CA, Jacobs BL. Age-dependent decline in hippocampal neurogenesis is not altered by chronic treatment with fluoxetine. Brain Res 2008, 1228:14-9.

[121] Kodama M, Fujioka T, Duman RS. Chronic olanzapine or fluoxetine administration increases cell proliferation in hippocampus and prefrontal cortex of adult rat. Biol Psychiatry 2004, 56:570-80.

[122] Nasrallah HA, Hopkins T, Pixley SK. Differential effects of antipsychotic and antidepressant drugs on neurogenic regions in rats. Brain Res 2010, 1354:23-9.

[123] Marcussen AB, Flagstad P, Kristjansen PE, Johansen FF, Englund U. Increase in neurogenesis and behavioural benefit after chronic fluoxetine treatment in Wistar rats. Acta neurologica Scandinavica 2008, 117:94-100.

[124] Huang GJ, Herbert J. Stimulation of neurogenesis in the hippocampus of the adult rat by fluoxetine requires rhythmic change in corticosterone. Biol Psychiatry 2006, 59:619-24.

[125] Sairanen M, Lucas G, Ernfors P, Castren M, Castren E. Brain-derived neurotrophic factor and antidepressant drugs have different but coordinated effects on neuronal turnover, proliferation, and survival in the adult dentate gyrus. J Neurosci 2005, 25:1089-94.

[126] Manev R, Uz T, Manev H. Fluoxetine increases the content of neurotrophic protein S100beta in the rat hippocampus. European journal of pharmacology 2001, 420:R1-2.

[127] Miller BH, Schultz LE, Gulati A, Cameron MD, Pletcher MT. Genetic regulation of behavioral and neuronal responses to fluoxetine. Neuropsychopharmacology 2008, 33:1312-22.

[128] Navailles S, Hof PR, Schmauss C. Antidepressant drug-induced stimulation of mouse hippocampal neurogenesis is age-dependent and altered by early life stress. J Comp Neurol 2008, 509:372-81.

[129] Kong H, Sha LL, Fan Y, Xiao M, Ding JH, Wu J, *et al.* Requirement of AQP4 for antidepressive efficiency of fluoxetine: implication in adult hippocampal neurogenesis. Neuropsychopharmacology 2009, 34:1263-76.

[130] Bai F, Bergeron M, Nelson DL. Chronic AMPA receptor potentiator (LY451646) treatment increases cell proliferation in adult rat hippocampus. Neuropharmacology 2003, 44:1013-21.

[131] Yoshimizu T, Chaki S. Increased cell proliferation in the adult mouse hippocampus following chronic administration of group II metabotropic glutamate receptor antagonist, MGS0039. Biochemical and biophysical research communications 2004, 315:493-6.

[132] Koo JW, Duman RS. Interleukin-1 receptor null mutant mice show decreased anxiety-like behavior and enhanced fear memory. Neurosci Lett 2009, 456:39-43.

[133] Jaako-Movits K, Zharkovsky T, Pedersen M, Zharkovsky A. Decreased hippocampal neurogenesis following olfactory bulbectomy is reversed by repeated citalopram administration. Cellular and molecular neurobiology 2006, 26:1559-70.

[134] Ekstrand J, Hellsten J, Wennstrom M, Tingstrom A. Differential inhibition of neurogenesis and angiogenesis by corticosterone in rats stimulated with electroconvulsive seizures. Progress in neuro-psychopharmacology & biological psychiatry 2008, 32:1466-72.

[135] Keilhoff G, Becker A, Grecksch G, Bernstein HG, Wolf G. Cell proliferation is influenced by bulbectomy and normalized by imipramine treatment in a region-specific manner. Neuropsychopharmacology 2006, 31:1165-76.

[136] Silva R, Mesquita AR, Bessa J, Sousa JC, Sotiropoulos I, Leao P, *et al.* Lithium blocks stress-induced changes in depressive-like behavior and hippocampal cell fate: the role of glycogen-synthase-kinase-3beta. Neuroscience. 2008, 152:656-69.

[137] Chen G, Masana MI, Manji HK. Lithium regulates PKC-mediated intracellular cross-talk and gene expression in the CNS *in vivo*. Bipolar disorders 2000, 2:217-36. Epub 2001/03/16.

[138] Katoh-Semba R, Asano T, Ueda H, Morishita R, Takeuchi IK, Inaguma Y, *et al.* Riluzole enhances expression of brain-derived neurotrophic factor with consequent proliferation of granule precursor cells in the rat hippocampus. FASEB journal : official publication of the Federation of American Societies for Experimental Biology 2002, 16:1328-30.

[139] Nakagawa S, Kim JE, Lee R, Malberg JE, Chen J, Steffen C, *et al.* Regulation of neurogenesis in adult mouse hippocampus by cAMP and the cAMP response element-binding protein. The Journal of neuroscience : the official journal of the Society for Neuroscience 2002, 22:3673-82.

[140] Larsen MH, Rosenbrock H, Sams-Dodd F, Mikkelsen JD. Expression of brain derived neurotrophic factor, activity-regulated cytoskeleton protein mRNA, and enhancement of adult hippocampal neurogenesis in rats after sub-chronic and chronic treatment with the triple monoamine re-uptake inhibitor tesofensine. European journal of pharmacology 2007, 555:115-21.

[141] Czeh B, Michaelis T, Watanabe T, Frahm J, de Biurrun G, van Kampen M, *et al.* Stress-induced changes in cerebral metabolites, hippocampal volume, and cell proliferation are prevented by antidepressant treatment with tianeptine. Proc Natl Acad Sci U S A 2001, 98:12796-801.

[142] Malberg JE, Eisch AJ, Nestler EJ, Duman RS. Chronic antidepressant treatment increases neurogenesis in adult rat hippocampus. The Journal of neuroscience : the official journal of the Society for Neuroscience 2000, 20:9104-10.

[143] Mostany R, Valdizan EM, Pazos A. A role for nuclear beta-catenin in SNRI antidepressant-induced hippocampal cell proliferation. Neuropharmacology 2008, 55:18-26.

CHAPTER 10

NEW STRATEGIES FOR THE TREATMENT OF MOOD DISORDERS: THE TRIPLE REUPTAKE INHIBITORS

GAËL QUESSEVEUR, BRUNO GUIARD*

Faculty of Pharmacy, University Paris South IV, Paris, France

Abstract: It has been proposed that triple reuptake inhibitors (TRIs) that enhance serotonin, norepinephrine and dopamine extracellular levels in the brain may produce greater antidepressant effects than single- or dual-acting agents. This hypothesis is mainly based on the observations that drugs stimulating dopaminergic neurotransmission produce antidepressant effects or attenuate some side effects observed with selective serotonin reuptake inhibitors. Although preclinical data clearly establish the beneficial effects of TRIs in animal paradigms used to screen antidepressant-like effects, there are two limitations of these studies. On one hand, the effects of TRIs have been tested mainly after acute administration. However, given the functional and reciprocal interactions between monoaminergic neurons, it is conceivable that counter-productive effects occur when the treatment is prolonged. On the other hand, the relevance of TRIs in antidepressant-like activity is based exclusively on the forced swim and tail suspension tests in naïve animals which do not reproduce the complex biological and psychological changes associated with depression. In human, clinical evidence for antidepressant activity of TRIs and more particularly their ability to produce a greater efficacy than currently available agents remains equivocal. The present chapter synthesizes the preclinical and clinical data emphasizing the interest of increasing dopaminergic activity with the other two monoamines in the treatment of major depression and related symptoms such as pain.

Keywords: Serotonin (5-HT), norepinephrine (NE), dopamine (DA), serotonin (SERT), norepinephrine (NET) and dopamine (DAT) transporters, depression, antidepressant drugs, triple serotonin/ norepinephrine/ dopamine reuptake inhibitors (TRI), animal models.

1. INTRODUCTION

The monoaminergic hypothesis of major depression (MD) stipulates that a deficit in brain monoaminergic neurotransmission in various brain areas including the frontal cortex, hippocampus, amygdala, hypothalamus would account for some signs and symptoms of the pathology [1]. For instance, abnormalities in the serotonin (5-HT) transmission are associated with impulsive, aggressive, and anxious behaviors [2], whereas alteration in noradrenergic transmission, with motor activity, attention, memory and arousal [3]. The role of dopamine (DA) on the other hand, attracted less attention in the mechanisms of action underlying MD. However, the observations that reserpine, which depletes catecholamines, lowers mood [4] or that an inhibition of tyrosine hydroxylase induces a worsening of depressive symptoms [5], strongly suggest that decreasing DA function may be of particular relevance. The fact that several symptoms observed in MD, including impaired motivation, concentration, and pleasure result from an attenuation of dopaminergic neurotransmission, strengthens this hypothesis [6].

In this context, it is not surprising that most antidepressants approved, act by enhancing extracellular brain 5-HT and/or NE levels. Selective serotonin reuptake inhibitors (SSRIs) increase the synaptic

***Address correspondence to Bruno P. Guiard:** Faculty of Pharmacy, University Paris South IV, Paris, France; E-mail: bruno.guiard@u-psud.fr

Disclosure: Part of information included in this chapter has been previously published as B.P. Guiard (2011). A New Class of Antidepressant Drugs in the treatment of Psychiatric Disorders: The Triple Reuptake Inhibitors, Psychiatric Disorders - Trends and Developments, Dr. Toru Uehara (Ed.), ISBN: 978-953-307-745-1, InTech

Bruno P Guiard and Eliyahu Dremencov (Eds)

availability of 5-HT by inhibiting the 5-HT transporter (SERT). This class of antidepressant is safer than the first generation agents, such as the tricyclics (TCAs) and monoamine oxidase inhibitors (MAOIs). Despite their therapeutic action, residual symptoms remain and may explain the fact that approximately 50% of depressive individuals do not respond adequately to these agents [7]. Moreover, for patients who respond, 2-4 weeks of treatment are required to achieve a clinically meaningful effect [8].

A growing body of literature suggests that antidepressants with more than one mechanism of action would be more effective than agents with a single pharmacological target [9]. The use of the dual serotonin/norepinephrine reuptake inhibitors (SNRIs) has been proposed as a relevant and frequent strategy in the management of non-response to SSRIs [10]. Indeed, when facing treatment resistance, the classic approach is to switch medications, ideally using an antidepressant with an additional therapeutic action [11]. Interestingly, in the STAR*D study, whereby citalopram-resistant patients were switched to the SNRI venlafaxine, remission rate was only of 25% [12]. Nevertheless, the dose of venlafaxine was too low and a significant proportion of patients in that study were on a SSRI regimen of venlafaxine. In contrast, when using a noradrenergic regimen of venlafaxine, the remission was twice that obtained with paroxetine [13].

Converging lines of evidence indicate that drugs enhancing dopaminergic neurotransmission can diminish anhedonia and improve cognition and motivation [6]. This is particularly important because symptoms of anhedonia respond poorly to SSRIs [14,15]. Clinical studies indicate that it is possible to achieve an antidepressant action by enhancing DA neurotransmission. This is supported by several reports of the augmenting action of the D2 receptor agonists such as pramipexole in treatment-resistant patients [16,17,18,19,20,21], and by the intrinsic antidepressant activity of these drugs in placebo-controlled trials [22]. Moreover, the dopamine reuptake inhibitor bupropion has also demonstrated antidepressant activities [23] and its use in combination with SSRIs enhances the antidepressant response in resistant patients [24]. It has been proposed that part of bupropion efficacy results from its capacity to attenuate SSRI-induced sexual or fatigue side effects.

Together, these clinical considerations, have given rise to a new class of antidepressants that simultaneously inhibit 5-HT, NE and DA reuptake with the hope to offer a clinically relevant advantage over single- or dual-acting agents [25]. Indeed, since the Triple Reuptake Inhibitors (TRIs) act by enhancing extracellular levels of 5-HT, NE and DA neurotransmissions in various brain regions, these antidepressants could exert their therapeutic activity by treating more symptoms of MD and/or by attenuating some side effects observed in response to traditional antidepressants. It is also possible that the better efficacy of TCAs than SSRIs represented an additional argument for the development of TRIs.

2. PRECLINICAL PROPERTIES OF TRIPLE REUPTAKE INHIBITORS

A number of compounds with the ability to bind and block all three monoamine transporters have been developed with the hope to produce greater symptomatic relief than single- or dual-acting agents. DOV Pharmaceutical is the first company having provided *in vitro* and *in vivo* preclinical data with their triple reuptake inhibitors DOV 216303, DOV21947 (amitifadine) and DOV 220075 (bicifadine). New molecules have followed such as NS2330 (tesofensine, GlaxoSmith-Kline/NeuroSearch), SEP225289 (Sepracor Inc.), CNS-1 and CNS-2 (Albany Molecular Research Institute Inc), PRC-025, PRC-050, PRC-200SS (Mayo Foundation), JNJ-7925476 (Johnson & Johnson Pharmaceutical Research & Development), WF-23 (Eli Lilly), JZAD-IV-22 (PsychoGenics) and more recently TP1 (Luye Pharmaceutical Group). Others compounds will undoubtedly emerge in a near future. During

2010-2011, the Structure-Activity Relationship (SAR), of at least eleven new TRIs, has been reported [26,27,28,29,30,31,32,33,34,35,36].

2.1. *IN VITRO* PROPERTIES OF TRIS

In vitro data suggest some pharmacodynamic differences among TRIs. Indeed, some of them, depending on their relative potencies at binding and/or inhibiting the three monoaminergic transporters display a balanced profile while others compounds (unbalanced), are characterized by their ability to block preferentially one transporter. It is thus possible to have a perfectly balanced TRI where the potencies at all three transporters are equal, however, the question that remains is whether optimal antidepressant effect requires the ideal rank order and the ideal relative potency towards three transporters? This question could be answered, at least in part, by correlating *in vitro* and *in vivo* data.

2.1.1. Binding properties of TRIs

In vitro binding properties of TRIs are extremely variable as shown in Table **1**. Despite distinct affinities towards monoaminergic transporters, TRIs such as DOV 21947, DOV 216303 or bicifadine appear quite balanced. Among these compounds, DOV 21947 displays, however, the highest affinity for all three transporters. The PRC compounds preferentially bind to the SERT and NET while displaying a relatively lower affinity for the dopamine transporter (DAT). Finally, compounds such as JNJ-7925476 or TP1 have a preferential binding affinity for one transporter, the SERT and DAT respectively. In general, the value of the constant affinity of TRIs is lower than that of SSRIs and NRIs at binding SERT, NET and/or DAT indicating that the novelty of TRIs lies in their "broad spectrum" activity rather than in their potency at blocking monoamines transporters [37].

TABLE 1

TRIs	In vitro binding (Ki or Kd in nM)			References
	SERT	NET	DAT	
DOV 21947[a]	100	260	210	[49]
DOV 216303[a]	190	380	190	[105]
Bicifadine[a]	1000	2000	2000	[47]
PRC200-SS[b]	2.3	0.6	18	[39]
PRC050[b]	6	0.4	120	[48]
PRC025[b]	6	19	100	[48]
JNJ-7925476[a]	0.9	16	5	[46]
TP1[a]	1023	2076	190	[92]

Table 1: **In vitro binding affinities of triple reuptake inhibitors (TRIs).** [a]Ki values are expressed in nM (Ki for inhibition of radioligand binding). [b]Kd values are expressed in nM and represent the equilibrium dissociation constant. The smaller the Kd or Ki values, the higher affinity of a drug is for the corresponding monoaminergic transporter.

2.1.2 In vitro functional activity of TRIs assessed from synaptosomal preparation

Inhibition of [^{3}H]-5-HT, [^{3}H]-NE or [^{3}H]-DA reuptake in synaptosomes is one of the most widespread methods to assess the *in vitro* potency of reuptake inhibitors and to predict their selectivity towards biogenic amines transporters. It is noteworthy that the profile of monoamines reuptake inhibition observed with PRC compounds parallels that of their binding properties with a preferential inhibition of [^{3}H]-5-HT and [^{3}H]-NE reuptake (Table **2**). This is, however, not the case with DOV 21947 and DOV 216303, which preferentially block [^{3}H]-5-HT and [^{3}H]-NE reuptake despite their balanced profile. It is thus possible that a significant reuptake of [^{3}H]-5-HT and [^{3}H]-NE is mediated through the DAT. Consistent with this hypothesis; heterologous reuptake mechanisms have been previously reported with monoaminergic systems. In particular, it has been shown that the clearance of NE from the extracellular space can occur through the DAT in the hippocampus [25]. With respect to TP1, it blocks the reuptake of all three monoamines with the same potency (Table **2)** despite its higher affinity for the SERT (Table **1**). Once again, this result may emphasize the importance of heterologous monoamine reuptake particularly in monoaminergic transporters-expressing HEK-293 cells. If these unexpected observations result from methodological issues in relation with the use of *in vitro* transfected cells, one would expect a higher degree of correlation *in vivo*.

TABLE 2

TRI	In vitro uptake (synaptosomes) (IC50, Kd or Ki in nM)			In vivo uptake (intracerebral microdialysis)			References
	SERT	NET	DAT	5-HT	NE	DA	
DOV 216303[a]	14	20	78	+++	++	++	[31,106, 107]
DOV 21947[a]	12	23	96	ND	ND	ND	[49]
Bicifadine[a]	117	55	910	+++	++	+++	[45,47]
PRC200-SS[c]	2	1.5	61	+	+++	++	[39]
PRC050[c]	12	1.2	43	ND	ND	ND	[48]
PRC025[c]	6	10	53	ND	ND	ND	[48]
JNJ-7925476[a]	1	1	2.6	+++	+++	+++	[46]
TP1 [a]	628	521	712	+++	++	+	[44]
JZAD-IV-22[a]	15	84	120	++	+++	+++	[31]

Table 2: **In vitro and in vivo functional activity of triple reuptake inhibitors (TRIs) from synaptosomes and intracerebral microdialysis.** [a]Values are expressed in IC50. [b,c]Values are Kd or Ki respectively expressed in nM. The smaller the Kd values, the higher inhibitory effect of a drug is for the corresponding monoaminergic transporter. In microdialysis experiments, signs "+" reflect the relative increase in 5-HT, NE and DA obtained with the highest acute dose used. ND: Not Determined.

2.2. IN VIVO PROPERTIES OF TRIS

2.2.1. In vivo functional activity of TRIs assessed by intracerebral microdialysis studies

In vivo intracerebral microdialysis in freely moving animals became a powerful neurochemical technique to sample extracellular levels of neurotransmitters and their major metabolites in the brain fluid [38]. As expected all TRIs tested increase extracellular monoamines levels. Nevertheless, depending on their pharmacological properties, the brain region studied and their relative equipment in monoamines transporters and, on the model used "naïve" *vs* depressed mice or rats, the effects of TRIs are quite different (Table **2**). In a recent study performed in control rats, PRC200-SS was shown to increase the extracellular levels of the three monoamines in the medial prefrontal cortex (mPFC) and the Nucleus accumbens (NAcc) [39]. In the mPFC, in agreement with its *in vitro* pharmacological profile, PRC200-SS significantly increased extracellular levels of 5-HT and NE with a more pronounced effect for NE. Nevertheless, PRC200-SS failed to modify the extracellular levels of DA in this brain region. This result is somewhat surprising given the good affinity of this compound for the DAT and the dense dopaminergic innervation or high expression of DAT in the mPFC reported in human [40]. Several hypotheses can be raised to explain such findings. First, it is possible that the lack of increase in cortical DA extracellular levels is related to a weak expression of DAT in the rodent mPFC (in comparison to human). Secondly, these data may result from an inhibitory effect of 5-HT and/or NE on the dopaminergic system. Indeed at somatodendritic levels, it has been proposed that both monoamines exert an inhibitory influence on DA neurons in the ventral tegmental area (VTA) [25]. For example, the 5-HT_{2C} receptor characterized by high levels of constitutive activity, inhibits tonic as well as evoked release of DA [41] by acting at least in part, in the VTA [42]. At nerve terminal, 5-HT_{2C} receptor also inhibits DA release in the nigrostrial and mesolimbic pathways but not in the frontal cortex [41]. Whether the lack of increase of DA in the mPFC is a disadvantage in the therapeutic activity of TRIs remains to be determined. However, this example emphasizes the fact that *even in vivo*, it can be difficult to predict the effects of TRIs due to functional and reciprocal interactions between monoaminergic neurons [43]. Others examples illustrate the fact that *in vivo,* the activity of TRIs does not necessarily reflect their *in vitro* property either in term of binding affinity or functional activity. Using microdialysis in the hypothalamus of freely moving rats, a recent study with TP1, showed that its acute oral administration significantly increased the extracellular concentrations of 5-HT, NE and DA with a marginal effect on DA despite its high affinity for the DAT compared to the SERT and NET [44]. As above-mentioned, the increase in 5-HT and NE levels might have attenuated the expected increase in DA in the synaptic cleft.

Finally, confirmation of the blocking activity of JNJ-7925476 and bicifadine on the SERT, NET and DAT has been provided. A preferential increase in DA with both compounds in the cortex and nucleus accumbens respectively has been detected compared to 5-HT and NE at the highest dose tested [45,46,47]. These results strongly contrast with *in vitro* data showing that JNJ-7925476 and bicifadine displayed a better *in vitro* binding affinity and blocking activity for the SERT [45,46,47].

2.2.2. Antidepressant-like activity of TRIs

The optimum preclinical profile for a TRI, defined as maximum antidepressant efficacy and minimum abuse liability, cannot be predicted accurately based on *in vitro* or *in vivo* neurochemical profiles alone. Therefore, the use of behavioral screening approach to supplement the neurochemical data for identifying TRIs with favorable *in vivo* profiles is of great interest.

2.2.2.1. In naïve animals

The most frequently paradigms used to screen the antidepressant-like activity of pharmacological agents are the forced swimming and the tail suspension tests (FST and TST, respectively). Behavioral data currently available, clearly demonstrated the antidepressant-like effect of TRIs that act by increasing the time of mobility and/or by reducing the time of immobility in the FST or the TST (Table **3**). Among the TRIs tested, JNJ-7925476 appears the most potent since a low dose of this agent (0.3 mg/kg; s.c.) produced significant antidepressant-like effects. In term of efficacy (i.e., maximal effect), compounds such as PRC200-SS (10mg/kg; i.p.), D-142 or D-161 produced a greater percentage of decrease in the time of immobility than the others TRIs (Table **3**). Interestingly, JNJ-7925476 and PRC200-SS display the highest affinity for the SERT and the NET suggesting that this double action is an important prerequisite to produce adequate antidepressant-like behavior. This can be surprising since microdialysis studies indicate that a high affinity to the SERT and the NET may prevent or attenuate the increase in extracellular levels of DA. The reasons of such discrepancy remain obscure and should draw attention for future investigations.

Since DA is known to enhance locomotor activity, the possibility cannot be excluded that TRIs increased the time of mobility in these various studies, through a psychostimulant effect. In various studies, however, TRIs did not modify locomotor activity at doses that produce antidepressant-like effects [39,44,46,48,49], thereby ruling out the possibility that the antidepressant-like activity detected does not appear to be from "false-positive" results.

2.2.2.2. In animal models of depression

An important drawback in the development of antidepressants is due to the fact that the new compounds are tested after acute administration in "naïve" non-depressed animals. Their chronic use in animal models is more appropriate and provide more informative results to determine whether or not a new pharmacological agents worth being tested in clinical trials. A recent study in bulbectomized rats provided some interesting results. In this model, a 14-day regimen of DOV 216303 normalized bulbectomy-induced hyperactivity in the open field, similar to the effect of imipramine at the same dose [50]. Inevitable, further studies in these animal models are required to precise the potential of TRIs and dissect their mechanism of action in pathological conditions.

TABLE 3

TRIs	**Doses, routes**	**Tests**	**Mobility (% of baseline increase)**	**Immobility (% of baseline decrease)**	**References**
DOV 216303	10 mg/kg; po 15 mg/kg; po 20 mg/kg; po	FST (mice)	ND ND ND	-20% (*) -20% (*) -40% (*)	[49]
DOV 21947	5 mg/kg; po 10 mg/kg; po 15 mg/kg; po 20 mg/kg; po	TST (mice)	ND ND ND ND	-25% (***) -40% (***) -40% (***) -55% (***)	[49]
	5 mg/kg; po 10 mg/kg; po 15 mg/kg; po 20 mg/kg; po	FST (rats)	ND ND ND ND	-20% (*) -25% (***) -30% (***) -40% (***)	
JNJ-7925476	0.3 mg/kg; po	TST (mice)	+115%	ND	[46]
PRC025	5 mg/kg; ip 10 mg/kg; ip	TST (mice)	+60% (*) +60% (*)	-40% (*) -40% (*)	[48]
	5 mg/kg; ip 10 mg/kg; ip	FST (rats)	+145% (*) +100% (*)	-40% (*) -30% (*)	
PRC200-SS (active enantiomere of PRC050)	5 mg/kg; ip 10 mg/kg; ip	TST (mice)	+80% (*) +70% (*)	-40% (*) -80% (*)	[48]
	5 mg/kg; ip 10 mg/kg; ip	FST (rats)	+110% (*) +165% (*)	-30% (*) -55% (*)	

PRC200-SS (active enantiomere of PRC050)	0.5 mg/kg; ip 1 mg/kg; ip 10 mg/kg; ip 1 mg/kg; ip 5 mg/kg; ip 10 mg/kg; ip	TST (mice) FST (rats)	+40% (*) +95% (**) +95% (**) +130% (*) +246% (*) +226% (*)	-40% (*) -90% (**) -90% (**) -45% (*) -85% (*) -75% (*)	[39]
D-142	2.5 mg/kg; ip 5 mg/kg; ip 10 mg/kg; ip 2.5 mg/kg; ip 5 mg/kg; ip 10 mg/kg; ip (*Subchronic*)	TST (mice) FST (rats)	ND	-7% -30% (**) -35% (**) -60% (**) -60% (**) -75% (**)	[108]
D-161	10 mg/kg; ip 15 mg/kg; ip 20 mg/kg; ip 10 mg/kg; ip 20 mg/kg; ip (*Subchronic*)	TST (mice) FST (rats)	ND	-20% (**) -35% (***) -65% (***) -75% (***) -70% (***)	[109]
JZAD-IV-22	15 mg/kg; ip 30 mg/kg; ip 60 mg/kg; ip 15 mg/kg; ip 30 mg/kg; ip 60 mg/kg; ip	TST (mice) FST (mice)	ND ND ND ND ND ND	-15% (ns) -30% (*) -35% (*) -20% (ns) -40% (*) -70% (*)	[31]
6-(3,4-dichlorophenyl)-1-[(methyloxy) methyl]-3-azabicyclo[4.1.0]heptane	3 mg/kg; ip 10 mg/kg; ip 30 mg/kg; ip	FST (mice)	ND ND ND	-30% (**) -70% (**) -90% (**)	[35]
1-(Aryl)-6-[alkoxyalkyl]-3-azabicyclo[3.1.0] hexanes and 6-(aryl)-6-[alkoxyalkyl]-3-azabicyclo[3.1.0]hexanes	1 mg/kg; ip 3 mg/kg; ip 10 mg/kg; ip	FST (mice)	ND ND ND	-20% (ns) -40% (*) -90% (**)	[110]
3-aryl-3-azolylpropan-1-amines	3 mg/kg; po 10 mg/kg; po	TST (mice) FST (mice)	ND ND	-60% (*) -15% (*)	[33]
4-(3,4-dichlorophenyl)-N-methyl-1,2,3,4-tetrahydronaphthalenyl amines (compound#10)	3 mg/kg; ip 10 mg/kg; ip 30 mg/kg; ip	TST (mice)	ND	-15% -20% (*) -50% (*)	[27]

N-methyl-1-(1-phenyl-cyclohexyl)methanamine (compound #1)	3 mg/kg; ip 10 mg/kg; ip 30 mg/kg; ip	TST (mice)	ND	-5% -10% -25% (*)	[28]
N-methyl-1-(1-phenyl-cyclohexyl)methanamine (compound #31)	3 mg/kg; ip 10 mg/kg; ip 30 mg/kg; ip	TST (mice)	ND	-10% -14% (*) -30% (*)	[29]
Aryl Octahydrocyclopenta[c] pyrrole (compound #26a)	3 mg/kg; ip 10 mg/kg; ip 30 mg/kg; ip	TST (mice)	ND	-10% -29% (*) -42% (*)	[30]
TP1	2 mg/kg; po 4 mg/kg; po 8 mg/kg; po 16 mg/kg; po 32 mg/kg; po	TST (mice)	ND	-15% -22% (*) -25% (*) -25% (*) -35% (*)	[44]
TP1	4 mg/kg; po 8 mg/kg; po 16 mg/kg; po 32 mg/kg; po	FST (mice)	ND	-10% -17% (*) -23% (*) -25% (*)	[44]
4-((((3S,6S)-6 Benzhydryltetrahydro-2H-pyran-3 yl)amino)methyl) phenol	10 mg/kg; ip	FST (rats)	ND	-75% (**)	[26]

Table 3: **Antidepressant-like activity of triple reuptake inhibitors (TRIs) assessed in the forced swimming and tail suspension tests.** Data are expressed in percentage of mobility or immobility relative to controls. Symbols: *, ** and *** represent statistical differences depicted in the corresponding article. Given the heterogeneity of protocols comparisons between studies, in term of intensity of effect, are not necessarily relevant. ND: Not Determined.

2.2.3. Impact of TRIs on neurogenesis

Beyond the monoamine hypothesis, it has been suggested that neural adaptive mechanisms may underlie antidepressant efficacy. Recently, a neurotrophic–neurogenic theory of depression and antidepressant action has been proposed, in which adult neurogenesis takes a part [51,52,53]. A number of studies have demonstrated that SSRIs such as fluoxetine or citalopram increase cell proliferation and neurogenesis in the dentate gyrus (DG) of the hippocampus of naive [54,55,56,57] or depressed rodents [58,59]. Changes in cell proliferation in the hippocampus have also been observed following olfactory bulbectomy, showing that various components of the limbic circuitry may exhibit alterations in neuroplasticity that can be reversed by monoaminergic antidepressants [60]. Growing evidence also suggest that catecholamines (NE and DA) also stimulate neurogenesis. For example, in addition to SSRIs, NRIs and SNRIs have been shown to increase the local expression of neurotrophic factors including BDNF [61,62,63] and adult hippocampus neurogenesis in the DG [57]. In a recent study aimed at comparing monoaminergic compounds with different pharmacological profiles (at doses that have been shown to produce antidepressant-like effects in behavioral models), it was demonstrated that sustained administration of the reuptake inhibitors venlafaxine and imipramine, increased BDNF mRNA expression after 7 and 14 days of administration respectively, while the SSRI fluoxetine had no effect [64]. It is thus possible that the activation of the serotonergic and noradrenergic neurotransmitter system activates different downstream cascades that are both able to increase the transcription of BDNF.

Whether or not this effect resulted from an additive effect on noradrenergic and serotonergic systems is unclear [65]. Importantly, the hippocampus receives a sparse dopaminergic innervation from the ventral tegmental area [66], raising the possibility that DA and related receptors play a limited role in the local regulation of BDNF expression and neurogenesis. However, dopaminergic denervation in animals causes a dramatic reduction in the number of proliferating cells in the hippocampus [67] while the stimulation of DA receptors with selective D_2 agonists has recently been shown to enhance neurogenesis in the DG of the hippocampus [67,68]. In a recent series of *in vivo* experiments, it has been shown that the Cytokine Ciliary Neurotrophic Factor (CNTF), abundant in astrocytes close to dopaminergic terminals, constitutes an endogenous regulatory component of D_2-receptor-dependent neurogenesis in DG [68,69] suggesting that TRIs might be stronger on neurotrophic factor gene expression, neural plasticity, and neurogenesis than SSRIs, NRIs and SNRIs. Using *in situ* hybridization, an initial study showed that treatment with the TRI NS2330 (Tesofensine), for 5 and 14 days had no effect on BDNF expression in the granular cell layer, while increasing its expression by 35 % in the CA3 after 14 days [64]. Furthermore, NS2330 stimulated the number of neuroD-positive cells after 14 days treatment and the nuclear marker of proliferation Ki67, confirming the antidepressant potential of this novel agent [64]. Although these results revealed a strong effect of NS2330, the net effect of blockade of each of the monoamine reuptake sites remains unknown. Further studies are truly necessary to dissect the contribution of each monoamine uptake target on the regulation of BDNF or others neurotrophic factors gene expression. It is possible that the stimulation of the expression of various neurotrophic factors such as BDNF and CNTF induced by the concomitant enhancement of central 5-HT, NE and DA transmission, might contribute to shorten the delay of action of traditional antidepressants drugs.

Importantly, there is little clinical evidence demonstrating the requirement of hippocampal neurogenesis is mediating the therapeutic activity of antidepressant drugs in MD. Perhaps the most prominent evidence comes from the observation that decreased levels of BDNF could contribute to hippocampal atrophy seen in depressed patients [70] whereas antidepressants, notably SSRIs, increase the peripheral levels of this neurotrophic substance [70,71]. Hence future studies in human can be expected to determine the real impact of neurogenesis in treatment response induced by monoaminergic antidepressants, although methodological limitations impede the parallel between clinical and preclinical observations.

2.2.4. Impact of TRIs on astro-glial cells

Interestingly, glia and more particularly astrocytes are now recognized as partners with neurons in many aspect of brain function such as neuronal plasticity. It is thus conceivable that these cells are involved in pathophysiology of MD. Both clinical and preclinical findings support this hypothesis. For example, post-mortem studies report a reduction in the density of glial fibrillary associated protein (GFAP) immunoreactive cells in several cortical regions including the prefrontal and cingulate areas from individuals with MD [72,73,74] but also in their amygdala or hippocampus [74,75]. These clinical observations are in agreement with recent findings obtained in rats showing that L-alpha-aminodipate-induced decrease in the density of astrocytes in the prefrontal cortex (PFCx) of adult rats, produced depressive-like behaviors similar to those induced by chronic unpredictable stress [76]. Monoaminergic antidepressants may exert part of their therapeutic effects by modulating directly or indirectly the activity of astrocytes, which express SERT, NET and DAT [77] but also monoaminergic receptors [78]. Consistent with this hypothesis, fluoxetine reverses the inhibition of glial cell proliferation in the medial PFCx of rats subjected to chronic psychosocial stress [79]. Although the mechanism of antidepressant on glia is still not clear, current researches focus on the possibility that this cell population constitutes a major source of neurotrophic factors available for the proliferation, maturation and differentiation of progenitor cells. Accordingly, *in vitro* studies demonstrated that tricyclic antidepressants and SSRIs stimulate GDNF and BDNF levels [80,81] suggesting that 5-HT and/or NE may stimulate the production of neurotrophic/growth factors. This observation has been extended recently to DA, which may favor the synthesis of basic FGF, BDNF or GDNF [82,83]. Thus, astrocytes stimulation by the activation of dopaminergic receptors could allow TRIs to produce more robust effects than single- or dual-acting agents.

3. CLINICAL EVIDENCE FOR ANTIDEPRESSANT ACTIVITY OF TRIPLE REUPTAKE INHIBITORS

3.1. COMBINATION OF SELECTIVE SEROTONIN REUPTAKE INHIBITOR WITH BUPROPION

Bupropion is an antidepressant with novel neurotransmitter properties (NE and DA reuptake inhibitor) that seems to augment SSRI or SNRI effectiveness and/or help relieve or reverse certain adverse events associated with these agents [84]. Although multiple case reports in the literature describe improvement in depressive symptoms with a combination of bupropion and an SSRI [24], some prospective open-label studies were designed to evaluate this strategy in depressed patients who had failed to achieve adequate response to an SSRI. In the largest of the prospective trials, Lam and collaborators [85] compared the combination of citalopram and bupropion in adults who failed to respond to at least 6 weeks' treatment with the monotherapy. Results showed that combination therapy was superior to mono-therapy and well tolerated [85]. The second prospective, randomized, open-label study from DeBattista reported that 54% of resistant patients experienced a remission with bupropion supporting the use of this agent in the augmentation of SSRIs [86]. Similar results have been recently obtained by combining bupropion with fluoxetine [10], escitalopram [87] or others SSRIs [88,89], thus encouraging the development of broad-spectrum antidepressants [49].

3.2. TRIPLE REUPTAKE INHIBITORS

3.2.1. In major depression

On the basis of preclinical and clinical data, particularly on the association of SSRIs with bupropion, TRIs are in process of development [90] and most are now in Phase II clinical trials. A small citalopram controlled trial of DOV 216303 in severely depressed patients yielded significant improvements in Hamilton Depression Rating Scale (HAM-D) scores in both groups at one- and two-week time points [91]. DOV Pharmaceutical has recently reported the results of a multi-centric, randomized, double-blind, placebo-controlled study with amitifadine (DOV 21947) in 61 patients with MD [92]. For the primary outcome measure, treatment with amitifadine was associated with a significantly greater improvement in the MADRS and CGI-I total score at week 6 compared with placebo. In addition, a significantly greater remission rate for the CGI-S was observed with amitifadine compared with placebo at week 6. This study also showed that amitifadine was efficacious in improving anhedonia, a core symptom of depression that is presumed to be related to a hypodopaminergia. Despite these encouraging data, further investigations failed to demonstrate the beneficial therapeutic effect of NS2359 and GSK372475 and the development of these compounds was stopped.

3.2.2. Other symptoms of MD triggered by TRIs: pain perception

MD is a medical condition that includes abnormalities of affect and mood, cognition, and physical functioning. In particular, as many as 75% of patients suffering from depression are found to report somatic symptoms, including various types of pain such as headaches, stomach pain, back pain, and vague, poorly localized pain [10]. A recent study has shown that responders who have not achieved adequate remission have significantly more somatic symptoms than remitters following 8 weeks of treatment with fluoxetine. These data may suggest that antidepressants that are particularly effective in the treatment of pain and painful physical symptoms may yield higher remission rates in MD [37]. In addition, it has been suggested that presence of pain may be an indicator of MD that may have poorer treatment outcome with an initial SSRI [93]. Acute and chronic pains may result from reduced levels of endogenous 5-HT, NE and DA activities, at both the spinal and supraspinal levels [94]. Indeed, pain is a bi-directional process of ascending and descending neuronal pathways involving monoaminergic systems whose activation may have an inhibitory influence on nociception. Thus, one would expect a better efficacy of dual-or triple-acting agents over selective 5-HT or NE reuptake inhibitors in analgesia [37]. Selected antidepressants suppress pain by diverse mechanisms and are now considered as an essential component of the therapeutic strategy for treatment of many types of persistent pain [95]. Their main mechanism of action involves reinforcement of the descending inhibitory pathways by increasing the amount of 5-HT and NE, but also DA in the synaptic cleft at both supraspinal and spinal levels [37]. Several open-label randomized controlled clinical trials, meta-analyses, and systematic reviews have confirmed the clinical efficacy of selected antidepressants in persistent pain conditions [96]. The potential interest of TRIs in the relief of pain has been corroborated by a recent preclinical study characterizing the antinociceptive effects of bicifadine in acute, persistent and chronic models of pain [47]. In this study, bicifadine potently suppressed pain responses in two models of acute inflammatory pain in both rats and mice. It also normalized the nociceptive threshold in the complete Freund's adjuvant model of persistent inflammatory pain and suppressed mechanical and thermal hyperalgesia and mechanical allodynia in the spinal nerve ligation model of chronic neuropathic pain. Mechanical hyperalgesia was also reduced by bicifadine in streptozotocin-induced neuropathic pain model [47]. Clinical studies have corroborated that bicifadine is an effective analgesic in the treatment of postoperative pain [97]. In a second study, the TRI NS7051, has shown comparable antinociceptive properties to tramadol confirming the interest of these antidepressants in the relief of pain [98]. The molecule has undergone several phase II and III trials for the treatment of pain, including acute postsurgical pain and chronic low back pain, and is being evaluated for painful diabetic neuropathy (clinical trial.gov).

3.2.3. Safety and Tolerability of TRIs

The adverse event profiles of TRIs have been studied in several Phase I investigations. In a dose-escalating, placebo-controlled, double blind, phase 1a trial, no adverse effects were observed at several-fold higher doses of DOV 216303 [99]. In a Phase 1b, 10 subjects were given either placebo (n=3) or drug (n=7) at 3 doses (25 mg b.i.d., 25 mg t.i.d. and 50 mg b.i.d.) for 10 days. No severe side effects were noted, although diarrhea, vomiting and nausea were observed. This is also the case with amitifadine, which was similar to that of placebo [92]. As expected, amitifadine was associated with a small increase in mean heart rate but within the physiologic range [92]. This pharmacodynamic effect was probably related to blockade of the NE transporter, which in turn activates noradrenergic receptors in the heart [100]. All these observations contrast with those reported in a study showing that more patients suffering from Parkinson's disease and treated with the TRI tesofensine (82%) than in the placebo group (74%), experienced adverse events such as a higher rate of nervous system disorders (dyskinesia and headache), gastrointestinal tract disorders (nausea and constipation), and psychiatric disorders (hallucinations and insomnia) [101]. Finally, weight loss has been observed as an adverse event in studies with tesofensine [102], prompting further research for the indication of obesity. This result is not surprising since DA and 5-HT activities are known to suppress feeding activity and produce anorexant effects in animal models [103]. However, such weight changes were not observed with amitifadine raising the possibility that the intensity of binding and/or inactivation of the distinct monoaminergic transporters are important parameters to anticipate adverse event profiles of TRIs.

4. CONCLUSION

Several evidence support the idea that TRIs may produce more robust antidepressant effects than single- or dual-acting agents mainly due to the dopaminergic component. Firstly, it is believed that the enhancement of dopaminergic neurotransmission will act on core or specific symptoms of mood disorders including anhedonia or pain respectively, which poorly respond to SSRIs. Hence, it is envisaged to adapt the treatment to the nature of depressive symptoms. Drugs with high affinities for the DAT could be more beneficial to patients having a loss of motivation and/or anhedonia. Secondly, TRIs will be inevitably useful to prevent adverse events (*e.g.,* sexual dysfunctions) commonly observed with SSRIs and/or SNRIs. Finally, preclinical data strongly suggest that an increase in brain DA may favor the activity of the serotonergic system. Indeed, anatomical and functional interactions exists between DA and 5-HT neurons [23,25] and it has been clearly demonstrated that the stimulation of D_2-like receptor increase the neuronal activity of DR 5-HT neurons. As an example, the sustained administration of the D_2-like receptor agonist increased by almost 40% the firing of 5-HT neurons [104]. This point is particularly important given that SSRIs alone reduce the firing of these 5-HT neurons after acute treatment while they only normalize the firing rate after chronic administration. Consequently, it can be anticipated that an optimal electrophysiological response (an increase in firing activity), will be achieved by combining a dopaminergic agent to conventional serotonergic antidepressants. Whether or not such enhancement of DR 5-HT neuronal activity is correlated to a greater antidepressant-(like) activity and neurogenic process has yet to be determined.

REFERENCES

[1] Katz MM, Bowden CL, Frazer A. Rethinking depression and the actions of antidepressants: Uncovering the links between the neural and behavioral elements. Journal of Affective Disorders 2010, 120: 16-23.

[2] Handley SL. 5-Hydroxytryptamine pathways in anxiety and its treatment. Pharmacol Ther 1995, 66: 103-148.

[3] Morilak DA, Frazer A. Antidepressants and brain monoaminergic systems: a dimensional approach to understanding their behavioural effects in depression and anxiety disorders. Int J Neuropsychopharmacol 2004, 7: 193-218.

[4] Nutt DJ. The role of dopamine and norepinephrine in depression and antidepressant treatment. J Clin Psychiatry 2006, 67 Suppl 6: 3-8.

[5] Miller HL, Delgado PL, Salomon RM, Heninger GR, Charney DS. Effects of alpha-methyl-para-tyrosine (AMPT) in drug-free depressed patients. Neuropsychopharmacology 1996, 14: 151-157.

[6] Dunlop BW, Nemeroff CB. The role of dopamine in the pathophysiology of depression. Arch Gen Psychiatry 2007, 64: 327-337.

[7] Berton O, Nestler EJ (2006). New approaches to antidepressant drug discovery: beyond monoamines. Nat Rev Neurosci 2006, 7: 137-151.

[8] Blier P. The pharmacology of putative early-onset antidepressant strategies. Eur Neuropsychopharmacol 2003, 13: 57-66.

[9] Blier P, Ward HE, Tremblay P, Laberge L, Hebert C, Bergeron R. Combination of antidepressant medications from treatment initiation for major depressive disorder: a double-blind randomized study. Am J Psychiatry 2010, 167: 281-288.

[10] Fava M. New approaches to the treatment of refractory depression. J Clin Psychiatry 2000, 61 Suppl 1: 26-32.

[11] Blier P, Blondeau C. Neurobiological bases and clinical aspects of the use of aripiprazole in treatment-resistant major depressive disorder. J Affect Disord 2011, 128 Suppl 1: S3-10.

[12] Rush AJ, Trivedi MH, Wisniewski SR, Stewart JW, Nierenberg AA, Thase ME, Ritz L, Biggs MM, Warden D, Luther JF, Shores-Wilson K, Niederehe G, Fava M; STAR*D Study team. Bupropion-SR, sertraline, or venlafaxine-XR after failure of SSRIs for depression. N Engl J Med 2006, 354: 1231-1242.

[13] Poirier MF, Boyer P. Venlafaxine and paroxetine in treatment-resistant depression. Double-blind, randomized comparison. Br J Psychiatry 1999, 175: 12-16.

[14] Shelton RC, Tomarken AJ. Can recovery from depression be achieved? Psychiatr Serv 2001, 52: 1469-1478.

[15] McCabe C, Mishor Z, Cowen PJ, Harmer CJ. Diminished neural processing of aversive and rewarding stimuli during selective serotonin reuptake inhibitor treatment. Biol Psychiatry 2010, 67: 439-445.

[16] Cassano P, Lattanzi L, Soldani F, Navari S, Battistini G, Gemignani A, Cassano GB. Pramipexole in treatment-resistant depression: an extended follow-up. Depress Anxiety 2004, 20: 131-138.

[17] Goldberg JF, Burdick KE, Endick CJ. Preliminary randomized, double-blind, placebo-controlled trial of pramipexole added to mood stabilizers for treatment-resistant bipolar depression. Am J Psychiatry 2004, 161: 564-566.

[18] Zarate CA, Jr., Payne JL, Singh J, Quiroz JA, Luckenbaugh DA, Denicoff KD, Charney DS, Manji HK. Pramipexole for bipolar II depression: a placebo-controlled proof of concept study. Biol Psychiatry 2004, 56: 54-60.

[19] Lattanzi L, Dell'Osso L, Cassano P, Pini S, Rucci P, Houck PR,Gemignani A, Battistini G, Bassi A, Abelli M, Cassano GB. Pramipexole in treatment-resistant depression: a 16-week naturalistic study. Bipolar Disord 2002, 4: 307-314.

[20] Perugi G, Toni C, Ruffolo G, Frare F, Akiskal H. Adjunctive dopamine agonists in treatment-resistant bipolar II depression: an open case series. Pharmacopsychiatry 2001, 34: 137-141.

[21] Sporn J, Ghaemi SN, Sambur MR, Rankin MA, Recht J, Sachs GS, Rosenbaum JF, Fava M. Pramipexole augmentation in the treatment of unipolar and bipolar depression: a retrospective chart review. Ann Clin Psychiatry 2000, 12: 137-140.

[22] Corrigan MH, Denahan AQ, Wright CE, Ragual RJ, Evans DL. Comparison of pramipexole, fluoxetine, and placebo in patients with major depression. Depress Anxiety 2000, 11: 58-65.

[23] Tremblay P, Blier P. Catecholaminergic strategies for the treatment of major depression. Curr Drug Targets 2006, 7: 149-158.

[24] Zisook S, Rush AJ, Haight BR, Clines DC, Rockett CB. Use of bupropion in combination with serotonin reuptake inhibitors. Biol Psychiatry 2006, 59: 203-210.

[25] Guiard BP, El Mansari M, Merali Z, Blier P. Functional interactions between dopamine, serotonin and norepinephrine neurons: an *in-vivo* electrophysiological study in rats with monoaminergic lesions. Int J Neuropsychopharmacol 2008, 11: 625-639.

[26] Gopishetty B, Hazeldine S, Santra S, Johnson M, Modi G, Ali S, Zhen J, Reith M, Dutta A. Further structure-activity relationship studies on 4-((((3S,6S)-6-benzhydryltetrahydro-2H-pyran-3-yl)amino)methyl)phenol: identification of compounds with triple uptake inhibitory activity as potential antidepressant agents. J Med Chem 2011, 54: 2924-2932.

[27] Shao L, Hewitt MC, Malcolm SC, Wang F, Ma J, Campbell UC, Spicer NA, Engel SR, Hardy LW, Jiang ZD, Schreiber R, Spear KL, Varney MA. Synthesis and pharmacological characterization of bicyclic triple reuptake inhibitor 3-aryl octahydrocyclopenta[c]pyrrole analogues. J Med Chem 2011, 54: 5283-5295.

[28] Shao L, Hewitt MC, Wang F, Malcolm SC, Ma J, Campbell JE, Campbell UC, Engel SR, Spicer NA, Hardy LW, Schreiber R, Spear KL, Varney MA. Discovery of N-methyl-1-(1-phenylcyclohexyl) ethanamine, a novel triple serotonin, norepinephrine and dopamine reuptake inhibitor. Bioorg Med Chem Lett 2011, 21: 1434-1437.

[29] Shao L, Hewitt MC, Wang F, Malcolm SC, Ma J, Campbell JE, Campbell UC, Engel SR, Spicer NA, Hardy LW, Schreiber R, Spear KL, Varney MA. Discovery of N-methyl-1-(1-phenylcyclohexyl) methanamine, a novel triple serotonin, norepinephrine, and dopamine reuptake inhibitor. Bioorg Med Chem Lett 2011, 21: 1438-1441.

[30] Shao L, Wang F, Malcolm SC, Ma J, Hewitt MC, Campbell UC, Bush LR, Spicer NA, Engel SR, Saraswat LD, Hardy LW, Koch P, Schreiber R, Spear KL, Varney MA. Synthesis and pharmacological evaluation of 4-(3,4-dichlorophenyl)-N-methyl-1,2,3,4-tetrahydronaphthalenyl amines as triple reuptake inhibitors. Bioorg Med Chem 2011, 19: 663-676.

[31] Caldarone BJ, Paterson NE, Zhou J, Brunner D, Kozikowski AP, Westphal KG, Korte-Bouws GA, Prins J, Korte SM, Olivier B, Ghavami A. The novel triple reuptake inhibitor JZAD-IV-22 exhibits an antidepressant pharmacological profile without locomotor stimulant or sensitization properties. J Pharmacol Exp Ther 2010, 335: 762-770.

[32] Carter DS, Cai HY, Lee EK, Iyer PS, Lucas MC, Roetz R, Schoenfeld RC, Weikert RJ. 2-Substituted N-aryl piperazines as novel triple reuptake inhibitors for the treatment of depression. Bioorg Med Chem Lett 2010, 20: 3941-3945.

[33] Lee KH, Park CE, Min KH, Shin YJ, Chung CM, Kim HH, Yoon HJ, Won-Kim, Ryu EJ, Shin YJ, Nam HS, Cho JW, Lee HY. Synthesis and pharmacological evaluation of 3-aryl-3-azolylpropan-1-amines as selective triple serotonin/norepinephrine/dopamine reuptake inhibitors. Bioorg Med Chem Lett 2010, 20: 5567-5571.

[34] Lucas MC, Weikert RJ, Carter DS, Cai HY, Greenhouse R, Iyer PS, Lin CJ, Lee EK, Madera AM, Moore A, Ozboya K, Schoenfeld RC, Steiner S, Zhai Y, Lynch SM. Design, synthesis, and biological evaluation of new monoamine reuptake inhibitors with potential therapeutic utility in depression and pain. Bioorg Med Chem Lett 2010, 20: 5559-5566.

[35] Micheli F, Cavanni P, Andreotti D, Arban R, Benedetti R, Bertani B, Bettati M, Bettelini L, Bononomi G, Braggio S, Carletti R, Checchia A, Corsi M, Fazzolari E, Fontana S, Marchioro C, Merlo-Pich E, Negri M, Oliosi B, Ratti E, Read KD, Roscic M, Sartori I, Spada S, Tedesco G, Tarsi L, Terreni S, Visentini F, Zoccho A, Zonzini L, Di Fabio R. 6-(3,4-dichlorophenyl)-1-[(methyloxy) methyl]-3-azabicyclo[4.1.0]heptane: a new potent and selective triple reuptake inhibitor. J Med Chem 2010, 53: 4989-5001.

[36] Schoedel KA, Meier D, Chakraborty B, Manniche PM, Sellers EM. Subjective and objective effects of the novel triple reuptake inhibitor tesofensine in recreational stimulant users. Clin Pharmacol Ther 2010, 88: 69-78.

[37] Hache G, Coudore F, Gardier AM, Guiard BP. Monoaminergic antidepressants in the relief of pain: potential utility of triple reuptake inhibitors (TRIs). Pharmaceuticals 2011, 4: 285-342.

[38] Benveniste H. Brain microdialysis. J Neurochem 1989, 52: 1667-1679.

[39] Liang Y, Shaw AM, Boules M, Briody S, Robinson J, Oliveros A, Blazar E, Williams K, Zhang Y, Carlier PR, Richelson E. Antidepressant-like pharmacological profile of a novel triple reuptake inhibitor, (1S,2S)-3-(methylamino)-2-(naphthalen-2-yl)-1-phenylpropan-1-ol (PRC200-SS). J Pharmacol Exp Ther 2008, 327: 573-583.

[40] Kuikka JT, Tiihonen J, Bergstrom KA, Karhu J, Hartikainen P, Viinamaki H, Lansimies E, Lehtonen J, Hakola P. Imaging of serotonin and dopamine transporters in the living human brain. Eur J Nucl Med 1995, 22: 346-350.

[41] Alex KD, Pehek EA. Pharmacologic mechanisms of serotonergic regulation of dopamine neurotransmission. Pharmacol Ther 2007, 113: 296-320.

[42] Prisco S, Esposito E. Differential effects of acute and chronic fluoxetine administration on the spontaneous activity of dopaminergic neurones in the ventral tegmental area. Br J Pharmacol 1995, 116: 1923-1931.

[43] Guiard BP, El Mansari M, Blier P. Prospect of a dopamine contribution in the next generation of antidepressant drugs: the triple reuptake inhibitors. Curr Drug Targets 2009,10: 1069-1084.

[44] Tian JW, Jiang WL, Zhong Y, Meng Q, Gai Y, Zhu HB, Hou J, Xing Y, Li YX. Preclinical pharmacology of TP1, a novel potent triple reuptake inhibitor with antidepressant properties. Neuroscience 2011, 196:124-130.

[45] Nicholson KL, Balster RL, Golembiowska K, Kowalska M, Tizzano JP, Skolnick P, Basile AS. Preclinical evaluation of the abuse potential of the analgesic bicifadine. J Pharmacol Exp Ther 2009, 330(1): 236-248.

[46] Aluisio L, Lord B, Barbier AJ, Fraser IC, Wilson SJ, Boggs J, Dvorak LK, Letavic MA, Maryanoff BE, Carruthers NI. *In-vitro* and *in-vivo* characterization of JNJ-7925476, a novel triple monoamine uptake inhibitor. Eur J Pharmacol 2008, 587: 141-146.

[47] Basile AS, Janowsky A, Golembiowska K, Kowalska M, Tam E, Benveniste M, Popik P, Nikiforuk A, Krawczyk M, Nowak G, Krieter PA, Lippa AS, Skolnick P, Koustova E. Characterization of the antinociceptive actions of bicifadine in models of acute, persistent, and chronic pain. J Pharmacol Exp Ther 2007, 321: 1208-1225.

[48] Shaw AM, Boules M, Zhang Y, Williams K, Robinson J, Carlier PR, Richelson E. Antidepressant-like effects of novel triple reuptake inhibitors, PRC025 and PRC050. Eur J Pharmacol 2007, 555: 30-36.

[49] Skolnick P, Popik P, Janowsky A, Beer B, Lippa AS. Antidepressant-like actions of DOV 21,947: a "triple" reuptake inhibitor. Eur J Pharmacol 2003, 461: 99-104.

[50] Breuer ME, Chan JS, Oosting RS, Groenink L, Korte SM, Campbell U, Schreiber R, Hanania T, Snoeren EM, Waldinger M, Olivier B. The triple monoaminergic reuptake inhibitor DOV 216,303 has antidepressant effects in the rat olfactory bulbectomy model and lacks sexual side effects. Eur Neuropsychopharmacol 2008, 18: 908-916.

[51] Sahay A, Drew MR, Hen R. Dentate gyrus neurogenesis and depression. Prog Brain Res 2007, 163: 697-722.

[52] Sahay A, Hen R. Adult hippocampal neurogenesis in depression. Nat Neurosci 2007, 10: 1110-1115.

[53] Duman RS, Monteggia LM. A neurotrophic model for stress-related mood disorders. Biol Psychiatry 2006, 59: 1116-1127.

[54] Marcussen AB, Flagstad P, Kristjansen PE, Johansen FF, Englund U. Increase in neurogenesis and behavioural benefit after chronic fluoxetine treatment in Wistar rats. Acta Neurol Scand 2008, 117: 94-100.

[55] Sairanen M, Lucas G, Ernfors P, Castren M, Castren E. Brain-derived neurotrophic factor and antidepressant drugs have different but coordinated effects on neuronal turnover, proliferation, and survival in the adult dentate gyrus. J Neurosci 2005, 25: 1089-1094.

[56] Santarelli L, Saxe M, Gross C, Surget A, Battaglia F, Dulawa S, Weisstaub N, Lee J, Duman R, Arancio O, Belzung C, Hen C. Requirement of hippocampal neurogenesis for the behavioral effects of antidepressants. Science 2003, 301: 805-809.

[57] Malberg JE, Eisch AJ, Nestler EJ, Duman RS. Chronic antidepressant treatment increases neurogenesis in adult rat hippocampus. J Neurosci 2000, 20: 9104-9110.

[58] David DJ, Samuels BA, Rainer Q, Wang JW, Marsteller D, Mendez I, Drew M, Craig DA, Guiard BP, Guilloux JP, Artymyshyn RP, Gardier AM, Gerald C, Antnijevic IA, Leonardo ED, Hen R. Neurogenesis-dependent and -independent effects of fluoxetine in an animal model of anxiety/depression. Neuron 2009, 62: 479-493.

[59] Malberg JE, Duman RS. Cell proliferation in adult hippocampus is decreased by inescapable stress: reversal by fluoxetine treatment. Neuropsychopharmacology 2003, 28: 1562-1571.

[60] Keilhoff G, Becker A, Grecksch G, Bernstein HG, Wolf G. Cell proliferation is influenced by bulbectomy and normalized by imipramine treatment in a region-specific manner. Neuropsychopharmacology 2006, 31: 1165-1176.

[61] Nibuya M, Morinobu S, Duman RS. Regulation of BDNF and trkB mRNA in rat brain by chronic electroconvulsive seizure and antidepressant drug treatments. J Neurosci 1995, 15: 7539-7547.

[62] Larsen MH, Hay-Schmidt A, Ronn LC, Mikkelsen JD. Temporal expression of brain-derived neurotrophic factor (BDNF) mRNA in the rat hippocampus after treatment with selective and mixed monoaminergic antidepressants. Eur J Pharmacol 2008, 578: 114-122.

[63] Russo-Neustadt AA, Alejandre H, Garcia C, Ivy AS, Chen MJ. Hippocampal brain-derived neurotrophic factor expression following treatment with reboxetine, citalopram, and physical exercise. Neuropsychopharmacology 2004, 29: 2189-2199.

[64] Larsen MH, Rosenbrock H, Sams-Dodd F, Mikkelsen JD. Expression of brain derived neurotrophic factor, activity-regulated cytoskeleton protein mRNA, and enhancement of adult hippocampal neurogenesis in rats after sub-chronic and chronic treatment with the triple monoamine re-uptake inhibitor tesofensine. Eur J Pharmacol 2007, 555: 115-121.

[65] Ivy AS, Rodriguez FG, Garcia C, Chen MJ, Russo-Neustadt AA. Noradrenergic and serotonergic blockade inhibits BDNF mRNA activation following exercise and antidepressant. Pharmacol Biochem Behav 2003, 75: 81-88.

[66] Scatton B, Simon H, Le Moal M, Bischoff S. Origin of dopaminergic innervation of the rat hippocampal formation. Neurosci Lett 1980, 18: 125-131.

[67] Hoglinger GU, Rizk P, Muriel MP, Duyckaerts C, Oertel WH, Caille I, Hirsch EC. Dopamine depletion impairs precursor cell proliferation in Parkinson disease. Nat Neurosci 2004, 7: 726-735.

[68] Yang P, Arnold SA, Habas A, Hetman M, Hagg T. Ciliary neurotrophic factor mediates dopamine D2 receptor-induced CNS neurogenesis in adult mice. J Neurosci 2008, 28: 2231-2241.

[69] Mori M, Jefferson JJ, Hummel M, Garbe DS. CNTF: a putative link between dopamine D2 receptors and neurogenesis. J Neurosci 2008, 28: 5867-5869.

[70] Sheline YI, Gado MH, Kraemer HC. Untreated depression and hippocampal volume loss. Am. J. Psychiatry (2003), 160: 1516-1518.

[71] Shen S, Duman R, Sanacora G. Serum brain-derived neurotrophic factor, depression, and antidepressant medications: meta-analyses and implications. Biological Psychiatry 2008, 64: 527-537.

[72] Rajkowska G, Miguel-Hidalgo JJ, Wei J, Dilley G, Pittman SD, Meltzer HY, Overholser JC, Roth BL, Stockmeier CA. Morphometric evidence for neuronal and glial prefrontal cell pathology in major depression. Biol Psychiatry 1999, 45: 1085-1098.

[73] Miguel-Hidalgo JJ, Baucom C, Dilley G, Overholser JC, Meltzer HY, Stockmeier CA, Rajkowska G. Glial fibrillary acidic protein immunoreactivity in the prefrontal cortex distinguishes younger from older adults in major depressive disorder. Biol Psychiatry 2000, 48: 861-873.

[74] Webster MJ, O'Grady J, Kleinman JE, Weickert CS. Glial fibrillary acidic protein mRNA levels in the cingulate cortex of individuals with depression, bipolar disorder and schizophrenia. Neuroscience 2005, 133: 453-461.

[75] Hamidi M, Drevets WC, Price JL. Glial reduction in amygdala in major depressive disorder is due to oligodendrocytes. Biol Psychiatry 2004, 55: 563-569.

[76] Banasr M, Duman RS. Glial loss in the prefrontal cortex is sufficient to induce depressive-like behaviors. Biol Psychiatry 2008, 64: 863-870.

[77] Inazu M, Takeda H, Ikoshi H, Sugisawa M, Uchida Y, Matsumiya T. Pharmacological characterization and visualization of the glial serotonin transporter. Neurochem Int 2001, 39: 39-49.

[78] Hertz L, Schousboe I, Schousboe A. Receptor expression in primary cultures of neurons or astrocytes. Prog Neuropsychopharmacol Biol Psychiatry 1984, 8: 521-527.

[79] Czeh B, Simon M, Schmelting B, Hiemke C, Fuchs E. Astroglial plasticity in the hippocampus is affected by chronic psychosocial stress and concomitant fluoxetine treatment. Neuropsychopharmacology 2006, 31: 1616-1626.

[80] Hisaoka K, Takebayashi M, Tsuchioka M, Maeda N, Nakata Y, Yamawaki S. Antidepressants increase glial cell line-derived neurotrophic factor production through monoamine-independent activation of protein tyrosine kinase and extracellular signal-regulated kinase in glial cells. J Pharmacol Exp Ther 2007, 321: 148-157.

[81] Allaman I, Fiumelli H, Magistretti PJ, Martin JL. Fluoxetine regulates the expression of neurotrophic/growth factors and glucose metabolism in astrocytes. Psychopharmacology (Berl) 2011, 216: 75-84.

[82] Forget C, Stewart J, Trudeau LE. Impact of basic FGF expression in astrocytes on dopamine neuron synaptic function and development. Eur J Neurosci 2006, 23: 608-616.

[83] Ohta K, Kuno S, Inoue S, Ikeda E, Fujinami A, Ohta M. The effect of dopamine agonists: the expression of GDNF, NGF, and BDNF in cultured mouse astrocytes. J Neurol Sci 2010, 291: 12-16.

[84] Stahl SM, Pradko JF, Haight BR, Modell JG, Rockett CB, Learned-Coughlin S. A Review of the Neuropharmacology of Bupropion, a Dual Norepinephrine and Dopamine Reuptake Inhibitor. Prim Care Companion J Clin Psychiatry 2004, 6: 159-166.

[85] Lam RW, Hossie H, Solomons K, Yatham LN. Citalopram and bupropion-SR: combining versus switching in patients with treatment-resistant depression. J Clin Psychiatry 2004, 65: 337-340.

[86] DeBattista C, Solvason HB, Poirier J, Kendrick E, Schatzberg AF. A prospective trial of bupropion SR augmentation of partial and non-responders to serotonergic antidepressants. J Clin Psychopharmacol 2003, 23: 27-30.

[87] Leuchter AF, Lesser IM, Trivedi MH, Rush AJ, Morris DW, Warden D, Fava M, Wisniewski SR, Luther JF, Perales M, Gaynes BN, Stewart JW. An open pilot study of the combination of escitalopram and bupropion-SR for outpatients with major depressive disorder. J Psychiatr Pract 2008, 14: 271-280.

[88] Gulrez G, Badyal DK, Deswal RS, Sharma A. Bupropion as an Augmenting Agent in Patients of Depression with Partial Response. Basic Clin Pharmacol Toxicol. 2011, 110: 227-230.

[89] Rosso G, Rigardetto S, Bogetto F, Maina G. A randomized, single-blind, comparison of duloxetine with bupropion in the treatment of SSRI-resistant major depression. J Affect Disord. 2011, 136: 172-176.

[90] Millan MJ. Dual- and triple-acting agents for treating core and co-morbid symptoms of major depression: novel concepts, new drugs. Neurotherapeutics 2009, 6: 53-77.

[91] Skolnick P, Krieter P, Tizzano J, Basile A, Popik P, Czobor P, Lippa A. Preclinical and clinical pharmacology of DOV 216,303, a "triple" reuptake inhibitor. CNS Drug Rev 2006, 12: 123-134.

[92] Tran P, Skolnick P, Czobor P, Huang NY, Bradshaw M, McKinney A, Fava M. Efficacy and tolerability of the novel triple reuptake inhibitor amitifadine in the treatment of patients with major depressive disorder: A randomized, double-blind, placebo-controlled trial. J Psychiatr Res. 2011, 46: 64-71

[93] Leuchter AF, Husain MM, Cook IA, Trivedi MH, Wisniewski SR, Gilmer WS, Luther JF, Fava M, Rush AJ. Painful physical symptoms and treatment outcome in major depressive disorder: a STAR*D (Sequenced Treatment Alternatives to Relieve Depression) report. Psychol Med 2010, 40: 239-251.

[94] Ren K, Dubner R. Descending modulation in persistent pain: an update. Pain 2002, 100: 1-6.

[95] Sawynok J, Esser MJ, Reid AR. Antidepressants as analgesics: an overview of central and peripheral mechanisms of action. J Psychiatry Neurosci 2001, 26: 21-29.

[96] Dharmshaktu P, Tayal V, Kalra BS. Efficacy of Antidepressants as Analgesics: A Review. J Clin Pharmacol. 2011, 52: 6-17.

[97] Krieter PA, Gohdes M, Musick TJ, Duncanson FP, Bridson WE. Pharmacokinetics, disposition, and metabolism of bicifadine in humans. Drug Metab Dispos 2008, 36: 252-259.

[98] Munro G, Baek CA, Erichsen HK, Nielsen AN, Nielsen EO, Scheel-Kruger J, Weikop P, Peters D. The novel compound (+/-)-1-[10-((E)-3-Phenyl-allyl)-3,10-diaza-bicyclo[4.3.1]dec-3-yl]-propan -1-one (NS7051) attenuates nociceptive transmission in animal models of experimental pain; a pharmacological comparison with the combined mu-opioid receptor agonist and monoamine reuptake inhibitor tramadol. Neuropharmacology 2008, 54: 331-343.

[99] Beer B, Stark J, Krieter P, Czobor P, Beer G, Lippa A, Skolnick P. DOV 216,303, a "triple" reuptake inhibitor: safety, tolerability, and pharmacokinetic profile. J Clin Pharmacol 2004, 44: 1360-1367.

[100] Roose SP, Miyazaki M. Pharmacologic treatment of depression in patients with heart disease. Psychosom Med 2005, 67 Suppl 1: S54-57.

[101] Rascol O, Poewe W, Lees A, Aristin M, Salin L, Juhel N, Waldhauser L, Schindler T; ADVANS study group. Tesofensine (NS 2330), a monoamine reuptake inhibitor, in patients with advanced Parkinson disease and motor fluctuations: the ADVANS Study. Arch Neurol 2008, 65: 577-583.

[102] Hauser RA, Salin L, Juhel N, Konyago VL. Randomized trial of the triple monoamine reuptake inhibitor NS 2330 (tesofensine) in early Parkinson's disease. Mov Disord 2007, 22: 359-365.

[103] Axel AM, Mikkelsen JD, Hansen HH. Tesofensine, a novel triple monoamine reuptake inhibitor, induces appetite suppression by indirect stimulation of alpha1 adrenoceptor and dopamine D1 receptor pathways in the diet-induced obese rat. Neuropsychopharmacology 2010, 35: 1464-1476.

[104] Chernoloz O, El Mansari M, Blier P. Sustained administration of pramipexole modifies the spontaneous firing of dopamine, norepinephrine, and serotonin neurons in the rat brain. Neuropsychopharmacology 2009, 34: 651-661.

[105] Skolnick P, Basile AS. Triple reuptake inhibitors ("broad spectrum" antidepressants). *CNS* Neurol Disord Drug Targets 2007, 6: 141-149.

[106] Chen Z, Skolnick P. Triple uptake inhibitors: therapeutic potential in depression and beyond. Expert Opin Investig Drugs 2007, 16: 1365-1377.

[107] Prins J, Westphal KG, Korte-Bouws GA, Quinton MS, Schreiber R, Olivier B, Korte SM. The potential and limitations of DOV 216,303 as a triple reuptake inhibitor for the treatment of major depression: a microdialysis study in olfactory bulbectomized rats. Pharmacol Biochem Behav 2011, 97: 444-452.

[108] Dutta AK, Gopishetty B, Gogoi S, Ali S, Zhen J, Reith M. The novel trisubstituted pyran derivative D-142 has triple monoamine reuptake inhibitory activity and exerts potent antidepressant-like activity in rodents. Eur J Pharmacol. 2011, 671: 39-44.

[109] Dutta AK, Ghosh B, Biswas S, Reith ME. D-161, a novel pyran-based triple monoamine transporter blocker: behavioral pharmacological evidence for antidepressant-like action. Eur J Pharmacol 2008, 589: 73-79.

[110] Micheli F, Cavanni P, Arban R, Benedetti R, Bertani B, Bettati M, Bettelini L, Bonanomi G, Braggio S, Checchia A, Davalli S, Di Fabio R, Fazzolari E, Fontana S, Marchioro C, Minick D, Negri M, Oliosi B, Read KD, Sartori I, Tedesco G, Tarsi L, Terreni S, Visentini F, Zocchi A, Zonzini L. 1-(Aryl)-6-[alkoxyalkyl]-3-azabicyclo[3.1.0]hexanes and 6-(aryl)-6-[alkoxyalkyl]-3-azabicyclo[3.1.0]hexanes: a new series of potent and selective triple reuptake inhibitors. J Med Chem 2010, 53: 2534-2551.

CHAPTER 11

NEW STRATEGIES FOR THE TREATMENT OF MOOD DISORDERS: VAGUS NERVE STIMULATION FOR THE TREATMENT OF RESISTANT DEPRESSION

STELLA MANTA*, MOSTAFA EL MANSARI, PIERRE BLIER

Laval University, Institut Universitaire en Santé Mentale de Québec (IUSMQ), Québec-City, Québec, Canada

Abstract: Depression is a severe psychiatric disorder, in which a third of patients do not achieve remission, despite the wide variety of therapeutic strategies that are currently available. Vagus nerve stimulation (VNS) has shown promise in treating resistant-depressed patients, and it has been approved as an adjunctive treatment for resistant depression. However, the mechanism of action by which VNS exerts its antidepressant effects has remained elusive. The present chapter was aimed first at introducing VNS, beginning from the anatomy of the vagus nerve, the surgical procedure of the stimulator implantation, and the rationale leading to the use of VNS for the treatment of resistant depression. A second goal of this chapter was to review what has been done so far in clinical and preclinical research, from neuroimaging, neurochemical, molecular and electrophysiological studies, in order to understand the mechanism of action of VNS. These studies reported an effect of VNS on brain regions, such as limbic structures, involved in mood regulation. Furthermore an influence of VNS on all three central monoamine systems (serotonin, norepinephrine, and, dopamine) implicated in the pathophysiology of depression and that are especially targeted by antidepressant medications has been revealed, contributing to the clinical efficacy of this approach. Finally, this chapter described the stimulation parameters of this therapy and the results of different studies aimed at characterizing the optimal VNS parameters to treat resistant depression and to potentially minimize and/or even prevent stimulation-related side effects, thus improving patients' quality of life.

Keywords: Serotonin (5-HT), norepinephrine (NE), depression, antidepressant drugs, electroconvulsive treatment (ECT), A, B, and C-fibes of vagus nerve, nucleus of the solitary tract (NTS) of medulla oblongata (MO), vagus nerve stimulation (VNS).

1. INTRODUCTION

Major depression is a severe psychiatric disorder which carries the greatest burden of all diseases, according to the World Health Organization, in middle and high income countries [1]. Despite a wide variety of treatments that exists for this pathology, half of all patients treated for depression still do not respond adequately to first-line monotherapy [2], and a third of patients will not achieve remission even after several treatment strategies [3]. Additional approaches are thus necessary to improve the treatment outcomes in treatment-resistant depression. As a result, brain stimulation became a good alternative in case of many failed pharmacotherapies. Among the neurostimulation methods, electroconvulsive therapy (ECT) has shown evidence of efficacy and has been used for many decades in the treatment of resistant-depression. More recently, vagus nerve stimulation (VNS), already used for refractory epilepsy, has shown promise in treating resistant-depressed patients who have failed to respond to at least four antidepressant trials and was approved as an adjunctive treatment for refractory depression.

***Address correspondence to Stella Manta**: Laval University, Institut Universitaire en Santé Mentale de Québec (IUSMQ), Québec-City, Québec, Canada; E-mail: stella.manta@hotmail.com

Bruno P Guiard and Eliyahu Dremencov (Eds)

2. THE VAGUS NERVE ANATOMY

The vagus nerve, also named cranial nerve X, is part of the cranial parasympathetic branch of the autonomic nervous system. The vagus nerves are composed of A-, B-, and C-fibers based on their diameter and myelination. The A-fibers are the largest and most myelinated vagal fibers with the lowest excitation threshold (0.02-0.2 mA). The myelinated B-fibers have a higher threshold to be excited (0.04-0.6 mA). Finally, the C-fibers are the smallest, unmyelinated, and with the highest excitation threshold (> 2 mA; [4, 5]). Thus, following a stimulation, A-fibers are recruited first followed by B-, and then C-fibers. Early animal studies of the therapeutic mechanisms of VNS for epilepsy indicated that activation of vagal C-fibers was not necessary for VNS to suppress seizures [6], suggesting the implication of only vagal A- and B-fibers in the action of VNS. This is consistent with the therapeutic parameters settings used in humans that are below the C-fibers activation threshold.

The parasympathetic efferents of the vagus nerve emerge from the dorsal vagal nucleus and nucleus ambiguus in the medulla and innervate striated muscles of the pharynx and larynx and also project to the heart, lung, stomach, intestines, liver, pancreas, and kidneys. The vagus nerves are asymmetric with respect to their cardiovascular efferents that regulate heart rate and blood pressure. The left vagus nerve innervates the ventricles while the right vagus nerve innervates more densely the atria. Vagus nerve stimulation therapy is thus conducted on the left vagus nerve to avoid effects on cardiac rhythms. Furthermore, the vagus nerve is in fact a mixed nerve composed predominantly of about 80% afferents fibers transmitting information to the brain [7].

The majority of vagal afferents synapse in the nucleus of the solitary tract (NTS) within the medulla and each vagus nerve innervates the NTS bilaterally. The NTS then, through indirect and direct projections, relays information in multiple brain regions that are implicated in mood regulation, seizure activity, and other functions [4]. Among these regions affected by vagus nerve afferences, and that are associated with psychiatric disorders are principally the locus coeruleus, raphe nuclei, amygdala, hypothalamus, thalamus, hippocampus, orbito-frontal cortex and cingulate gyrus (Figure **1**) [8-10]. It was therefore clear that altering input from the vagus nerve could have far reaching effects in these brain areas as well as in structures innervated by these areas.

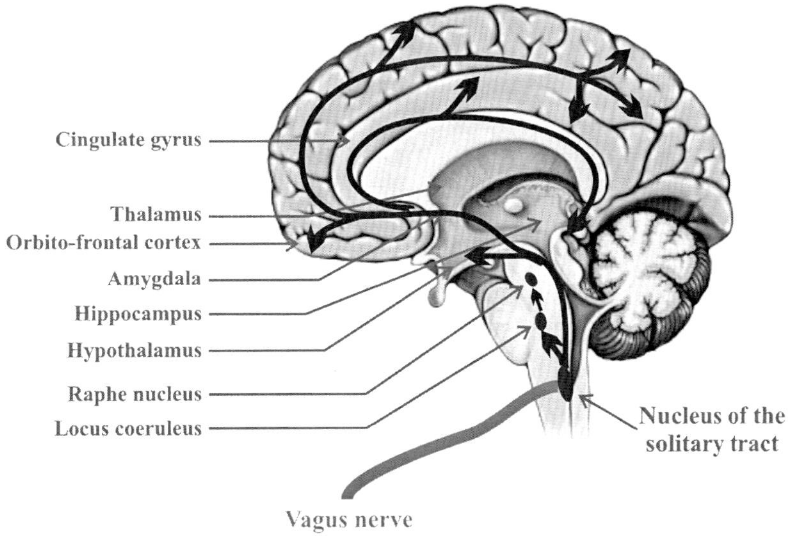

Figure 1. The VNS therapy system and implantation location.

3. THE VAGUS NERVE STIMULATION

3.1. THE PROCEDURE

The VNS therapy is accomplished through a surgical procedure most commonly performed by a neurosurgeon under general or local anesthesia. The surgery, that lasts 30 minutes to 1 hour, consists of implanting subcutaneously a pulse generator, which looks like a pacemaker, in patient's upper left chest. Two helical electrodes are wrapped around the left vagus nerve after making an incision at the level of the neck and are then connected to the pulse generator *via* a subcutaneous tunnel (Figure **2**). After one or two weeks of recovery, the device is turned on and can be programmed non-invasively using a programming wand (held over the chest wall at the location level of the generator) that communicates information from a hand-held PDA *via* telemetry. The different parameters of stimulation that can be modified are the current intensity in milliamperes, the frequency of stimulation in hertz, the pulse width (PW) in μseconds, and the ON and OFF periods of stimulation. The device can also be turned ON or OFF temporarily and magnetically. Indeed, patients are given a magnet that is able to shut off the generator when held over it and when the magnet is removed the pulse generator restarts automatically with the same parameters settings as before the interruption. This manipulation permit patients to momentarily prevent the side effects related to the stimulation such as voice tremor during public speaking or mild shortness of breath during heavy exercising [10]. The pulse generator works with a battery the life of which depends on the generator model, stimulation parameters, lead impedance, and use of the magnet. The most recent model, the demipulse Model 103, has an average expected longevity of 6 to 8 years, after then it needs to be replaced.

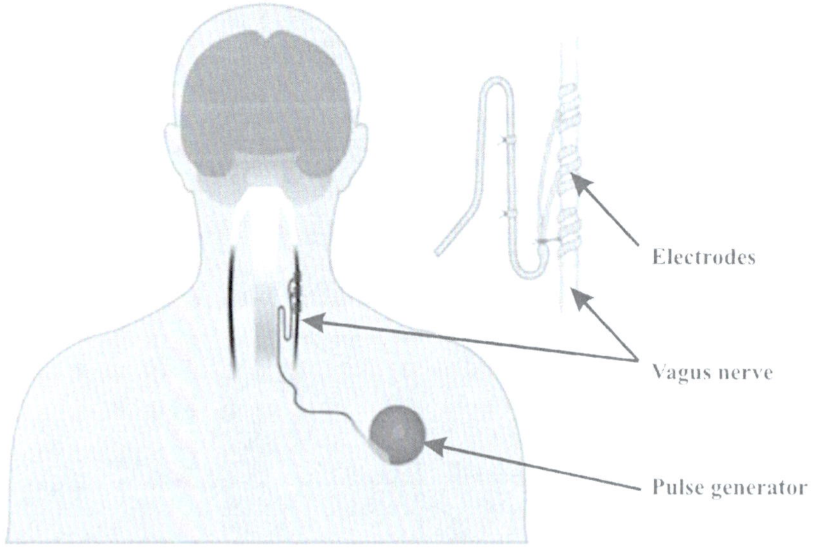

Figure 2. Shematic projections of vagal afferents in the nucleus of the solitary tract which relays information in many brain regions including the locus coeruleus, raphe nucleus, hypothalamus, hippocampus, amygdala, thalamus, orbito-frontal cortex and cingulated gyrus.

3.2. VNS AND EPILEPSY

The history of VNS began in the nineteenth century when an American neurologist, James L. Corning, found that applying a pressure on the carotid artery associated with transcutaneous vagus nerve stimulation could stop seizure. These techniques were, however, not adopted by other neurologists and abandoned in the late 19th century [11]. Then in 1938, Bailey and Bremer reintroduced the notion of VNS by showing a synchronized activity in the orbital cortex of the cat elicited by stimulation of the vagus [12]. In 1951, VNS was shown to evoke a slow-wave response in the anterior rhinal sulcus and in the amygdala of awake cats [13]. Cortical and subcortical electroencephalographic (EEG) changes were noticed in animals undergoing afferent vagal stimulation [14, 15]. Finally, in 1985, Zabara showed that VNS stopped experimental motor seizures in dogs [16] and the first human implant of the VNS device to treat intractable epilepsy was reported in 1988 [17], followed by many others human studies.

Two single-blind pilot studies were conducted on 14 patients with medically refractory partial seizures treated by VNS. A decrease in seizure frequency was reported with both short-term and long-term VNS delivery and with very few side effects, primarily limited to hoarseness and tingling sensation at the electrode site when the stimulator was activated [18]. At that time, two multicenter randomized double-blind studies [19, 20] were started in patients with resistant epilepsy with a total of 313 completers. These studies were also aimed at investigating high (30 Hz, 500 μseconds PW, and 30 seconds ON-5 minutes OFF) versus low (1 Hz, 130 μseconds PW, and 30 seconds ON-90 to 180 minutes OFF) stimulation paradigms over a 12- to 16-week period. Both studies showed a higher impact of high frequency VNS group with about 30 % decrease in seizure frequency compared to baseline, while the low frequency VNS group showed only 10 to 15% reduction. As a result, VNS therapy was approved as an adjunctive treatment for refractory epilepsy in Europe in 1994 and in the United States and Canada in 1997.

Long-term studies then showed an increase efficacy of VNS over time with more patients reaching 50 % or more seizure reduction after 2 or 3 years of treatment, whereas adverse events became less common [21]. VNS therapy then became a well established treatment for refractory epilepsy and there are now over 50 000 people implanted worldwide. Interestingly, soon after the approval of VNS for epilepsy, preliminary reports found a mood improvement in patients with epilepsy receiving VNS and even in those with no reduction of seizure, thus leading to the investigation of the potential efficacy of VNS to treat resistant-depression [22, 23].

4. VNS IN THE TREATMENT OF RESISTANT-DEPRESSION

4.1. RATIONALE

The idea of investigating VNS in the treatment of resistant-depression was based on several factors. First, as reported previously, the positive effects of VNS on the mood of patients with epilepsy, with no correlation with their improvement of seizure, was an important clue [22, 23]. These findings were also relevant with the common use of anticonvulsivant medications (such as carbamazepine, valproate or lamotrigine) as mood stabilizers and/or antidepressant in bipolar disorders [24, 25]. Furthermore, neuroimaging studies reported that VNS was able to alter the functional activity of cortical and subcortical brain regions and particularly limbic structures [26]. Other findings reported an effect of VNS on brain regions associated with norepinephrine [27] and serotonin [28] (the locus coeruleus and dorsal raphe, respectively) which are two keys neurotransmitters implicated in the pathophysiology of depression and that are targeted by antidepressant medications. Thus, both basic and clinical evidence provided a rationale for the use of VNS in the treatment of mood disorders.

4.2. CLINICAL STUDIES

The first open label multicenter trial of VNS for depression enrolled 30 patients with severe non psychotic treatment-resistant depression who had failed at least two robust antidepressant medications, and who had a current major depressive episode (MDE) longer than 2 years in duration or the patients had to have more than 4 MDEs in their lifetime (Table **1**). The patients were monitored during 10

Study	Authors	Type	Nb of patients	Duration	Response rate*	Remission rate*
	Rush *et al*, 2000	Open label	30	10 weeks	**40 %**	**17 %**
	Marangell *et al*, 2002	Open label	30	12 months	**46 %**	**29 %**
D-01	Sackeim *et al*, 2001	Open label	59	10 weeks	**31 %**	**15 %**
	Nahas *et al*, 2005	Open label	59	12 months	**44 %**	**27 %**
				24 months	**42 %**	**22 %**
D-02	Rush *et al*, 2005a	Randomized Double-blind acute phase trial	112 active VNS	10 weeks	Active VNS **15.2 %**	-
			110 Sham		Sham group **10 %**	-
	Rush *et al*, 2005b	Open label	202	12 months	**27 %**	**16 %**
D-03	Shlaepfer *et al*, 2008	Open label	74	3 months	**37 %**	**17 %**
				12 months	**53 %**	**33 %**
	Bajbouj *et al*, 2010	Open label	49	24 months	**53 %**	**39 %**
D-04	George *et al*, 2005	Open label	205 VNS +TAU	12 months	**27 %**	-
			124 TAU		**13 %**	-

* Response and remission rates are according to the 24 or 28-item HDRS
VNS = Vagus nerve stimulation
TAU = Treatment as usual

Table 1: VNS studies in treatment-resistant depression.

weeks, with the device at stable stimulation settings for the last 8 weeks. The response was determined as showing a ≥ 50 % decrease in depression scores compared to the pre-trial level using the 28-item Hamilton Rating Depression Scale (HDRS28), the 10-item Montgomery-Åsberg Depression Rating Scale (MADRS), and the Clinical Global Impression-Severity (CGI-S) and -Improvement (CGI-I) indices. Interestingly, the response rates reached 40 % by the HDRS28 and CGI and 50 % on the MADRS, while the remission rate was 17 % based on the HDRS28 [29]. Given the small sample size, these findings were preliminary but were suggesting an antidepressant effect of VNS in treatment-resistant depression.

Additional larger studies then quickly followed. Sackeim and colleagues in 2001 extended the previous open pilot study to include 30 additional patients. The response rate of the combined studies (labeled D-01), after 10 weeks of VNS, was 31 % for the HDRS28, 34 % for the MADRS, and 37 % according to the CGI [30]. The study was also investigating the profile of side effects which were principally voice alteration or hoarseness that were generally mild, well tolerated, and related to the current intensity of the stimulation. Patients could also experience coughing and shortness of breath (dyspnea) during exercise and pain in the neck, again related to output current intensity. However, side effects that are usually associated with antidepressant medications such as sexual dysfunction, dry mouth, urinary retention, and weight gain were not noticed with VNS. In contrast to ECT, which has adverse cognitive effects, VNS is more associated with cognitive improvements [30].

As the previous studies were somewhat short-term and considering the increased efficacy of VNS over time in patients with epilepsy [21], the patients from the acute, open-label phase were then followed for 2 years. After 1 year follow-up, the HDRS28 response rates increased from 31% at 3 months to 44 % and the remission rates from 15 % after 3 months of VNS to 27 % after 12 months [31, 32]. After 2 years of VNS, the response and remission rates were not significantly changed, but the benefits achieved after 12 months of VNS were largely sustained while side effects of the therapy were diminished [32].

Similar results were then obtained recently in the D-03 multicenter European study after 3, 12, and 24 months of VNS in patients with treatment-resistant major depressive disorders. The percentage of patients that met the criteria for response on the HDRS28 was 37 % after 3 months of VNS delivery, 53 % after 12 and 24 months while the percentage of patients that fulfilled the remission criteria was 17 % after 3 months of VNS, increased to 33 % after 12 months, and reached 39 % after 24 months [33, 34].

The positive results of the open-label studies supported the probable antidepressant effects of VNS. Thus, a subsequent randomized, sham-controlled double-blind trial of VNS (labeled D-02) was conducted in 2005 by Rush and colleagues [35]. The study design was similar to that of the original study and compared adjunctive VNS (stimulator turned on) with sham (stimulator left off) treatment in 235 outpatients with nonpsychotic major depressive disorder (n=210) or in the depressed phase of bipolar disorder (n=25). However, at the end of the 10-week stimulation period, no statistical significant difference was found between the group undergoing active VNS, with a 15 % response rate, and in the sham group, with a 10 % response rate. A significant improvement in the 30-item Inventory of Depressive Symptomatology Self-Report was nevertheless significantly improved in the active VNS versus sham group (17 % and 7 %, respectively). This study thus failed to yield definitive evidence of short-term efficacy for adjunctive VNS in treatment resistant depression. Possible explanations for the failure of VNS to separate from sham might have been an inadequate dosing of the VNS compared to D-01 and D-03 and also an inadequate duration of the trial. Thus, after 3 months, the patients in the sham arm had the stimulators turned on for 12 months and the patients already with active VNS were given 9 additional months of treatment. During that period, both antidepressant treatments and VNS could be adjusted. That study demonstrated a response rate of 27 % and a remission rate of 16 %, revealing a statistically significant reduction in depressive symptoms and suggesting a potential long-term, growing benefit in treatment resistant-depression [36]. To determine whether these benefits were attributable to VNS or to changes in depression treatments, the previous reports that described the effects of 12-month VNS plus treatment as usual (VNS+TAU) was compared with a treatment-resistant depression group receiving only TAU (D-04 study). Both groups received similar TAU (drugs and ECT) during follow-up. Response rates, according to the 24-item HDRS were 27 % for VNS+TAU and 13 % for TAU thus showing that VNS+TAU was associated with a greater antidepressant benefit over 12 months [37]. It is also interesting to note that despite the wide range of treatment options available for depression, the response rates, remission rates, and quality-of-life of most patients with a substantial degree of treatment-resistance have a very low probability of sustained treatment response, even after 2 years when receiving TAU that includes any therapeutic strategies [38]. For example, when remission is achieved with ECT, the relapse rate in the following 12 months is estimated to be 60-70% among patients who have not responded to one or more adequate antidepressant trials [39]. In contrast, among the 30 % of patients responding to VNS within the first year, approximately two-thirds maintained clinical benefit through 21 months of follow-up which is a remarkably high rate regarding the treatment-resistance of the patients involved [40].

As a result, VNS, which had already been accepted in Canada and Europe since 2001, was finally approved by the US Food and Drug Administration in 2005 as an adjunctive therapy for the treatment of nonpsychotic unipolar or bipolar depressed patients that have failed to respond to at least four antidepressant trials. Afterward, the studies that followed, as well clinical or preclinical, were mostly aimed at understanding the mechanism of action by which acts VNS in treating resistant-depression.

4.3. MECHANISM OF ACTION

The mechanisms of action of VNS for the treatment of resistant-depression are still not completely understood but diverse clues, from imaging or neurochemical and electrophysiological studies, are regularly added to the scheme to provide a global idea of how that therapy works.

4.3.1. Neuroimaging.

Functional neuroimaging studies have been widely used as an investigative tool for shedding light on how VNS works in epilepsy and depression by identifying the brain regions affected by VNS therapy.

Before the study of VNS for treatment of resistant-depression, positron emission tomography (PET) imaging already demonstrated significant blood flow decreases, equivalent to reductions in the metabolic activity, in limbic structures such as the amygdala, the hippocampus, and cingulate gyrus [26]. These brain limbic structures are involved in mood regulation, as shown by PET imaging, in depressed patients treated with antidepressants. Indeed, chronic treatment and clinical response to antidepressants have been shown to be associated with a reciprocal pattern of subcortical and limbic decreases and cortical increases in brain glucose metabolism [41, 42]. A smaller PET study on four patients with resistant-depression reported the increase induced by acute VNS in regional cerebral blood flow in cortical areas such as the bilateral orbitofrontal cortex, bilateral anterior cingulated cortex, and right superior and medial frontal cortex [43]. Longer-term effects of VNS for depression were also investigated. Single photon emission computed tomography (SPECT) after 4 weeks of VNS revealed a reduction in regional cerebral blood flow in the limbic system and associated regions, particularly the hippocampus, amygdala, subgenual and ventral anterior cingulum, posterior orbitofrontal cortex and interior inferior temporal lobes similar to that ocerved in pharmacological studies [44]. The only increase in blood flow from that study was found in the middle frontal gyrus, a region that is activated in responders in some pharmacological studies [41, 44, 45]. After 10 weeks of VNS, blood flow was also shown by SPECT to be increase in the dorsolateral/ventromedial prefrontal cortex, which was associated to an improvement of depression [46].

Functional magnetic resonance imaging (fMRI), which has a high spatial and temporal resolution, has also been used to study patients with depression treated with VNS. Changes following acute VNS were observed in hypothalamus, orbitofrontal cortex, amygdala, hippocampus, medial prefrontal cortex and cingulated gyrus [47]. Several fMRI studies were also used to investigate acute immediate regional brain activity changes with different stimulation parameters [48, 49].

4.3.2. Neurochemical, molecular and electrophysiological studies

The antidepressant effects of VNS have been shown in patients with resistant-depression but understanding the mechanisms of action of this therapy for depression could be enhanced by animal studies. Thus, rats undergoing VNS were tested in the forced-swim test (FST) which is a standard validated predictor of clinical antidepressant action [50]. The significant reduction of the immobility time in the FST model in rats receiving VNS demonstrated the antidepressant-like effects of VNS in animals [51, 52].

Many findings suggesting the role for VNS in the treatment of resistant-depression were supported by alterations in brain regions affected by VNS that are associated with the norepinephrine (NE) and serotonin (5-HT) systems such as the locus coeruleus (LC) and dorsal raphe nucleus (DRN), respectively. Indeed, lesioning the LC, which is the main source of NE, has been shown to suppress the seizure-attenuating effect of VNS in rats, suggesting the major implication of NE in the therapeutic action of VNS to suppress seizure [27]. The 5-HT metabolite, 5-hydroxyindoleacetic acid (5-HIAA), was increased by 33 % in the cerebrospinal fluid (CSF) of patients undergoing 3 months of VNS [28]. Another study conducted on 21 treatment-resistant depressed patients did not reveal significant changes in CSF NE, 5-HIAA after 12 or 24 weeks of active VNS versus sham group but, interestingly, a significant VNS-associated increase in CSF homovanillic acid (HVA), the metabolite of dopamine (DA) was reported [53]. Higher levels of extracellular DA are also been reported, using *in vivo* microdialysis in rats, after chronic VNS in the prefrontal cortex and nucleus accumbens, which plays an important role in reward and hedonia [54]. This was of interest because DA has also been suggested to be implicated in the pathophysiology of depression [55] and lower concentrations of DA and its metabolite HVA had been reported in the CSF of depressed patients [56, 57].

Regarding NE and 5-HT systems in animal studies, acute VNS was shown to produce an increase of the biomarker of short-term neuronal activation c-fos in several rat brain regions including the LC but not the DRN. In contrast, an activation of the DRN was revealed by an enhancement of another gene product specific to delayed and persistent neuronal activation, delta fosB, only after prolonged VNS treatment [51]. These data were consistent with electrophysiological studies that previously showed that one hour of VNS increases the basal firing activity of LC NE neurons and secondarily that of DRN 5-HT neurons but only after 14 days [58, 59]. An additional increase in firing rates of 5-HT neurons after three months of VNS was also reported [58] and reflected the effect seen in clinical depression studies in which mean HDRS for Depression scores tend to decrease progressively over time, suggesting a time-dependent improvement [31-33]. The robust effect of VNS on NE system was also revealed by the *in vivo* microdialysis technique, showing an significant increase in extracellular NE levels in the hippocampus and prefrontal cortex after acute or chronic VNS [54, 60-62].

The effects of VNS on the 5-HT system had appeared to be indirect and mediated through its effect in enhancing the firing rate and pattern of NE neurons since a lesion of LC NE neurons, by the noradrenergic toxin DSP-4, completely prevented the increase of 5-HT neuronal firing rate after chronic VNS [63]. A proposed mechanism is that this effect was mediated through the vagus nerve projections to the NTS, which in turn projects to the LC. The LC would then modify the firing rate of 5-HT neurons through its monosynaptic input to the DRN *via* α 1-adrenergic receptors which have their degree of activation enhanced following chronic VNS [63]. The resulting increase in DRN 5-HT neuronal firing rate would then affect postsynaptic projection areas and importantly the hippocampus. Indeed, the hippocampus is a structure that appears central in the mediation of the therapeutic effect of various classes of antidepressant treatments [64, 65]. More specifically, the degree of activation of postsynaptic 5-HT 1A receptors in this brain region is enhanced after long-term administration of a variety of antidepressant strategies, including electroconvulsive shock [65, 66]. After long-term VNS, the tonic activation of these hippocampal 5-HT 1A postsynaptic receptors has also been reported to be enhanced, translating into an increased 5-HT transmission in the rat hippocampus following VNS [63].

Still at the hippocampus level, a two-day VNS delivery increased the dentate gyrus BrdU-incorporation, which reflects an increase in progenitor proliferation [67]. Chronic VNS was then recently found to prevent the decrease of the number of BrdU positive cells in the dentate gyrus in a validated model of depression, the olfactory bulbectomized rats [68]. As well, acute VNS was found to increase the expression of brain derived neurotrophic factor (BDNF) and fibroblast growth factor in that area (Figure **3**) [60]. Chronic VNS was then shown to induce long-lasting increases in the amount of BDNF immunoreactivity [69]. Interestingly, both of the previous factors are important modulators of hippocampal plasticity and neurogenesis that are also required for the behavioural effects of antidepressants [64].

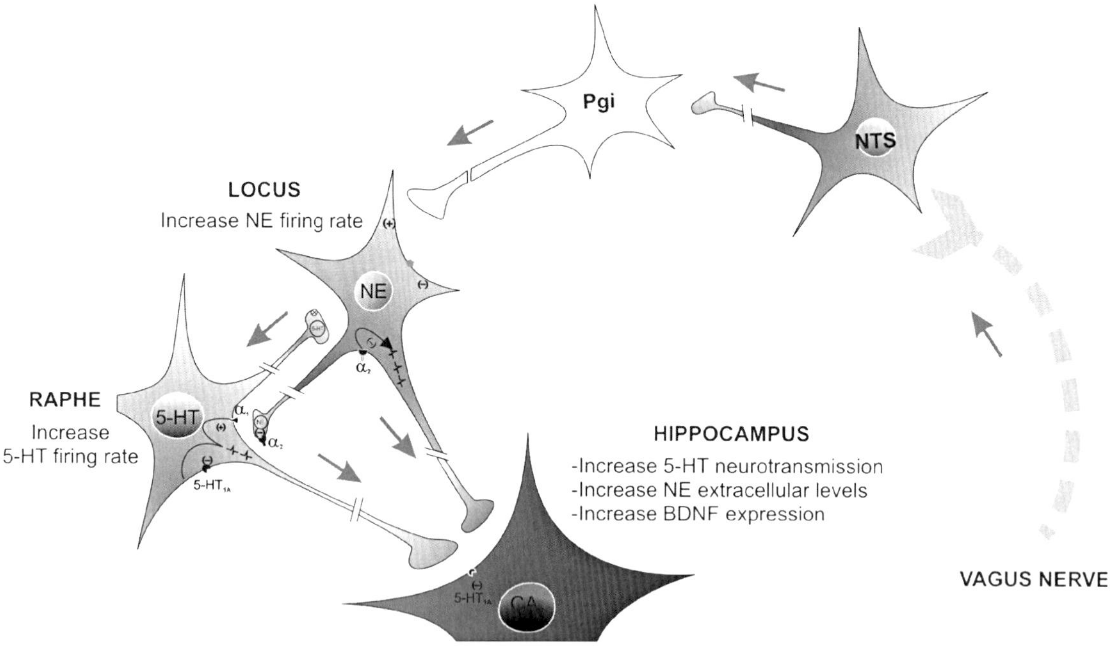

Figure 3. Putative mechanisms of VNS in resistant-depression.
The vagus nerve sends afferents to the nucleus tractus solitarius (NTS), which in turn projects to the locus coeruleus (LC) through the nucleus paragigantocellularis (PgI). The LC, which has an increased firing activity, would then modify the firing rate of 5-HT neurons through its monosynaptic input to the raphe *via* excitatory α 1-adrenoceptors. This will lead to a net enhancement of 5-HT transmission in the hippocampus.

VNS therapy has also been shown to influence sleep. Sleep disturbances are part of the diagnostic criteria in the DSM-IV for major depressive disorder with more than 80 % of depressed inpatients and 40 to 60 % of outpatients reporting troubles in initiating and maintaining sleep, as well as feeling fatigued upon awakening [70]. The effect of VNS on sleep EEG in depression showed an improvement in sleep architecture with sleep EEG rhythms restored to near normal after VNS treatment [71].

Thus, even if the mechanism of action of VNS in treating resistant-depression is still not completely understood, both preclinical and clinical studies reported many changes following VNS and notably in brain regions, and neurotransmitters that are especially targeted by antidepressant medications.

4.4. STIMULATION PARAMETERS

The device is multi-programmable and stimulation parameters include output current (in mA), frequency (in Hz), pulse width (in μsec), and stimulation periods that can be modified for each patient to maximize the effectiveness of VNS on disease state.

In 1992, an animal study was conducted in dogs using EEG and EMG to determine the most effective parameters for epilepsy [72]. These parameters were then employed in the initial clinical trials for epilepsy [19, 20] and also adopted for clinical trials in patients with depression [16, 29, 30, 73].

Reports from clinical studies suggested that modifying stimulation parameters could increase the efficacy of VNS in refractory patients and/or modify its effects on brain functions. Indeed, using neuroimaging techniques in depressed patients, VNS was shown to activate brain regions to a greater extent when applied at 20 Hz than at 5 Hz [48]. As well, using the same technique, a pulse width of 130 μseconds has been reported to be insufficient for activation of certain regions compared to the 250 or 500 μsecond ones [49].

To date, typical therapeutic settings to treat resistant-depression range from 1.0 to 1.5 mA for the output current, the frequency is usually 20 Hz, the pulse width range from 250 to 500 μsec and the recommended ON time is 30 seconds followed by 5 minutes OFF [74].

Even if VNS has proven to be efficient in about a third of treatment-resistant depressed patients, further studies are still necessary to further improve the success rate of this therapy. Thus, electrophysiological experiments have been conducted on the rat brain to test whereby variations of the standard parameters currently used in the clinic could better increase the firing activity of 5-HT neurons. These experiments indicated that the optimal VNS parameters that activate 5-HT neurons were the ones routinely used in the clinic to treat resistant depression and that increasing to much the charge deliver to nerve led to a loss of the effects of VNS in increasing 5-HT neuronal firing [75]. A subsequent study, using the same paradigm, showed that 12 hours of stimulation per day or 30 seconds stimulation every 10 or 15 minutes, as well as stimulation in a burst mode (that were the equivalent of a global stimulation of 1 or 2 Hz in terms of total number of pulses) were as effective as standard parameters to increase 5-HT neuronal firing rate [76]. Even if these experiments did not reveal a further augmentation of the firing rate of 5-HT neurons, these new parameters could be interesting in the clinic to potentially minimize and/or even prevent side effects, which are related to the stimulation in VNS-responsive patients. To date, these parameters have not been yet tested in the clinic.

4.5. OTHER CLINICAL APPLICATIONS

Beside its proven efficacy and use for resistant epilepsy and depression, VNS was proposed to have potential for treatment for other clinical conditions. Indeed, VNS may play a role in pain modulation

[77, 78], be effective in enhancing cognition in patients with Alzheimer's disease [79, 80], be beneficial in the treatment of migraines [81, 82], and obesity [83]. VNS could also be implicated in improvement of cerebellar tremor and dysphagia in multiple sclerosis [84]. This variety of possible application for VNS reflects the wide range of functions of the vagus nerve and need to be further investigated.

5. CONCLUSION

Even if VNS therapy is an approved adjunctive treatment for resistant-depression, further research is still needed to further improve the response and remission rates of patients or further improve their quality of life, maybe by targeting stimulation parameters.

The reason why this therapy is effective in patients that have failed to respond to many antidepressant strategies is still not fully understood but many studies have been and are being conducted to elucidate the mechanism of action by which VNS exerts its antidepressant effects. Understanding entirely the mechanism of action of VNS could also eventually lead to clues toward novel ways to treat depression.

REFERENCES

[1] World Health Organization. The global burden of diseases. 2004 Update. WHO press. 2008, part 4:40-51.

[2] Hirschfeld RM, Montgomery SA, Aguglia E, Amore M, Delgado PL, Gastpar M, Hawley C, Kasper S, Linden M, Massana J, Mendlewicz J, Moller HJ, Nemeroff CB, Saiz J, Such P, Torta R, Versiani M. Partial response and nonresponse to antidepressant therapy: current approaches and treatment options. J Clin Psychiatry 2002, 63:826-37.

[3] Rush AJ, Trivedi MH, Wisniewski SR, Nierenberg AA, Stewart JW, Warden D, Niederehe G, Thase ME, Lavori PW, Lebowitz BD, McGrath PJ, Rosenbaum JF, Sackeim HA, Kupfer DJ, Luther J, Fava M. Acute and longer-term outcomes in depressed outpatients requiring one or several treatment steps: a STAR*D report. Am J Psychiatry 2006, 163:1905-17.

[4] Henry TR. Therapeutic mechanisms of vagus nerve stimulation. Neurology 2002, 59:S3-14.

[5] Woodbury DM, Woodbury JW. Effects of vagal stimulation on experimentally induced seizures in rats. Epilepsia 1990, 31 Suppl 2:S7-19.

[6] Krahl SE, Senanayake SS, Handforth A. Destruction of peripheral C-fibers does not alter subsequent vagus nerve stimulation-induced seizure suppression in rats. Epilepsia 2001, 42:586-9.

[7] Foley JO, Dubois F. Quantitative studies of the vagus nerve in the cat. I: The ratio of sensory and motor studies. J Comp Neurol 1937, 67:49-67.

[8] Rutecki P. Anatomical, physiological, and theoretical basis for the antiepileptic effect of vagus nerve stimulation. Epilepsia 1990, 31 Suppl 2:S1-6.

[9] Van Bockstaele EJ, Peoples J, Telegan P. Efferent projections of the nucleus of the solitary tract

to peri-locus coeruleus dendrites in rat brain: evidence for a monosynaptic pathway. J Comp Neurol 1999, 412:410-28.

[10] George MS, Rush AJ, Sackeim HA, Marangell LB. Vagus nerve stimulation (VNS): utility in neuropsychiatric disorders. Int J Neuropsychopharmacol 2003, 6:73-83.

[11] Lanska DJ. J.L. Corning and vagal nerve stimulation for seizures in the 1880s. Neurology 2002, 58:452-9.

[12] Bailey P, Bremer F. A Sensory Cortical Representation of the Vagus Nerve. Journal of Neurophysiology 1938, 1:405-12.

[13] Dell P, Olson R. [Secondary mesencephalic, diencephalic and amygdalian projections of vagal visceral afferences]. C R Seances Soc Biol Fil 1951, 145:1088-91.

[14] Zanchetti A, Wang SC, Moruzzi G. The effect of vagal afferent stimulation on the EEG pattern of the cat. Electroencephalogr Clin Neurophysiol 1952, 4:357-61.

[15] Chase MH, Sterman MB, Clemente CD. Cortical and subcortical patterns of response to afferent vagal stimulation. Exp Neurol 1966, 16:36-49.

[16] George MS, Sackeim HA, Rush AJ, Marangell LB, Nahas Z, Husain MM, Lisanby S, Burt T, Goldman J, Ballenger JC. Vagus nerve stimulation: a new tool for brain research and therapy. Biol Psychiatry 2000, 47:287-95.

[17] Penry JK, Dean JC. Prevention of intractable partial seizures by intermittent vagal stimulation in humans: preliminary results. Epilepsia 1990, 31 Suppl 2:S40-3.

[18] Uthman BM, Wilder BJ, Penry JK, Dean C, Ramsay RE, Reid SA, Hammond EJ, Tarver WB, Wernicke JF. Treatment of epilepsy by stimulation of the vagus nerve. Neurology 1993, 43:1338-45.

[19] Ben-Menachem E, Manon-Espaillat R, Ristanovic R, Wilder BJ, Stefan H, Mirza W, Tarver WB, Wernicke JF. Vagus nerve stimulation for treatment of partial seizures: 1. A controlled study of effect on seizures. First International Vagus Nerve Stimulation Study Group. Epilepsia 1994, 35:616-26.

[20] Handforth A, DeGiorgio CM, Schachter SC, Uthman BM, Naritoku DK, Tecoma ES, Henry TR, Collins SD, Vaughn BV, Gilmartin RC, Labar DR, Morris GL, 3rd, Salinsky MC, Osorio I, Ristanovic RK, Labiner DM, Jones JC, Murphy JV, Ney GC, Wheless JW. Vagus nerve stimulation therapy for partial-onset seizures: a randomized active-control trial. Neurology 1998, 51:48-55.

[21] Morris GL, 3rd, Mueller WM. Long-term treatment with vagus nerve stimulation in patients with refractory epilepsy. The Vagus Nerve Stimulation Study Group E01-E05. Neurology 1999, 53:1731-5.

[22] Elger G, Hoppe C, Falkai P, Rush AJ, Elger CE. Vagus nerve stimulation is associated with mood improvements in epilepsy patients. Epilepsy Res 2000, 42:203-10.

[23] Harden CL, Pulver MC, Ravdin LD, Nikolov B, Halper JP, Labar DR. A Pilot Study of Mood in Epilepsy Patients Treated with Vagus Nerve Stimulation. Epilepsy Behav 2000, 1:93-9.

[24] Post RM, Ketter TA, Denicoff K, Pazzaglia PJ, Leverich GS, Marangell LB, Callahan AM,

George MS, Frye MA. The place of anticonvulsant therapy in bipolar illness. Psychopharmacology (Berl) 1996, 128:115-29.

[25] Calabrese JR, Bowden CL, Sachs GS, Ascher JA, Monaghan E, Rudd GD. A double-blind placebo-controlled study of lamotrigine monotherapy in outpatients with bipolar I depression. Lamictal 602 Study Group. J Clin Psychiatry 1999, 60:79-88.

[26] Henry TR, Bakay RA, Votaw JR, Pennell PB, Epstein CM, Faber TL, Grafton ST, Hoffman JM. Brain blood flow alterations induced by therapeutic vagus nerve stimulation in partial epilepsy: I. Acute effects at high and low levels of stimulation. Epilepsia 1998, 39:983-90.

[27] Krahl SE, Clark KB, Smith DC, Browning RA. Locus coeruleus lesions suppress the seizure-attenuating effects of vagus nerve stimulation. Epilepsia 1998, 39:709-14.

[28] Ben-Menachem E, Hamberger A, Hedner T, Hammond EJ, Uthman BM, Slater J, Treig T, Stefan H, Ramsay RE, Wernicke JF, *et al.* Effects of vagus nerve stimulation on amino acids and other metabolites in the CSF of patients with partial seizures. Epilepsy Res 1995, 20:221-7.

[29] Rush AJ, George MS, Sackeim HA, Marangell LB, Husain MM, Giller C, Nahas Z, Haines S, Simpson RK, Jr., Goodman R. Vagus nerve stimulation (VNS) for treatment-resistant depressions: a multicenter study. Biol Psychiatry 2000, 47:276-86.

[30] Sackeim HA, Rush AJ, George MS, Marangell LB, Husain MM, Nahas Z, Johnson CR, Seidman S, Giller C, Haines S, Simpson RK, Jr., Goodman RR. Vagus nerve stimulation (VNS) for treatment-resistant depression: efficacy, side effects, and predictors of outcome. Neuropsychopharmacology 2001, 25:713-28.

[31] Marangell LB, Rush AJ, George MS, Sackeim HA, Johnson CR, Husain MM, Nahas Z, Lisanby SH. Vagus nerve stimulation (VNS) for major depressive episodes: one year outcomes. Biol Psychiatry 2002, 51:280-7.

[32] Nahas Z, Marangell LB, Husain MM, Rush AJ, Sackeim HA, Lisanby SH, Martinez JM, George MS. Two-year outcome of vagus nerve stimulation (VNS) for treatment of major depressive episodes. J Clin Psychiatry 2005, 66:1097-104.

[33] Bajbouj M, Merkl A, Schlaepfer TE, Frick C, Zobel A, Maier W, O'Keane V, Corcoran C, Adolfsson R, Trimble M, Rau H, Hoff HJ, Padberg F, Muller-Siecheneder F, Audenaert K, van den Abbeele D, Matthews K, Christmas D, Eljamel S, Heuser I. Two-year outcome of vagus nerve stimulation in treatment-resistant depression. J Clin Psychopharmacol 2010, 30:273-81.

[34] Schlaepfer TE, Frick C, Zobel A, Maier W, Heuser I, Bajbouj M, O'Keane V, Corcoran C, Adolfsson R, Trimble M, Rau H, Hoff HJ, Padberg F, Muller-Siecheneder F, Audenaert K, Van den Abbeele D, Stanga Z, Hasdemir M. Vagus nerve stimulation for depression: efficacy and safety in a European study. Psychol Med 2008, 38:651-61.

[35] Rush AJ, Marangell LB, Sackeim HA, George MS, Brannan SK, Davis SM, Howland R, Kling MA, Rittberg BR, Burke WJ, Rapaport MH, Zajecka J, Nierenberg AA, Husain MM, Ginsberg D, Cooke RG. Vagus nerve stimulation for treatment-resistant depression: a randomized, controlled acute phase trial. Biol Psychiatry 2005, 58:347-54.

[36] Rush AJ, Sackeim HA, Marangell LB, George MS, Brannan SK, Davis SM, Lavori P, Howland

R, Kling MA, Rittberg B, Carpenter L, Ninan P, Moreno F, Schwartz T, Conway C, Burke M, Barry JJ. Effects of 12 months of vagus nerve stimulation in treatment-resistant depression: a naturalistic study. Biol Psychiatry 2005, 58:355-63.

[37] George MS, Rush AJ, Marangell LB, Sackeim HA, Brannan SK, Davis SM, Howland R, Kling MA, Moreno F, Rittberg B, Dunner D, Schwartz T, Carpenter L, Burke M, Ninan P, Goodnick P. A one-year comparison of vagus nerve stimulation with treatment as usual for treatment-resistant depression. Biol Psychiatry 2005, 58:364-73.

[38] Dunner DL, Rush AJ, Russell JM, Burke M, Woodard S, Wingard P, Allen J. Prospective, long-term, multicenter study of the naturalistic outcomes of patients with treatment-resistant depression. J Clin Psychiatry 2006, 67:688-95.

[39] Sackeim HA, Prudic J, Devanand DP, Decina P, Kerr B, Malitz S. The impact of medication resistance and continuation pharmacotherapy on relapse following response to electroconvulsive therapy in major depression. J Clin Psychopharmacol 1990, 10:96-104.

[40] Sackeim HA, Brannan SK, Rush AJ, George MS, Marangell LB, Allen J. Durability of antidepressant response to vagus nerve stimulation (VNS). Int J Neuropsychopharmacol 2007, 10:817-26.

[41] Mayberg HS, Brannan SK, Tekell JL, Silva JA, Mahurin RK, McGinnis S, Jerabek PA. Regional metabolic effects of fluoxetine in major depression: serial changes and relationship to clinical response. Biol Psychiatry 2000, 48:830-43.

[42] Drevets WC, Bogers W, Raichle ME. Functional anatomical correlates of antidepressant drug treatment assessed using PET measures of regional glucose metabolism. Eur Neuropsychopharmacol 2002, 12:527-44.

[43] Conway CR, Sheline YI, Chibnall JT, George MS, Fletcher JW, Mintun MA. Cerebral blood flow changes during vagus nerve stimulation for depression. Psychiatry Res 2006, 146:179-84.

[44] Zobel A, Joe A, Freymann N, Clusmann H, Schramm J, Reinhardt M, Biersack HJ, Maier W, Broich K. Changes in regional cerebral blood flow by therapeutic vagus nerve stimulation in depression: an exploratory approach. Psychiatry Res 2005, 139:165-79.

[45] Kennedy SH, Evans KR, Kruger S, Mayberg HS, Meyer JH, McCann S, Arifuzzman AI, Houle S, Vaccarino FJ. Changes in regional brain glucose metabolism measured with positron emission tomography after paroxetine treatment of major depression. Am J Psychiatry 2001, 158:899-905.

[46] Kosel M, Brockmann H, Frick C, Zobel A, Schlaepfer TE. Chronic vagus nerve stimulation for treatment-resistant depression increases regional cerebral blood flow in the dorsolateral prefrontal cortex. Psychiatry Res 2011, 191:153-9.

[47] Bohning DE, Lomarev MP, Denslow S, Nahas Z, Shastri A, George MS. Feasibility of vagus nerve stimulation-synchronized blood oxygenation level-dependent functional MRI. Invest Radiol 2001, 36:470-9.

[48] Lomarev M, Denslow S, Nahas Z, Chae JH, George MS, Bohning DE. Vagus nerve stimulation (VNS) synchronized BOLD fMRI suggests that VNS in depressed adults has frequency/dose dependent effects. J Psychiatr Res 2002, 36:219-27.

[49] Mu Q, Bohning DE, Nahas Z, Walker J, Anderson B, Johnson KA, Denslow S, Lomarev M, Moghadam P, Chae JH, George MS. Acute vagus nerve stimulation using different pulse widths produces varying brain effects. Biol Psychiatry 2004, 55:816-25.

[50] Lucki I. The forced swimming test as a model for core and component behavioral effects of antidepressant drugs. Behav Pharmacol 1997, 8:523-32.

[51] Cunningham JT, Mifflin SW, Gould GG, Frazer A. Induction of c-Fos and DeltaFosB immunoreactivity in rat brain by Vagal nerve stimulation. Neuropsychopharmacology 2008, 33:1884-95.

[52] Krahl SE, Senanayake SS, Pekary AE, Sattin A. Vagus nerve stimulation (VNS) is effective in a rat model of antidepressant action. J Psychiatr Res 2004, 38:237-40.

[53] Carpenter LL, Moreno FA, Kling MA, Anderson GM, Regenold WT, Labiner DM, Price LH. Effect of vagus nerve stimulation on cerebrospinal fluid monoamine metabolites, norepinephrine, and gamma-aminobutyric acid concentrations in depressed patients. Biol Psychiatry 2004, 56:418-26.

[54] Manta S, El Mansari M, Debonnel G, Blier P. Electrophysiological and neurochemical effects of long-term vagus nerve stimulation on the rat monoaminergic systems. Int J Neuropsychopharmacol 2012:1-12.

[55] Dunlop BW, Nemeroff CB. The role of dopamine in the pathophysiology of depression. Arch Gen Psychiatry 2007, 64:327-37.

[56] Lambert G, Johansson M, Agren H, Friberg P. Reduced brain norepinephrine and dopamine release in treatment-refractory depressive illness: evidence in support of the catecholamine hypothesis of mood disorders. Arch Gen Psychiatry 2000, 57:787-93.

[57] Mitani H, Shirayama Y, Yamada T, Kawahara R. Plasma levels of homovanillic acid, 5-hydroxyindoleacetic acid and cortisol, and serotonin turnover in depressed patients. Prog Neuropsychopharmacol Biol Psychiatry 2006, 30:531-4.

[58] Dorr AE, Debonnel G. Effect of vagus nerve stimulation on serotonergic and noradrenergic transmission. J Pharmacol Exp Ther 2006, 318:890-8.

[59] Groves DA, Bowman EM, Brown VJ. Recordings from the rat locus coeruleus during acute vagal nerve stimulation in the anaesthetised rat. Neurosci Lett 2005, 379:174-9.

[60] Follesa P, Biggio F, Gorini G, Caria S, Talani G, Dazzi L, Puligheddu M, Marrosu F, Biggio G. Vagus nerve stimulation increases norepinephrine concentration and the gene expression of BDNF and bFGF in the rat brain. Brain Res 2007, 1179:28-34.

[61] Raedt R, Clinckers R, Mollet L, Vonck K, El Tahry R, Wyckhuys T, De Herdt V, Carrette E, Wadman W, Michotte Y, Smolders I, Boon P, Meurs A. Increased hippocampal noradrenaline is a biomarker for efficacy of vagus nerve stimulation in a limbic seizure model. J Neurochem 2011, 117:461-9.

[62] Roosevelt RW, Smith DC, Clough RW, Jensen RA, Browning RA. Increased extracellular concentrations of norepinephrine in cortex and hippocampus following vagus nerve stimulation in the rat. Brain Res 2006, 1119:124-32.

[63] Manta S, Dong J, Debonnel G, Blier P. Enhancement of the function of rat serotonin and norepinephrine neurons by sustained vagus nerve stimulation. J Psychiatry Neurosci 2009, 34:272-80.

[64] Santarelli L, Saxe M, Gross C, Surget A, Battaglia F, Dulawa S, Weisstaub N, Lee J, Duman R, Arancio O, Belzung C, Hen R. Requirement of hippocampal neurogenesis for the behavioral effects of antidepressants. Science 2003, 301:805-9.

[65] Blier P, de Montigny C. Current advances and trends in the treatment of depression. Trends Pharmacol Sci 1994, 15:220-6.

[66] Haddjeri N, Blier P, de Montigny C. Long-term antidepressant treatments result in a tonic activation of forebrain 5-HT1A receptors. J Neurosci 1998, 18:10150-6.

[67] Revesz D, Tjernstrom M, Ben-Menachem E, Thorlin T. Effects of vagus nerve stimulation on rat hippocampal progenitor proliferation. Exp Neurol 2008, 214:259-65.

[68] Gebhardt N, Bar KJ, Boettger MK, Grecksch G, Keilhoff G, Reichart R, Becker A. Vagus nerve stimulation ameliorated deficits in one-way active avoidance learning and stimulated hippocampal neurogenesis in bulbectomized rats. Brain Stimul 2012.

[69] Biggio F, Gorini G, Utzeri C, Olla P, Marrosu F, Mocchetti I, Follesa P. Chronic vagus nerve stimulation induces neuronal plasticity in the rat hippocampus. Int J Neuropsychopharmacol 2009, 12:1209-21.

[70] Armitage R. The effects of antidepressants on sleep in patients with depression. Can J Psychiatry 2000 45:803-9.

[71] Armitage R, Husain M, Hoffmann R, Rush AJ. The effects of vagus nerve stimulation on sleep EEG in depression:a preliminary report. J Psychosom Res 2003, 54:475-82.

[72] Zabara J. Inhibition of experimental seizures in canines by repetitive vagal stimulation. Epilepsia 1992, 33:1005-12.

[73] George MS, Sackeim HA, Marangell LB, Husain MM, Nahas Z, Lisanby SH, Ballenger JC, Rush AJ. Vagus nerve stimulation. A potential therapy for resistant depression? Psychiatr Clin North Am 2000, 23:757-83.

[74] Labiner DM, Ahern GL. Vagus nerve stimulation therapy in depression and epilepsy: therapeutic parameter settings. Acta Neurol Scand 2007, 115:23-33.

[75] Manta S, Dong J, Debonnel G, Blier P. Optimization of vagus nerve stimulation parameters using the firing activity of serotonin neurons in the rat dorsal raphe. Eur Neuropsychopharmacol 2009, 19:250-5.

[76] Manta S, El Mansari M, Blier P. Novel Attempts to Optimize Vagus Nerve Stimulation Parameters on Serotonin Neuronal Firing Activity in the Rat Brain. Brain Stimul 2012, 5:422-9.

[77] Bohotin C, Scholsem M, Bohotin V, Franzen R, Schoenen J. Vagus nerve stimulation attenuates heat- and formalin-induced pain in rats. Neurosci Lett 2003, 351:79-82.

[78] Bohotin C, Scholsem M, Multon S, Martin D, Bohotin V, Schoenen J. Vagus nerve stimulation in awake rats reduces formalin-induced nociceptive behaviour and fos-immunoreactivity in trigeminal nucleus caudalis. Pain 2003, 101:3-12.

[79] Sjogren MJ, Hellstrom PT, Jonsson MA, Runnerstam M, Silander HC, Ben-Menachem E. Cognition-enhancing effect of vagus nerve stimulation in patients with Alzheimer's disease: a pilot study. J Clin Psychiatry 2002, 63:972-80.

[80] Merrill CA, Jonsson MA, Minthon L, Ejnell H, H CsS, Blennow K, Karlsson M, Nordlund A, Rolstad S, Warkentin S, Ben-Menachem E, Sjogren MJ. Vagus nerve stimulation in patients with Alzheimer's disease: Additional follow-up results of a pilot study through 1 year. J Clin Psychiatry 2006, 67:1171-8.

[81] Hord ED, Evans MS, Mueed S, Adamolekun B, Naritoku DK. The effect of vagus nerve stimulation on migraines. J Pain 2003, 4:530-4.

[82] Mauskop A. Vagus nerve stimulation relieves chronic refractory migraine and cluster headaches. Cephalalgia 2005, 25:82-6.

[83] Pardo JV, Sheikh SA, Kuskowski MA, Surerus-Johnson C, Hagen MC, Lee JT, Rittberg BR, Adson DE. Weight loss during chronic, cervical vagus nerve stimulation in depressed patients with obesity: an observation. Int J Obes (Lond) 2007, 31:1756-9.

[84] Marrosu F, Maleci A, Cocco E, Puligheddu M, Barberini L, Marrosu MG. Vagal nerve stimulation improves cerebellar tremor and dysphagia in multiple sclerosis. Mult Scler 2007, 13:1200-2.

Index

D

E

O

P

R

S

T

V

Made in United States
North Haven, CT
04 November 2026

21719584R00166